Scar Management: Practical Dermatology

Scar Management: Practical Dermatology

Edited by Asher Hill

STATES
ACADEMIC PRESS
www.statesacademicpress.com

States Academic Press,
109 South 5th Street,
Brooklyn, NY 11249, USA

Visit us on the World Wide Web at:
www.statesacademicpress.com

ISBN: 978-1-63989-478-9

Cataloging-in-Publication Data

Scar management : practical dermatology / edited by Asher Hill.
p. cm.
Includes bibliographical references and index.
ISBN 978-1-63989-478-9
1. Scars. 2. Burns and scalds. 3. Dermatology. I. Hill, Asher.
RD94 .S33 2022
617.1--dc23

Table of Contents

Preface

Scars are unavoidable and occur during a remodeling phase of wound healing when the fibrous tissue replaces normal tissue. Scar tissue is made up of the same protein as the tissue which it replaces, but the composition of the fibers of the protein is different. The collagen fibers of the normal tissue are present in a random basketweave formation, while the collagen fibers after fibrosis are cross-linked and form a pronounced alignment in a single direction. The collagen alignment of the scar tissue usually has an inferior functional quality as compared to the randomized alignment of the normal collagen. The various studies that are constantly contributing towards advancing technologies of scar management are examined in this book in detail. From theories to research to practical applications, case studies related to all contemporary topics of relevance to this field have been included herein. Those in search of information to further their knowledge will be greatly assisted by this book.

This book is a result of research of several months to collate the most relevant data in the field.

When I was approached with the idea of this book and the proposal to edit it, I was overwhelmed. It gave me an opportunity to reach out to all those who share a common interest with me in this field. I had 3 main parameters for editing this text:

1. Accuracy - The data and information provided in this book should be up-to-date and valuable to the readers.

2. Structure - The data must be presented in a structured format for easy understanding and better grasping of the readers.

3. Universal Approach - This book not only targets students but also experts and innovators in the field, thus my aim was to present topics which are of use to all.

Thus, it took me a couple of months to finish the editing of this book.

I would like to make a special mention of my publisher who considered me worthy of this opportunity and also supported me throughout the editing process. I would also like to thank the editing team at the back-end who extended their help whenever required.

Editor

1

Other Scar Types: Optimal Functional and Aesthetic Outcome of Scarring in Cleft Patients

Wouter B. van der Sluis, Nirvana S. S. Kornmann, Robin A. Tan, and Johan P. W. Don Griot

Contents

Background

Cleft lip and palate are facial and oral malformation due to failures in the embryologic craniofacial development during early pregnancy. They occur in approximately 1 in 750/1000 births in Europe, which makes it the most common congenital craniofacial abnormality. Different variations in phenotype of this malformation exist. It can occur unilateral (left or right) or bilateral, with involvement of lip and/or alveolus and/or palate and can be microform, incomplete, or complete. Unilateral cleft lip and palate are the most common type, whereby the upper lip, the orbicularis muscle, the alveolar bone, the floor of the nose, and the hard and soft palate are interrupted, creating an open communication between nasopharynx and oropharynx.

Patients with a cleft lip and palate are treated in specialized cleft centers by a multidisciplinary team, consisting of geneticists; (plastic) surgeons; orthodontists; dentists; ear, nose, and throat (ENT) doctors; speech and language therapists; and psychologists. All surgical interventions aimed at closure of the cleft lip and palate induce restriction of maxillary growth. Surgical timing, staging, and techniques differ between treatment centers. The lip is usually closed at 3–6 months after birth and the soft palate at 6–12 months. In some cleft centers, the hard palate is closed before 12 months after birth in either a one-stage or two-stage procedure. Other cleft centers prefer to close the hard palate later in life, at 18 months to 3 years, or during the closure of the alveolar gap at the age of 8–11 years.

Having cleft lip and/or palate has a noteworthy impact on quality of life and psychosocial functioning. Postoperative scarring is a common cause of patient dissatisfaction. The degree of postoperative scarring in cleft patients is associated with symptoms of anxiety, depression, and a lower self-esteem. For cleft surgeons, every possible measure to optimize functional and aesthetic outcome is important.

◘ Table Short overview of the "surgical treatment of cleft patients" protocol of the Amsterdam University Medical Center

Unilateral cleft lip and palate	Bilateral cleft lip and palate	Cleft palate
3 months: Lip closure	3 months: Lip closure	
9 months: Palatography	9 months: Palatography	9 months: Palatography
7–9 years: If necessary, hard palate closure If necessary, orthognathic surgery	7–9 years: If necessary, hard palate closure if necessary, orthognathic surgery	7–9 years: Hard palate closure
>15 years If necessary, secondary corrections	>15 years If necessary, secondary corrections	>15 years If necessary, secondary corrections
>17 years If necessary, rhinoplasty	>17 years If necessary, rhinoplasty	

Objectives of Cleft Lip Surgery

The goal of cleft lip surgery is to close the lip separation, provide optimal function in terms of speech, mastication, dental protection, breathing and feeding, and provide an aesthetically pleasing facial scar and optimal shape of nose and nostril. The visible facial scar and its effect on nose and lip aesthetics are a daily reminder to the patient of its underlying cause. Over the years, different surgical techniques have been described regarding surgical closure of the cleft lip. The ideal technique should create a balanced lip, allow for easy adjustments, and produce a favorable scar pattern combined with a symmetrical shape of the nose. Closure of a cleft lip, also called "cheilorrhaphy," is a functional and aesthetic reconstruction of the upper lip, orbicularis muscle, nasal floor, and ala.

Treatment Protocol

As stated above, surgical timing, staging, and techniques differ between treatment centers. In ◘ Table 7.1, a short overview of the "surgical treatment of cleft patients" protocol of the Amsterdam University Medical Center is provided.

Cleft Lip Reconstruction: Surgical Techniques

Precise surgical technique and adequate aligning of anatomical structures is important for the postoperative aesthetic result and scar formation. Patients with a cleft lip have, besides the obvious interrupted upper lip, a typical flared nostril and a septum deviation. As stated above, different surgical techniques are used to reconstruct this defect, each with its pros and cons. Though many approaches exist, the Millard (rotation advancement) and Fisher (anatomic subunit) approaches are historically most frequently performed.

Unilateral Cleft Lip

Millard Lip Closure

Since the 1950s, the Millard rotation advancement technique for surgical lip closure was the most popular among cleft surgeons. It consists of downward rotation of the medial cleft component and a lateral lip advancement flap. The majority of the scar can be placed at the philtral column. A disadvantage of this approach is that the superior part of the scar crosses the philtrum perpendicularly at the columellar base. Various modifications of the traditional Millard technique have been developed to overcome this disadvantage.

Fisher Lip Closure

In 2005, Fisher published his lip closure technique, in which the anatomical subunit principles guide lip repair. In this technique, a circumferential incision at the cleft side of the columella is continued to the Cupid's bow top in a straight manner. This mirrors the unaffected philtral ridge. To lengthen the medial flap, small inlet incisions are frequently necessary. To prevent upper lip shortening, a triangular flap above the cutaneous roll can be incorporated (◘ Figs. 7.1, 7.2, and 7.3).

Bilateral Cleft Lip

"Bilateral cleft lip" can manifest in different ways, in which symmetrical complete bilateral

cleft lip–cleft palate is the most prevalent. When looking at the lip alone, the bilateral symmetrical complete variant accounts for 50% of cases, bilateral incomplete for 25%, and asymmetrical bilateral (complete/incomplete) for 25%. A one-stage surgical approach is advocated in most centers.

The Millard–Mulliken technique is frequently employed. A cranially based philtrum flap is created, the gap is closed, and orbicularis oris continuity and lip continuity are restored. Ideally, both scars are positioned symmetrically at the philtral ridge.

In several cleft centers these surgical techniques are combined with preoperative nasoalveolar molding (NAM). The aim of NAM is to improve the shape and form of the alveolar wall and nose and to bring the divided lip together with an orthodontic plate, nasal spring, and tape (Plaatje). In our center NAM is only used in cases with bilateral cleft lips. Furthermore, a nasal conformer is used in unilateral cases to improve the shape of the affected nostril postoperative.

Additional Measures to Improve Scarring

Visible facial scarring after cleft lip repair is inevitable. There are however some perioperative measures that can be taken to minimize scar morbidity in terms of hypertrophy and contraction.

Perioperative Botulinum Toxin

After surgical correction of the lip and philtrum, the underlying orbicularis oris muscle contracts in a direction perpendicular to the cutaneous scar. This results in accentuation of dynamic rhytides, which may slowly result in widening of the surgical scar. Some surgical teams temporarily paralyze the orbicularis oris muscle, by intraoperatively injecting it with botulinum toxin. Several studies showed a beneficial effect on postoperative scar width; however, the sample size is relatively small in most studies, and objective assessment tools are scarcely employed.

Sutureless Skin Closure

Using (too many) cutaneous sutures in a facial wound may cause a foreign body reaction and subsequent suboptimal scarring. The possibility of visible crosshatching of sutures is unappealing.

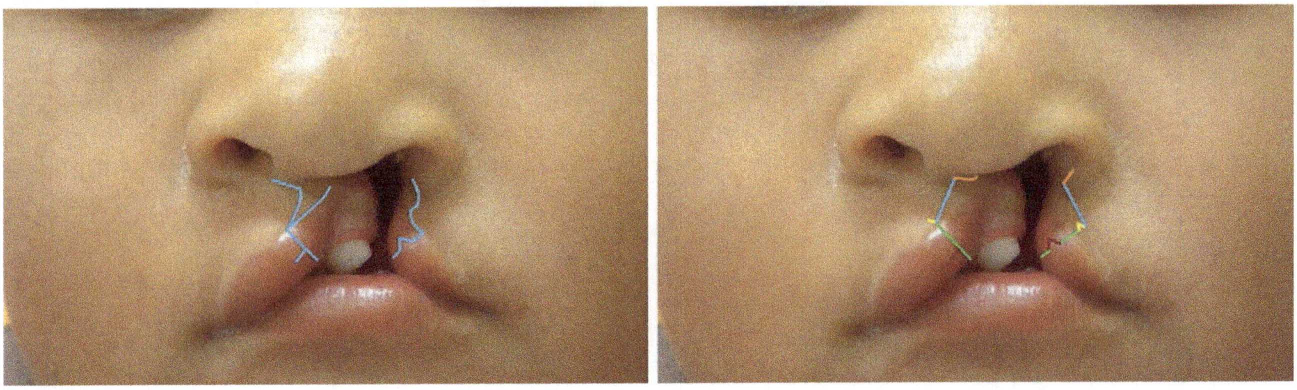

◘ **Fig.** Preoperative planning for Millard (left) and Fisher (right) lip closure

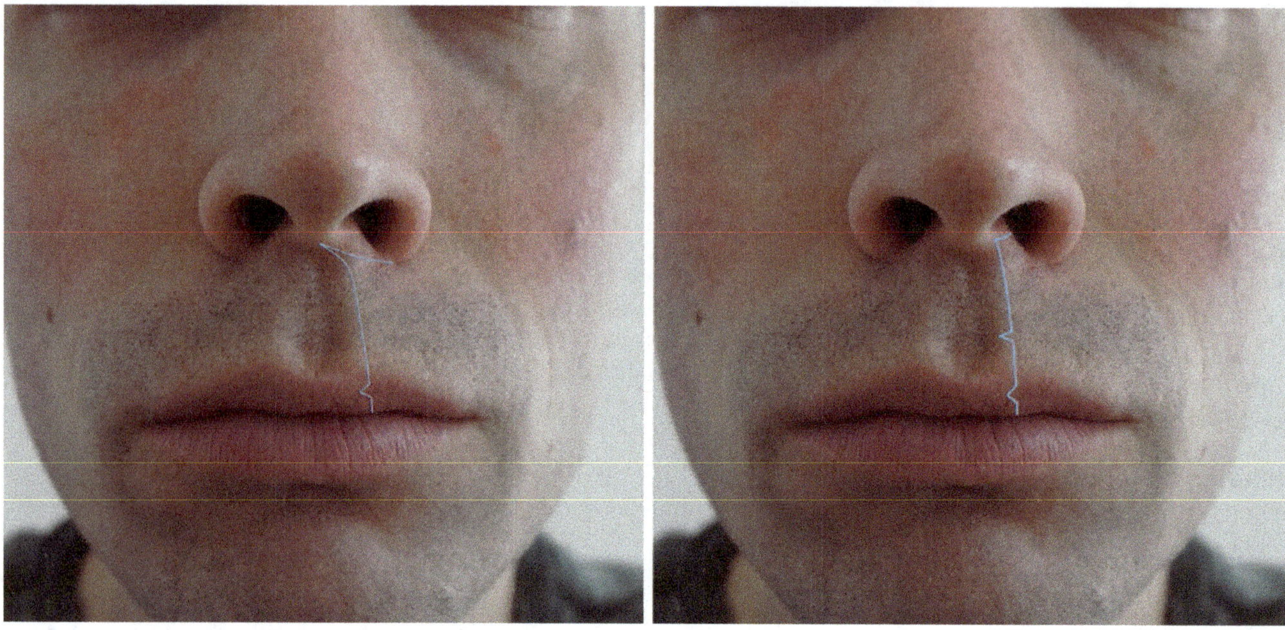

Fig. Postoperative scar pattern after Millard (left) and Fisher (right) lip closure. Note, different surgeons use different modifications of both techniques

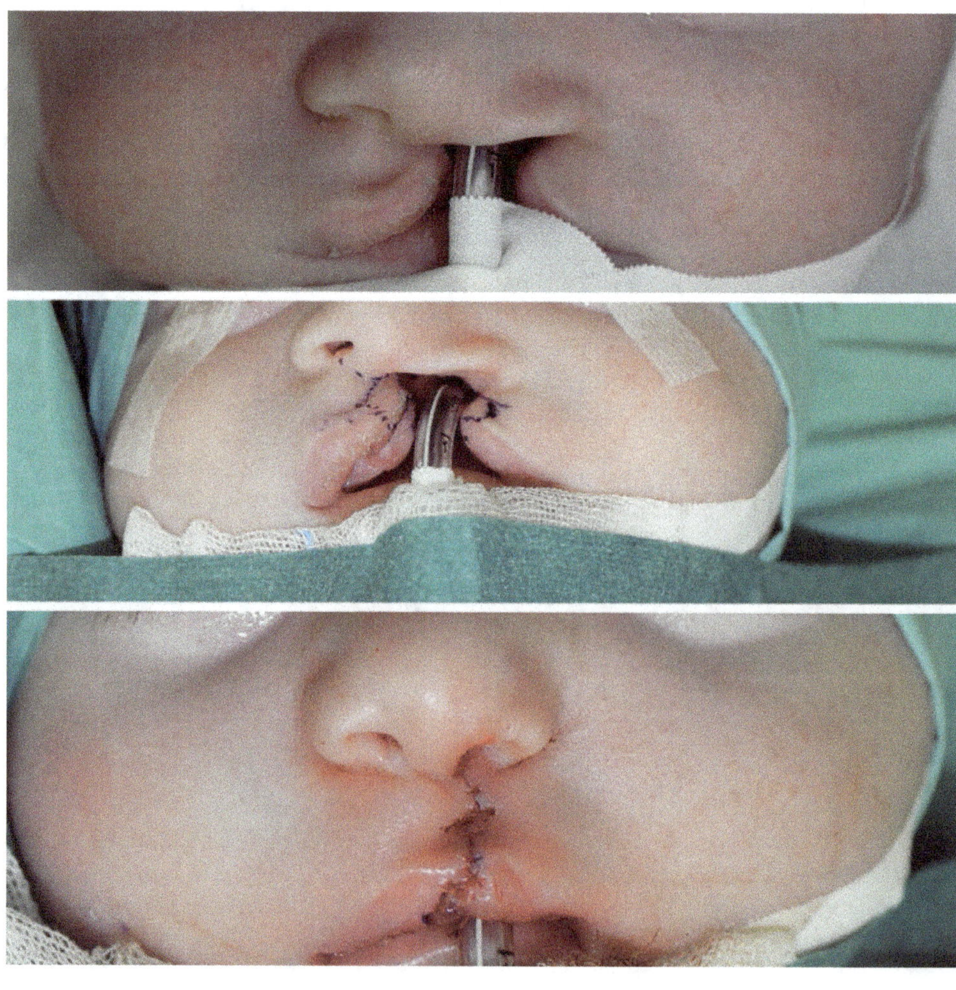

Fig. Preoperative (upper), planning (middle), and direct postoperative (lower) result of the Fisher lip closing technique in a patient with complete unilateral cleft lip and palate

Some advocate the use of sutureless skin closure, in which the cutaneous layer approximation is performed using surgical glue, such as butyl cyanoacrylate or amcrylate. An additional advantage is that is generally faster to perform, which reduces intraoperative time. No large, prospective comparative studies are performed on this subject.

Silicone Application

Topical silicone application is used for treating/preventing hypertrophic scars in different body locations. This is also the case for cheiloplasty scars. To which extent hypertrophic cheiloplasty scars can be treated/prevented with this application is unknown. Side effects of this treatment comprise skin rash and fusibility problems, such as loss of adhesiveness. Using silicone gel seems to be non-inferior to silicone sheeting.

Postoperative Laser Therapy

Use of carbon dioxide fractional laser, sometimes combined with intense pulsed light treatment, in the direct postoperative phase is shown to improve scars in terms of pliability and color. Though proven safe, pain during the session and crust formation are frequently reported.

Hair Transplantation

In male cleft patients, limited or missing moustache growth may be noticeable in the scarred area, especially in men with dark hair and ample hair growth. Hair graft transplantation can be performed; however, the poor vascularization of scar tissue poses a problem, because this is not a good bed for graft survival. Some use fat grafting of the scar before hair transplantation to optimize graft survival.

Secondary Cleft Lip Reconstruction

Secondary cleft lip reconstruction is frequently performed due to scar contracture, which has a negative impact on lip, philtrum, and nose aesthetics. The exact incidence of secondary lip correction is unknown and dependent on many factors, for example, patient factors, treatment protocol, access to health care services, etc. In the Western world, the estimated incidence is 40–60%. Conservative management of these cases is seldom successful. Surgical correction typically employs use of the Rose–Thompson effect (in which a scar is lengthened by using concave excisions of the scar, which is subsequently closed in a straight line), one or multiple Z-plasties, or a combination of these strategies. Some perform fat grafting of the scar to loosen it and provide more length. Remaining volume deficiencies, for example, volume deficiencies of the lip, can be restored in the same procedure with lipofilling or dermal fat grafts.

Evaluation of Aesthetic Outcome

One of the goals in the treatment of cleft lip (and palate) repair is improving nasolabial aesthetics by restoring symmetry and proportion of the nose and lip. Traditionally, aesthetic assessment is performed by symmetry measurements with a caliper. The last two decades, several scoring systems have been proposed for a simpler and quicker assessment. Most of these scoring systems use two-dimensional (2D) photographs in combination with Likert or visual analog (VAS) scales. The most frequently used method is the Asher–McDade (AMD) system, which utilizes a five-point Likert scale ranging from "excellent" to "very poor" to grade four anatomical nasal and lip structures. In 2016, the Cleft Aesthetic Rating Scale (CARS) was developed as a new tool to allow rapid assessment of the nose and lip separately.

The majority of assessment methods are focusing on symmetry and on the shape of the nose and lip, whereas the scar appears to be of secondary importance. In 2010, the Patient and Observer Scar Assessment Scale (POSAS) was proposed to assess the scar after cleft lip repair. Nevertheless, it remains unknown to which extend visible scarring plays a role in facial aesthetics after cleft surgery.

To determine the aesthetic outcome in a more objective way, measurements using three-dimensional (3D) photographs seem to be promising nowadays. These methods show a high reliability, but these techniques require expertise and costly equipment and are therefore not readily available worldwide. To compromise, computer-based programs, like SymNose, have been developed. These programs allow symmetry measurements on 2D images of the nose and lip by tracing the outline of the upper lip and the lower border of the nose. By reflecting the left side of the midline over the right, the percentage mismatch of the nonoverlapping area is calculated.

However, an internationally accepted assessment method for the aesthetic evaluation of cleft lips is still not available.

Palatal Scarring

Palatal Closure

Both the hard palate and soft palate can be involved in palatal clefts, resulting in a gap from anterior to posterior, affecting the maxilla, the mucosa, the levator veli palatini muscle, the tensor veli palatini muscle, and uvula muscle. An open communication between the nasopharynx and oropharynx prevents the infant to create an intraoral negative pressure, which is mandatory for productive suckling during (breast)feeding. A positive oropharyngeal pressure and elevation of the palate allows for the normal articulation of the oral consonants, most notably the oral stop-plosives, [p, t, k, b, d, g] in English. This can only be achieved by partitioning the oropharynx from the nasopharynx. Therefore, the aim of palatal closure, also called "palatography" or "palatoplasty," is functional reconstruction of structures that are necessary for feeding and speech development early in life. Different types of palatoplasties have been described to close the soft and the hard palate whereby several surgical considerations must be addressed. The most important anatomical structure, which should not be harmed during surgery is the greater palatine neurovascular bundle, proceeding through the greater palatine foramen through the lateral posterior hard palate. It is essential to obtain a tension-free closure of the palatal flaps, preventing compression or stretching of the neurovascular bundle. Releasing incisions may be necessary to achieve complete closure from anterior to posterior.

Timing of Palatal Closure

Impaired maxillary growth and an abnormal speech development are common findings in

patients after repaired cleft lip and palate. Delayed closure of the palate beyond 12 years or no closure at all minimizes abnormal facial growth, yet early closure of the palate, that is, before 12 months after birth, is necessary for normal speech development. Studies on speech development, maxillary growth, and timing of palatal closure show different results due to confounding variables as surgical technique, surgeon's experience level, and lack of standardized speech outcome or standardized indications for secondary maxillary surgery. Therefore, consensus on the optimal timing of palatal closure has not yet been reached.

Maxillary Growth

Impaired maxillary growth in cleft patients often results in typical features as crowding, lateral crossbite, and open bite. The exact pathophysiology of abnormal facial growth after cleft lip and palate repair remains unclear. It is a widely accepted hypothesis that abnormal maxillary growth has an iatrogenic cause and is secondary to surgical intervention due to scarring. However, other studies suggest that intrinsic maxillary underdevelopment contribute to impaired facial growth as well. It is most likely that a combination of intrinsic and iatrogenic factors is responsible, making it mandatory for a surgeon to minimize scarring in the oral cavity.

Speech Development

Due to a congenital short palate, hypernasal speech, and nasal air emission during speech are common findings in children after a cleft palate repair. Hypernasality and nasal air leakage are often the result of velopharyngeal insufficiency, which means that the velopharyngeal valve does not close completely and consistently during the production of oral sounds. As scarring tissue tends to contract in longitudinal direction, the palate frequently becomes even shorter or movement of the soft palate becomes inadequate, preventing the soft palate to make contact with the pharyngeal wall. Several techniques have been described to create more length of the palate, such as the V–Y pushback repair (Veau–Wardill–Kilner), the buccal mucosal flap, the double opposing Z-plasty (Furlow), or the lengthening of the soft palate with a pharyngoplasty.

Conclusion

Cleft lip and palate scars influence lip, philtrum, and nose aesthetics, as well as speech and growth of the maxilla. Optimal scar management can be divided in surgical (precise surgical technique, planning, and adequate aligning of anatomical structures) and nonsurgical methods (botulinum toxin, silicone application, carbon dioxide fractional laser).

Take-Home Message

- Cleft lip and palate are facial and oral malformation due to failures in the embryologic craniofacial development during early pregnancy.
- The goal of cleft lip surgery is to close the lip separation; provide optimal function in terms of speech, mastication, dental protection, breathing and feeding; and provide an aesthetically pleasing facial scar.
- Cleft lip scars influence lip, philtrum, and nose aesthetics.
- Optimal scar management can be divided in surgical (precise surgical technique, planning, and adequate aligning of anatomical structures).
- And nonsurgical methods (botulinum toxin, silicone application, carbon dioxide fractional laser).
- In secondary lip correction, cleft surgeons typically make use of the Rose–Thompson effect, one or multiple Z-plasties, or a combination of these strategies.

2

Fetal Wound Healing

Magda M. W. Ulrich

Contents

Background

Wound healing is a complex and tightly regulated process and can be divided in three different overlapping phases: the inflammatory phase, the proliferation phase, and the remodeling phase. The first phase begins directly after wounding and is characterized by hemostasis and inflammation. Platelets play an important role in the formation of the blood clot to stop the bleeding, and through the secretion of chemokines, they recruit different inflammatory cells such as neutrophils and monocytes to the wound. The inflammatory cells clean the wound by phagocytosis of invading microorganisms and damaged tissue. The inflammatory cells also secrete chemotactic signals which attract fibroblasts and endothelial cells to the wound which, together with the inflammatory cells, form the granulation tissue. This is the proliferation phase during which the destroyed tissue is replaced. During this phase, the keratinocytes migrate over the granulation tissue to form a new epidermis to close the skin defect.

The last phase in wound healing is the remodeling phase which is characterized by a decrease in cellularity and vascularity by apoptosis and an increase of synthesis and deposition of the components of the extracellular matrix (ECM). In adults, this process results is scar formation, whereas in fetal skin, complete regeneration of the skin, including the formation of skin appendices such as hairs and sebaceous and sweat glands, takes place.

Since the 1950, studies on scarless healing in fetal skin in animals have been published, and in the late 1970s of the last century, the first publications appeared describing scarless healing of fetal skin wounds in humans. Since then, several experimental studies on this subject have been published. From experimental animal and human studies it is known that scarless healing only occurs during the first period of gestation. Human fetuses lose the ability of skin regeneration around 22 weeks of gestation.

Animal experiments in which adult, late gestational, and early gestational fetal skin were transplanted on early gestational fetuses showed clear differences in wound healing outcome. Incision wounds created in these transplants showed scar formation in adult and late gestational fetal skin, whereas the wound created in the fetal skin resulted in complete regeneration [1]. These experiments show not only that this phenomenon is an intrinsic property of the fetal skin itself but also that scarless healing is not triggered by the intrauterine environment. Interestingly, the wounds at the fetal-adult interface also healed without scar formation implicating that direct contact of a wound with fetal skin is sufficient to induce regeneration of the tissue [2].

Several mechanisms have been suggested to be responsible for the scarless healing in fetal skin, e.g., a diminished inflammatory reaction, differences in composition and architecture of the extracellular matrix, and mechanical load in fetal skin. Furthermore, fetal skin differs from adult skin in many factors commonly associated with scar formation such as proteolytic activity and TGF-β secretion and sensitivity. This chapter will discuss the different mechanisms during the three phases of wound healing proposed in the literature to be involved in scarless healing.

Inflammation

Several studies have shown that the inflammatory response to injury is strongly reduced in fetal skin wounds, and induction of the local inflammation causes scar formation in early fetal skin.

The inflammatory reaction involves recruitment of inflammatory cells which produce inflammatory mediators such as growth factors and cytokines. The growth factors and cytokines subsequently recruit more inflammatory cells.

Inflammation in adult wound healing starts off with a pro-inflammatory cytokine and immune cell response and the activation of the acute phase response. During this period, invading microorganisms and injured tissue are cleared from the wound bed. Subsequently, the inflammatory reaction is skewed to an anti-inflammatory profile which initiates the healing response. Although the exact role of inflammatory cells in scar formation is not entirely elucidated, it is evident that they play an important role in the derailed wound healing process leading to scar formation. It was shown that in severely scarred wounds such as burn wounds, the acute (pro-) inflammatory status is continued for a very long time.

Cells involved in the pro-inflammatory reaction are neutrophils and the M1 subtype macrophages, while macrophages of the M2 subtypes and regulatory T cells are anti-inflammatory, pro-healing cells.

Platelets are the first cells involved in the induction of the inflammatory reaction. The platelets are activated and aggregate during the coagulation phase forming the hemostatic plug. The activated platelets release cytokines such as platelet-derived growth factor (PDGF), interleukins (IL) 1 and 6, and transforming growth factor beta (TGF-β) into the wound environment. It was shown that fetal platelets aggregate poorly when exposed to higher levels of hyaluronic acid, a component of the extracellular matrix, which is more abundantly expressed in fetal skin than in adult skin, and subsequently release lower levels of platelet-derived cytokines.

The lower platelet-derived cytokines are most likely responsible for the reduced inflammatory cell infiltration, such as neutrophils, macrophages, and lymphocytes, seen in fetal wounds at early gestational age [3].

Not only recruitment of inflammatory cells from the circulation to the fetal wound is reduced, but also the number of resident macrophages, mast cells, Langerhans cells, dendritic cells and T cells in uninjured fetal skin is reduced. Moreover, the immune cells present in the fetal skin have the anti-inflammatory, pro-healing phenotype as fetal skin contains higher numbers of regulatory T cells and macrophages of the M2 phenotype. In addition, chemoattractant cytokines such as CCL17, CCL21, and CCL27 involved in recruitment of T cells and dendritic cells are reduced in fetal skin [4].

Although the inflammatory growth factor TGF-β plays an important role in scar formation, it is also involved in the resolution of the inflammatory reaction. In fetal skin, high levels of all the components of the TGF-β pathway are present, and moreover, the pathway seems to be highly activated. This highly activated TGF-β pathway might also result in fast suppression of the pro-inflammatory reaction in fetal wounds [4].

These findings indicate that indeed the (pro-)inflammatory immune reactions is reduced in fetal wound healing. However, the inflammatory component cannot be the key link to scarless healing since wounding of transplanted adult sheep skin to a sheep fetus resulted in scar formation despite the diminished inflammatory state of the fetus itself and the intrauterine environment.

Extracellular Matrix

The extracellular matrix of fetal skin is distinctly different than adult skin matrix. Early gestational fetal skin contains higher amounts of collagen type III, fibronectin EIIIA, and hyaluronic acid (HA) and is deficient in elastin. Similar expression profiles for ECM components were demonstrated for the (adult) oral mucosa, a tissue also known for reduced scar formation.

Although collagen type I is the major component in both adult and fetal skin, in fetal skin, collagen type III/collagen type I ratio is higher compared to adult skin. The higher levels of collagen type III have effects on the ECM organization and collagen fiber diameter. Downregulation of collagen type III expression results in increased scar formation and differentiation of fibroblasts into myofibroblasts, the main cell type involved in scar formation [5].

The properties of the ECM network do not depend only on the presence and percentage of the different collagen subtypes and other ECM components but also on cross-linking of the ECM components. Increased cross-linking results in ECM accumulation and increased rigidity. In fetal skin, most of the collagen fibers are not cross-linked [5]. One of the enzymes involved in collagen and elastin cross-linking is lysyl oxidase (LOX). Early gestational fetal wounds show reduced LOX expression in comparison to late gestational wounds.

Other important components of the ECM which are differentially expressed between fetal and adult skin are glycosaminoglycans (GAGs) and proteoglycans. The GAGs like hyaluronic acid (HA) contain long polysaccharide chains which can absorb large amounts of water and are important for hydration of the skin and determine the viscoelasticity of the skin. HA is thought to play an important role in regulation of the inflammatory reaction during wound healing. However, its effect is dependent on the length of the polysaccharides. High-molecular-weight (HMW) HA suppresses the inflammatory reaction, while low-molecular-weight (LMW) HA fragments are immunostimulatory and induce the inflammatory reaction [6].

Expression of HA in fetal skin is high and during wound healing the expression is induced in adults. The positive effect in fetal wound healing might be related to the balance between HMW and LMW HA, which may be caused by differential expression of enzymes synthesizing HA (hyaluronan synthases) and enzymes degrading HA (hyaluronidases) between adult and fetal tissue. It was shown that addition of hyaluronidases to fetal wounds can induce fibroplasia, collagen deposition, and neovascularization, processes involved in scar formation.

Besides the abovementioned component, elastin is also an important component of the ECM. This protein is responsible for connective tissue pliability in the adult dermis; however, it is absent in early gestational skin, and its role in scarless wound healing is not clear [7] (◘ Fig.).

Angiogenesis

Several studies have shown that reduced angiogenesis during adult wound healing reduces scar formation. However, indisputable evidence that this also plays a role during fetal wound healing has not been provided although several studies suggested lack of strong neovascularization and reduced proangiogenic factors in fetal wounds.

Angiogenesis is much more prominent in adult wound healing compared to fetal wound healing. Early in adult wound healing, a dense capillary bed is created. However, this capillary tangle lacks the assembly of a functional network which is able to provide nutrition and oxygen to the wound bed [8].

It was shown that HA degradation products induce angiogenesis; therefore, the reduced synthesis of hyaluronidases not only has a positive effect on suppression of the inflammatory reaction but also reduces the exaggerated neovascularization seen in adult wounds.

However, this could also be attributed to reduced levels of angiogenic growth factors such as basic fibroblast growth factor and PDGF. Addition of angiogenic factors such as hyaluronidase and PDGF to fetal wounds was shown to induce angiogenesis and lead to scar formation.

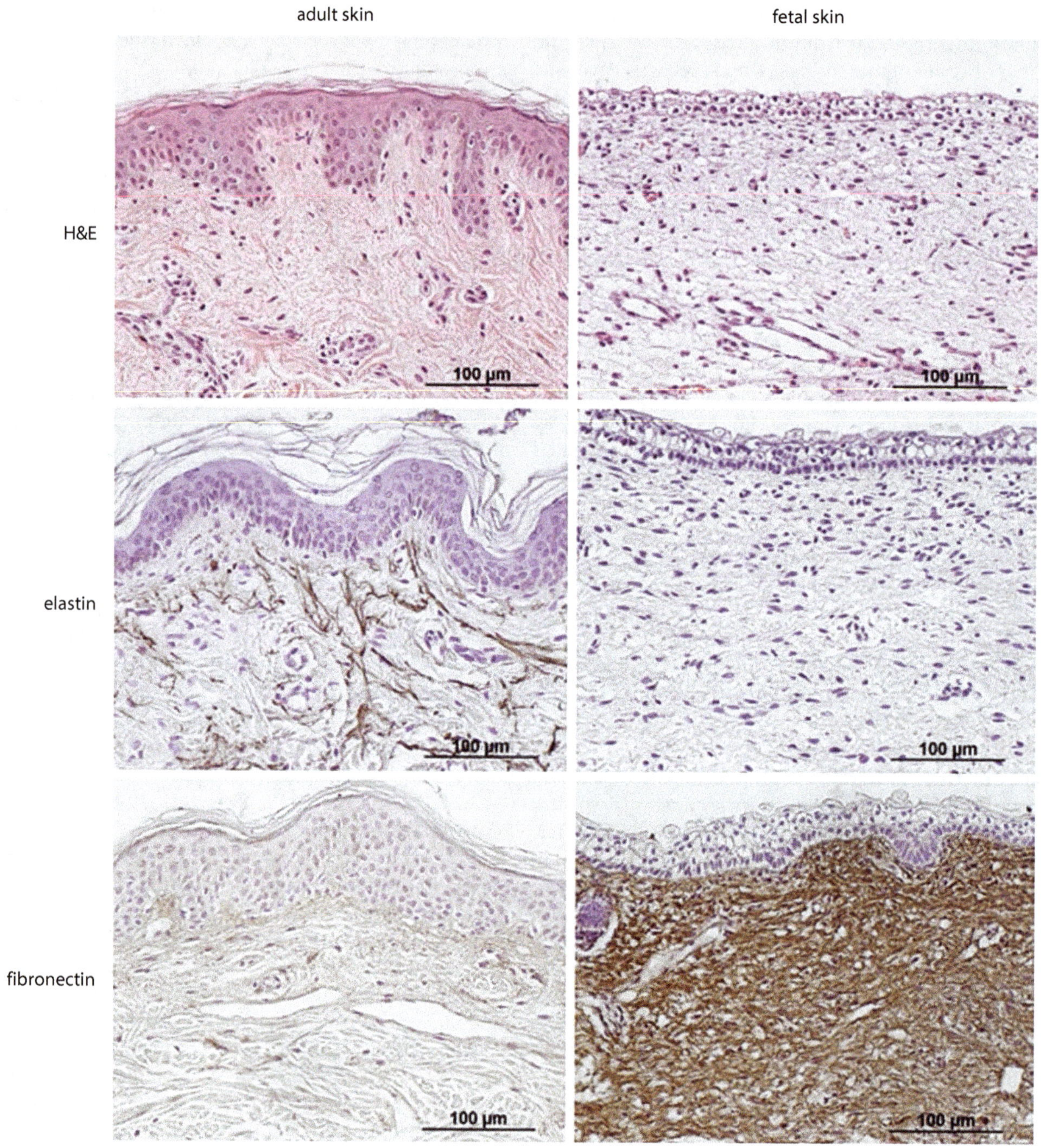

Fig. Expression of different ECM components in adult and fetal skin. The specific ECM components are stained in brown

Keratinocytes

One of the factors thought to play a role in scar formation is delayed wound closure by reepithelialization. Wound closure in fetal wounds is much faster in comparison to adult wounds.

Fetal keratinocytes not only have a higher proliferation rate; also the mechanism of reepithelialization was found to be distinctly different between adult and fetal wounds. In adult wound healing reepithelialization, the basal keratinocytes at the wound edge undergo morphological changes. They form actin containing cytoplasmic elongations called lamellipodia through which they crawl over the extracellular matrix of the wound bed. To be able to migrate, the cells lose their ECM binding structures (hemidesmosomes) and the cell-cell binding sites (desmosomes). Fetal keratinocytes do not form lamellipodia but form an actin myosin II containing cables through the front keratinocytes at the wound edge [9]. This cable runs from cell to cell most likely through the adherens junctions, another form of cell-cell junction similar to the desmosome. The cable is formed within hours after wounding and by contraction pulls the keratinocytes together to close the wound.

Integrins may also play a role in faster reepithelialization in fetal wound healing. Integrins are heterodimeric transmembrane receptors which can bind to specific ECM components. Different combinations of the subunit determine the specificity for the different ECM components, and they determine cellular processes like cell proliferation and migration. In the fetus, it was shown that specific integrins were rapidly upregulated upon wounding and that this occurred much faster than in adult keratinocytes.

It is evident that there is an interaction between keratinocytes and fibroblasts in the dermis. In vitro experiments have shown that fetal keratinocytes suppress proliferation, myofibroblast differentiation, and ECM production, in fibroblasts derived from hypertrophic scar, whereas fetal keratinocytes promote proliferation and migration in fetal and adult healthy skin-derived fibroblasts.

Fibroblasts

Fibroblasts are the main cell type of the dermis; they produce the ECM and therefore play an important role in wound healing and scar formation. During wound healing, this cell type differentiates into myofibroblasts. These latter cells produce high levels of ECM components and contain the contractile protein alpha smooth muscle actin (αSMA) which is involved in tissue contraction seen in scar formation. The transition to a myofibroblast population in the wound healing environment and especially the persistence of this cell population are seen as the most important contributor to scar formation. Transforming growth factor beta (TGF-β) plays an important role in this process. However, TGF-β also plays an important role during embryonic and fetal development and thus is abundantly present in the fetus. TGF-β is stored as an inactive compound in the ECM. In order to execute its role in the many processes this growth factor is involved in, it has to be activated which ultimately leads to the induction of various genes including genes involved in fibrosis and the process of scar formation. It was shown that all of the components are abundantly present in the fetal skin. In addition, the TGF-β pathway was also shown to be highly activated in healthy fetal skin in comparison to adult skin, but this does not result in fibrotic skin or scar formation. It was suggested that differential expression in TGF-β isoforms plays a crucial role in this. TGF-β1 and TGF-β2 are thought to be profibrotic, whereas TGF-β3 has antifibrotic properties. However, this segmentation is not completely indisputable. The balance between the profibrotic and antifibrotic TGF-β isoforms in fetal skin is shifted in comparison to adult skin: 99.5%:0.5% in adult to 97.4%:2.6% in fetal skin. However, the absolute concentrations of all TGF-β isoforms are much higher in fetal skin in comparison to adult skin.

Several differences were observed between fetal skin fibroblasts and adult dermal fibroblasts: The fetal cells migrated much faster than adult fibroblasts and exhibited a "hyperactive morphology." They produced higher amounts of extracellular matrix components. Furthermore, fetal cells produced a larger contraction effect when cultured in fibroblast-populated collagen lattices compared to adult fibroblasts.

As in fetal keratinocytes, it was shown that fetal fibroblasts express different integrins which results in higher proliferation and migration rates. Inhibition of one of the specific fetal integrins resulted in a more adultlike fibroblast phenotype.

Stimulation of fetal fibroblasts in vitro also induced myofibroblast differentiation and shows higher contraction of fibroblast-seeded collagen matrices [4].

Studies in which fetal skin cells have been applied to burn wounds show improved wound healing. Since it was shown that the fetal cells were not incorporated into the newly formed skin, it is thought that the cells secrete growth factors or in any other form interact with the host organism to accelerate wound healing.

Mechanical Forces

Mechanical forces, extracellular as well as intracellular, play an important role in skin homeostasis as it directs cell function and activity through a process called mechanotransduction. In this process, the composition, viscoelasticity, and stiffness of the ECM play an important role. Adult skin contains thick collagen bundles mainly consisting of type I fibrils, whereas fetal skin contains thin collagen fibers which are high in collagen type III fibrils and show reduced resting stress.

Through adhesion molecules on the surface of the skin, the integrins, the ECM is connected to the cytoskeleton of the cell. The link between the ECM and the cytoskeleton is a dynamic complex, called focal adhesions (FA), which are constantly assembled and disassembled. The FA are able to direct not only cell function such as gene expression but also cellular adhesion and cell migration. Fibroblasts exposed to mechanical stress form supermature FA displaying a specific composition of FA proteins such as paxilin (Pax). Fetal fibroblasts were shown to have reduced FA protein expression among which Pax and different integrin subunits [4].

Also from clinical data, there is evidence that mechanical stress plays an important role in scar formation. Collagen fibers in the ECM of the skin are aligned in a specific pattern depending on the location of the body. This pattern forms the so-called Langer lines and determines the direction of the tension in the skin. From surgery, it is known that incisions made parallel to these lines heal with less scar formation than incisions perpendicular to the Langer lines, suggesting that mechanical load to the wound influences scar formation [10]. In fetal skin, the ECM is organized in a loose reticular network of collagen, while in adult skin, there are thicker more compact collagen fibers. In fetal wound healing, the same reticular ECM network is formed indistinguishable from the unaffected surrounding, whereas in adult wound healing, the collagen fibers are arranged in dense parallel bundles [11].

Remodeling

The last phase in wound healing is the remodeling phase. During this phase, cellularity decreases by apoptosis, and the degradation of the excessive extracellular matrix takes place. In adult wound healing, the predominant type III collagen is replaced by type I collagen. However, in fetal recovered skin, type III collagen remains the main subtype.

The deposition of extracellular matrix is an interplay between synthesis and degradation of the components of the ECM. Matrix metalloproteinases (MMPs) and tissue inhibitors of metalloproteinases (TIMPs) play an important role in this process. The MMP family consists of more than 20 members which are able to degrade most of the components of the ECM with different specific activities toward the different components. The process of ECM degradation is controlled by specific tissue inhibitors of metalloproteinases (TIMPs). Currently, four TIMPs have been identified which possess varying affinity to specific MMPs. An imbalance between MMPs and TIMPs affects the deposition of ECM. In scarring, reduced collagen degradation as a result of reduced MMP expression and increased TIMP expression causes accumulation of ECM components. Early gestational fetal skin and middle gestational fetal skin express lower MMP and TIMP levels than late gestational skin and adult skin. During fetal wound healing, several MMPs were increased in early gestational fetal wounds, whereas later during gestation, when wounds heal with scar formation, MMP levels were reduced, and TIMP levels were increased [12]. This later finding may explain the accumulation of ECM seen in scar formation.

Skin Appendix Formation

Early gestational wound healing results not only in restoration of the dermis and epidermis but also in the regeneration of skin appendages such as hair follicles and sebaceous and sweat glands.

Hair follicles contain several stem cell niches and play an important role in adult wound healing. In partial-thickness wounds in which part of the hair follicle is still intact, healing can occur without scar formation.

Hair follicle development during embryogenesis starts, depending on the anatomical location, between weeks 9 and 15. One could envision that early gestational skin contains stem cells and still has the mechanisms available to induce skin appendage development and create the stem niches but that these stem cells can also regenerate the skin. It was shown that allogeneic cells derived from fetal skin could enhance burn wound healing and reduce scar formation.

Conclusions

The fact that adult skin in an intrauterine environment still heal with scar formation despite the low inflammatory milieu, the presence of fetal growth factors, and even fetal cells able to migrate into the adult tissue shows that the processes leading to scarless healing or scar formation cannot be attributed to single individual mechanisms, cells, or other factors but that it is a result of complex of interconnected processes.

Take-Home Messages

- Early to midgestational skin wounds result in skin regeneration instead of scar formation.
- The exact mechanism behind scarless healing is still unknown.
- Several mechanisms have been indicated: reduced inflammation, altered cytokine profile, and different ECM composition.
- The process of scarless healing is a result of a complex of interconnected processes.
- Several characteristics of fetal skin are shared with oral mucosa which is also known for its reduced scar formation.

References

1. West DC, Shaw DM, Lorenz P, Adzick NS, Longaker MT. Fibrotic healing of adult and late gestation fetal wounds correlates with increased hyaluronidase activity and removal of hyaluronan. Int J Biochem Cell Biol. 1997;29(1):201–10. Epub 1997/01/01.
2. Sullivan KM, Meuli M, MacGillivray TE, Adzick NS. An adult-fetal skin interface heals without scar formation in sheep. Surgery. 1995;118(1):82–6. Epub 1995/07/01.
3. Wilgus TA. Regenerative healing in fetal skin: a review of the literature. Ostomy Wound Manage. 2007;53(6):16–31; quiz 2–3. Epub 2007/06/26.
4. Walraven M. Cellular and molecular mechanisms involved in scarless wound healing in the fetal skin. Amsterdam: VU university medical center; 2016. https://research.vu.nl/ws/portalfiles/portal/42155796/complete+dissertation.pdf.
5. Moore AL, Marshall CD, Barnes LA, Murphy MP, Ransom RC, Longaker MT. Scarless wound healing: Transitioning from fetal research to regenerative healing. Wiley Interdiscip Rev Dev Biol. 2018;7(2):e309. Epub 2018/01/10.
6. Ghatak S, Maytin EV, Mack JA, Hascall VC, Atanelishvili I, Moreno Rodriguez R, et al. Roles of proteoglycans and glycosaminoglycans in wound healing and fibrosis. Int J Cell Biol. 2015;2015:834893. Epub 2015/10/09.
7. Li M, Zhao Y, Hao H, Han W, Fu X. Theoretical and practical aspects of using fetal fibroblasts for skin regeneration. Ageing Res Rev. 2017;36:32–41. Epub 2017/02/28.
8. DiPietro LA. Angiogenesis and wound repair: when enough is enough. J Leukoc Biol. 2016;100(5):979–84. Epub 2016/11/02.
9. Redd MJ, Cooper L, Wood W, Stramer B, Martin P. Wound healing and inflammation: embryos reveal the way to perfect repair. Philos Trans R Lond B Biol Sci. 2004;359(1445):777–84.
10. Barnes LA, Marshall CD, Leavitt T, Hu MS, Moore AL, Gonzalez JG, et al. Mechanical forces in cutaneous wound healing: emerging therapies to minimize scar formation. Adv Wound Care. 2018;7(2):47–56. Epub 2018/02/03.
11. Lo DD, Zimmermann AS, Nauta A, Longaker MT, Lorenz HP. Scarless fetal skin wound healing update. Birth Defects Res C Embryo Today. 2012;96(3):237–47. Epub 2012/10/31.
12. Chen W, Fu X, Ge S, Sun T, Sheng Z. Differential expression of matrix metalloproteinases and tissue-derived inhibitors of metalloproteinase in fetal and adult skins. Int J Biochem Cell Biol. 2007;39(5):997–1005. Epub 2007/04/06.

3

Ethical Considerations: Scar Management

Clarisse Ganier and Sonia Gaucher

Contents

The purpose of this chapter is to provide an overview and potential answers to the ethical considerations of the clinical management of patient scars. We will focus on two main aspects of this subject:

1. Is there truly a need to invoke ethics when the clinician is faced with managing a patient's scar?
2. What are the dilemmas that a clinician will confront in their daily practice when managing a patient's scar?

Is there Truly a Need to Invoke Ethics When the Clinician Is Faced with Managing a Patient's Scar?

The motivation for the clinical management of a patient's scar from both the patient's perspective and the clinician's perspective is clear: first, to improve the appearance of the scar and, second, if needed, to improve any functional impairment that the scar may have caused. If successful, these goals will enhance the beauty and function of the patient's skin and improve the patient's quality of life. Therefore, like all therapies or procedures in medicine, the ethical considerations of scar management are based upon balancing the risks and benefits of any treatment.

There are multiple causes of scars – scars generated by unintended accidents, iatrogenic scars from surgical procedures, and even self-inflected voluntary scars created by the patient. The constant among these, regardless of the reason(s) of the scar, is that the skin has been injured and has undergone the known phases of wound healing – clotting with platelet aggregation and activation, inflammation, reepithelialization, fibroplasia, neovascularization, granulation tissue formation, and then a long period of tissue remodeling with fibrosis and scarring. The scar is actually a witness to these events of "reparative" wound healing, rather than "regenerative" non-scarring wound healing that is seen in newts and lower animals.

Each cultural group has its own concept of beauty and of what it considers to be normal or aberrant. Moreover, the judgment of what is normal or not may be interpreted differently, not only by the society but also by the individuals. That is why when a patient bears a scar, it may take on different meanings, depending upon the societal and individual context of the scar.

Sometimes, a skin scar can carry a highly positive message. For example, the scar could be proudly exhibited as a testimony of some glorious actions such as the mark of a successful warrior exploit or survival from a savage assault. A voluntarily induced scar could also represent a ritualistic marking that symbolizes both social allegiance and beauty. Examples include scarifications and tattoos.

Conversely, a skin scar could represent an echo of an emotional scar. In these situations, the meaning of the scar is well beyond a simple previous threat to the integrity of the body envelope. Rather, the scar becomes a permanent remembrance a traumatic event. The scar may represent and even support the revival of the patient's spirit after a painful traumatic episode. The possibility of recognizing an aesthetic prejudice, which could be temporary and/or permanent, in the context of a judicial expertise, testifies to this aspect.

On the other hand, for patients whom are strictly compliant to societal standards and societal points of view of beauty, a scar in a visible location on the patient's body may cause loss of self-esteem and self-confidence, regardless of its origin.

Another potential context of scar management would be a patient who generates and accumulates self-inflicted scars and psychologically believes that the healed scars form sort of protective bandage.

Therefore, there is no single approach to the management of these various complex situations, except for the underlying understanding that patients who are scarred require attention, and a physician who listens to them assesses the proper context of the scar and considers carefully what the patient desires.

What Are the Dilemmas that a Clinician Will Confront in Their Daily Practice When Managing a Patient's Scar?

At the same time, the surgeon may be pleased to observe a minimal scar as the result from his/her surgical procedure and may be faced with the disappointed patient who wants the scar to disappear completely.

In many cases – and especially after surgery – scars can make the physician feels uncomfortable, because the scar is an obvious evidence of the physician's work and reminds the physician of his or her limitations and shortcomings. Totally scarless surgery is not possible. Beyond the disease that the patient would like to forget and beyond the pain and suffering that the patient went through, the physician needs to understand the disappointment and distress of the patient when he/she learns that the scar is permanent and cannot be erased.

Experience has taught us that objective criteria (surface area, surface texture, color, thickness, degree of fibrosis etc.) are not always sufficient to assess adequately a scar and its functional and psychological repercussions. A too fast clinical examination and judgment may lead to the conclusion that the patient's request for scar revision is superfluous, unnecessary, or even unreasonable. To avoid misunderstanding of the patient's feeling and desire for scar revision, the physician must look beyond the simple appearance of the scar and has to harken back to the patient's own history including his or her trauma and the context of the scar. A large discrepancy between the perspective of the patient and the perspective of the physician might be an early indication of psychological difficulties and a call for further clinical attention [1].

When the patient adamantly demands scar revision by surgical intervention, it often comes from the patient's point of view (and/or experience) that less invasive solutions (topical steroids, silicone membranes, laser treatment, etc.) are not satisfactory.

The origin of surgical ethics is uncertain [2, 3]. Reviews and studies on skin scar ethics are scarce [4]. Most of the articles involve issues related to the ethics of burn scars [5], the ethics in plastic surgery [6], or the ethics in major surgery [7]. Nevertheless, some reviews highlight the current problems associated with emerging approaches for scar management such as the use of fetal cells in skin regeneration [8].

According to Miles Little publications [9, 10], surgical ethics have generally been framed as general medical ethics applied to surgical situations. There are five categories of experience and relationship, which are especially important in surgery field. These include (i) rescue, (ii) proximity, (iii) ordeal, (iv) aftermath, and (v) presence. The sense of rescue and of relational proximity, the ordeal, and aftermath of surgery are things that the patient experiences. Understanding these feelings allow surgeons to know what may be asked of them in an ethical point of view. Recognition of the reality and validity of each category in the surgical process highlights the importance of presence that is the acts by which the surgeon demonstrates that he is present to the patient throughout the surgical process and its consequences. While communication skill trainings may never completely compensate for insensitivity, the ideal of presence as a virtue and as a duty can be taught by precept and by mentors.

As Albert Einstein said "If you always do what you always did, you will always get what you always got." Because each scar, each patient, and each context are unique, the search for an adequate and appropriate surgical solution constantly forces us to innovate. Innovation in surgery has contributed to progress in medicine and has enhanced the overall patient's quality of life. Nevertheless, surgical innovation itself also raises numerous ethical issues, such as patient safety, informed consent, the proper use of healthcare resources, and conflicts of interest – especially in the case of developing new devices by an industry-physician partnership. None of these challenges are specific to surgery field, nor to scars, but there are features about surgery and scars that complicates the identification and resolution of these issues [11, 12]. Therefore, it is important, from an ethical point of view, to consider that innovation is not only the key to progress but also the greatest challenge to our professionalism [13].

Take Home Message

Given that scar treatment needs to balance risks and benefits for the patient, it's impossible to define a skin scar by its physical appearance only.

References

1. Hoogewerf CJ, Van Baar ME, Middelkoop E, Van Loey NE. Patient reported facial scar assessment: directions for the professional. Burns. 2014;40(2):347–53.
2. Namm JP, Siegler M, Brander C, Kim TY, Lowe C, Angelos P. History and evolution of surgical ethics: John Gregory to the twenty-first century. World J Surg. 2014;38(7):1568–73.
3. Pellegrini CA, Ferreres A. Surgical ethics symposium "ethical dilemmas in surgical practice". World J Surg. 2014;38(7):1565–6.
4. Ferreres A, Angelos P. Surgical ethics symposium: ethical dilemmas in surgical practice. World J Surg. 2014;38(7):1567.
5. Teven CM, Gottlieb LJ. The four-quadrant approach to ethical issues in burn care. AMA J Ethics. 2018;20(6):595–601.
6. Sterodimas A, Radwanski HN, Pitanguy I. Ethical issues in plastic and reconstructive surgery. Aesthet Plast Surg. 2011;35(2):262–7.
7. Wall AE. Ethics in global surgery. World J Surg. 2014;38(7):1574–80.
8. Li Q, Zhang C, Fu X. Will stem cells bring hope to pathological skin scar treatment? Cytotherapy. 2016;18(8):943–56.
9. Little M. The fivefold root of an ethics of surgery. Bioethics. 2002;16(3):183–201.
10. Little M. Invited commentary: is there a distinctively surgical ethics? Surgery. 2001;129(6):668–71.
11. Johnson J, Rogers W. Innovative surgery: the ethical challenges. J Med Ethics. 2012;38(1):9–12.
12. Miller ME, Siegler M, Angelos P. Ethical issues in surgical innovation. World J Surg. 2014;38(7):1638–43.
13. Angelos P. Ethics and surgical innovation: challenges to the professionalism of surgeons. Int J Surg. 2013;11(S1):S2–5.

4

Long-Pulsed 1064 nm Nd:YAG Laser Treatment for Keloids and Hypertrophic Scars

Rei Ogawa

Contents

Background

Keloids and hypertrophic scars are fibroproliferative disorders of the skin that are caused by abnormal healing of injured or irritated skin [1]. Both disorders have similar histological features: the epidermis and the papillary layer of the dermis are almost normal apart from slight inflammation, and the only abnormality is in the reticular layer of the dermis [2]. While keloids typically exhibit marked hyalinized collagen deposition as a result of prolonged and strong inflammation, this feature is less pronounced in hypertrophic scars [3]. Thus, it is possible that hypertrophic scars and keloids are manifestations of the same fibroproliferative skin disorder and just differ in the intensity and duration of inflammation. These features may in turn be influenced by genetic, systemic, and local risk factors. It is possible that keloids arise largely as a result of genetic and systemic factors that promote massive and extended inflammation, while hypertrophic scars are more likely to be due to local factors. Genetic factors may include single nucleotide polymorphisms [4, 5], while systemic factors may include hypertension [6, 7], pregnancy [8, 9], hormones, and cytokines. The most important local factor is skin tension on the edges of the scar [10–12].

Our understanding of the pathogenesis of keloids and hypertrophic scars has improved markedly in the last 10 years, and these previously intractable scars are now regarded as being treatable. This has dramatically improved the quality of life of patients with these heavy scars [3]. There are many therapeutic options for keloids and hypertrophic scars, including surgery, radiation, corticosteroids, 5-fluorouracil, cryotherapy, laser therapy, anti-allergy agents, anti-inflammatory agents, bleaching creams, and make-up therapies. In terms of laser therapy, we have used long-pulsed 1064 nm Nd:YAG laser (Cutera Inc., Brisbane, CA) to treat keloids and hypertrophic scars and have reported its indications and limitations previously [13, 14].

Laser Therapies for Keloids and Hypertrophic Scars

Pulsed dye laser (PDL) has long been the therapy of choice for cutaneous vascular diseases, including telangiectasia, hemangioma, and vascular malformations [15–17]. It has also been used to treat keloids and hypertrophic scars because they have more blood vessels than normal skin. However, although PDL is effective for vascular diseases that affect the superficial skin layers (i.e., the epidermis and the papillary layer of the dermis), it does not penetrate deep enough to reach the deep dermal regions (i.e., the reticular layer of the dermis). Thus, PDL is not particularly effective for keloids and hypertrophic scars. By contrast, 1064 nm Nd:YAG laser reaches more deeply than PDL. As a result, it is increasingly being used to treat keloids and hypertrophic scars [13, 18–21]. It has been suggested that it acts by suppressing neovascularization and the dilatation of blood vessels.

Long-pulsed (not Q-switched) 1064 nm Nd:YAG laser plays an important role in our treatment algorithms for keloids and hypertrophic scars. This laser was developed for the treatment of vascular diseases, including inflammatory scars that exhibit neovascularization. It is also used to remove hair and to rejuvenate the skin [13]. The depth that is reached is determined by the spot size, the laser power, and the fluence: the larger the spot size, power, or fluence, the deeper the laser beam penetrates. Therefore, a large spot size and/or power are used for deep targets such as hair follicles and the blood vessels in the reticular layer of the dermis. However, since larger power increases the risk of cutaneous burn injury, the power should be determined on a case-by-case basis.

Indications and Limitations of Long-Pulsed 1064 nm Nd:YAG Laser for Keloids and Hypertrophic Scars

Keloid and hypertrophic scar development is due to chronic inflammation of the dermis during the course of wound healing. This associates with prolonged angiogenesis and collagen production. As mentioned above, long-pulsed 1064 nm Nd:YAG laser treatment may effectively treat keloid and hypertrophic scars because it reduces their vascularity. This reduction in vascularity may in turn decrease cytokine or growth factor levels in the tissue, which then promote collagen deposition. This notion is supported by the ability of several vascularity-suppressing treatments to improve inflammation and thereby ameliorate abnormal scars. One such treatment may be compression therapy, which is widely used with heavy scars, especially for hypertrophic scars that arise from burn wounds. This therapy may force the collapse of blood vessels in the scar, thereby decreasing cytokine or growth factor levels in the tissue. Moreover, it has been suggested that radiation therapy is effective for keloids because it suppresses angiogenesis. However, studies elucidating the mechanisms underlying long-pulsed 1064 nm Nd:YAG laser treatment efficacy in abnormal scars are warranted.

Our previous study [13] suggests that repeated tension on the edges of scars that is imposed by body movements prolongs scar inflammation: we observed that the patterns of mechanical force distribution around keloids

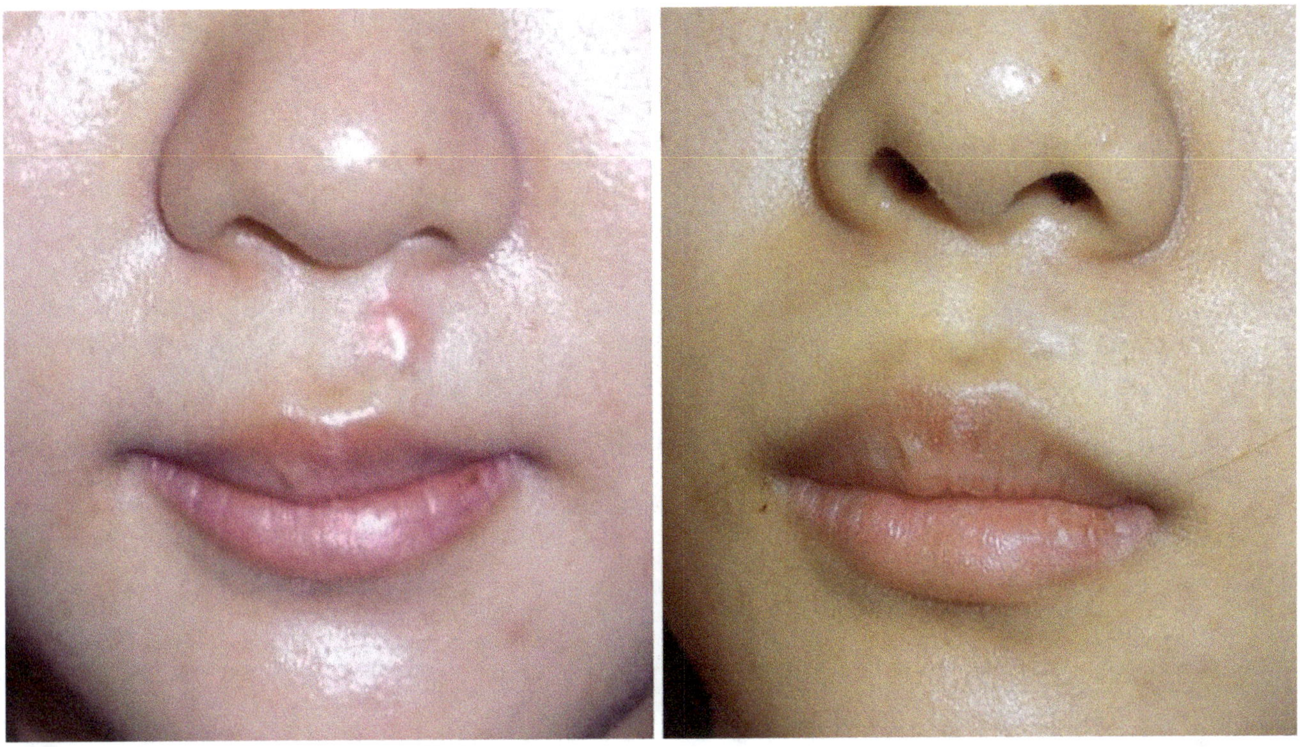

Fig. Upper lip hypertrophic scar. Left: before treatment. Right: 1 year after treatment. Two years before her referral to our clinic, a 20-year-old female received an abrasion injury to her upper lip that turned into a hypertrophic scar. Long-pulsed 1064 nm Nd:YAG laser was used at the following settings: 5 mm spot diameter, 65–70 J/cm^2, 25 ms, and 2 Hz. After 1 year of this treatment, the scar continued to exhibit a textural difference, but its redness and elevation had improved. (This figure is cited from Ref. [13] with approval from the publisher.)

and hypertrophic scars are largely consistent with the shape of the scar. In particular, our study suggests that keloids grow into the direction of the dominant prevailing skin tension. This mechanism explains why keloids on different regions of the body adopt specific shapes, such as the butterfly on the shoulder, the dumbbell on the upper arm, and the crab's claw on the anterior chest. These observations suggest that, if scars will continue to be subjected to strong tension due to the daily movements of the body, long-pulsed 1064 nm Nd:YAG laser will not be successful. Indeed, our experience suggests that scars on less stretched areas (i.e., the face and anterior lower leg) respond better to this therapy than scars on highly stretched areas (i.e., the anterior chest wall and scapula). We also found that (1) less inflamed scars (i.e., the typical hypertrophic scar) (Figs. 32.1, 32.2, and 32.3) respond better than highly inflamed scars (i.e., the typical keloid) (Figs. 32.4, 32.5, and 32.6); (2) thinner scars respond better than thick scars; (3) small scars respond better than large scars; (4) single scars respond better than multiple scars (Fig. 32.7); and (5) if even a little scar redness and induration remains after long-pulsed 1064 nm Nd:YAG laser treatment, these scars are highly likely to recur.

Treatment Settings of Long-Pulsed 1064 nm Nd:YAG Laser for Keloids and Hypertrophic Scars

The laser should generally be applied to the skin surface with the following standard treatment settings: a spot diameter of 5 mm, an energy density of 75 J/cm^2, an exposure time per pulse of 25 ms, and a repetition rate of 2 Hz. However, in the case of the face (Figs. 32.1 and 32.2) or pediatric patients, the treatment should start with a lower energy density (60–70 J/cm^2) to reduce the possibility of a burn injury. The best way to prevent such burn injuries is to cool the tip or air-cool the targeted skin before and immediately after irradiation. Each session should consist of three passes unless the patient feels strong pain at the second pass; in this case, the session should be stopped. Even if the patient feels no pain after the third pass, the session should be stopped. Local anesthesia is not necessary. However, if the patient expresses concern, anesthesia cream or tape can be used. The intervals between the sessions should generally be 2–4 weeks depending on the patient's schedule.

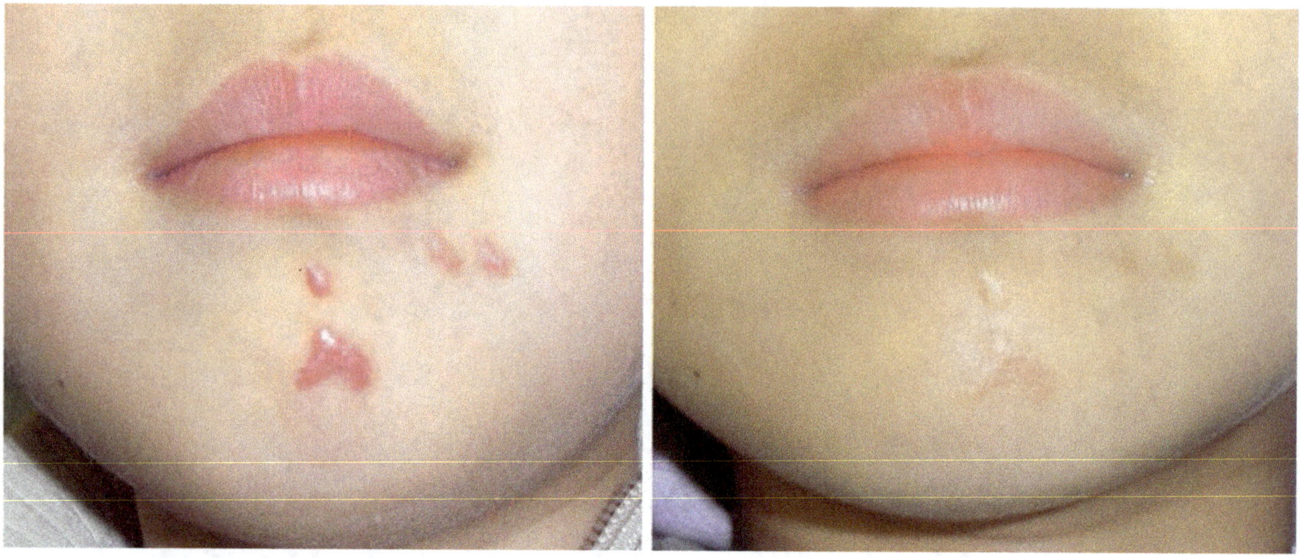

Fig. Lower lip hypertrophic scar. Left: before treatment. Right: 1 year after treatment. One year before her referral to our clinic, an 11-year-old female received an abrasion injury to her lower lip that developed into hypertrophic scars. Long-pulsed 1064 nm Nd:YAG laser was used at the following settings: 5 mm spot diameter, 60–70 J/cm^2, 25 ms, and 2 Hz. After 1 year of treatment, the scars continued to display textural differences and elevation, but there was clear improvement in their redness. (This figure is cited from Ref. [13] with approval from the publisher. © All rights reserved)

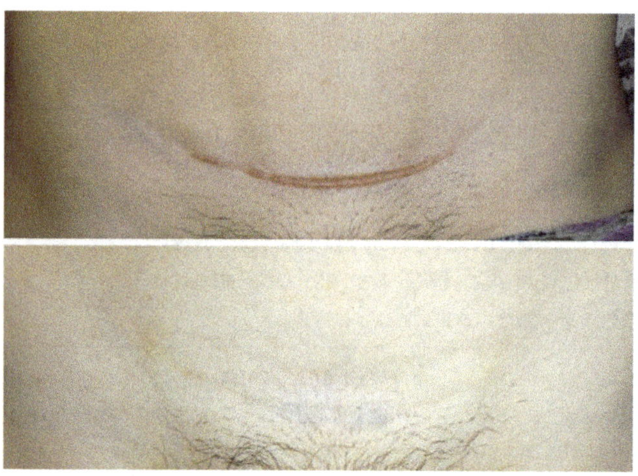

Fig. Abdomen hypertrophic scar. Upper: before treatment. Lower: 1 year after treatment. Four years before her referral to our clinic, a 50-year-old female developed hypertrophic scars on her abdomen after uterine myoma surgery. Long-pulsed 1064 nm Nd:YAG laser was used at the following settings: 5 mm spot diameter, 75 J/cm^2, 25 ms, and 2 Hz. After 1 year of treatment, the scar had almost disappeared. (This figure is cited from Ref. [13] with approval from the publisher. © All rights reserved)

Steroid tape is often used to decrease the inflammation in keloids and hypertrophic scars; this practice is particularly common in Japan and several other countries [22]. We use fludroxycortide tape (Drenison®, Dainippon Sumitomo Pharma Co., Ltd., Tokyo, Japan) with or without 1064-nm Nd:YAG laser (Cutera Inc., Brisbane, CA, USA) to treat pathological scars, including keloids and hypertrophic scars in recent years [23]. A retrospective cohort study [23] was performed to determine whether adding contact mode 1064-nm Nd:YAG laser therapy to conservative therapy (steroid tape) reduces the treatment time for hypertrophic Caesarean-section scars. In the results, combination of Nd:YAG laser and steroid tape treatment effectively decreased the total treatment time of hypertrophic Caesarean- section scars [23].

Follow-Up of Keloids and Hypertrophic Scars

It is important that patients with keloids and hypertrophic scars who undergo sequential treatments are followed up over the long term and that they are appropriately educated about scar management [3]. This is true regardless of the treatment that is being used. This is because, if patients develop pathological scars in the first place, they may be particularly prone to recurrence or the development of new pathological scars in

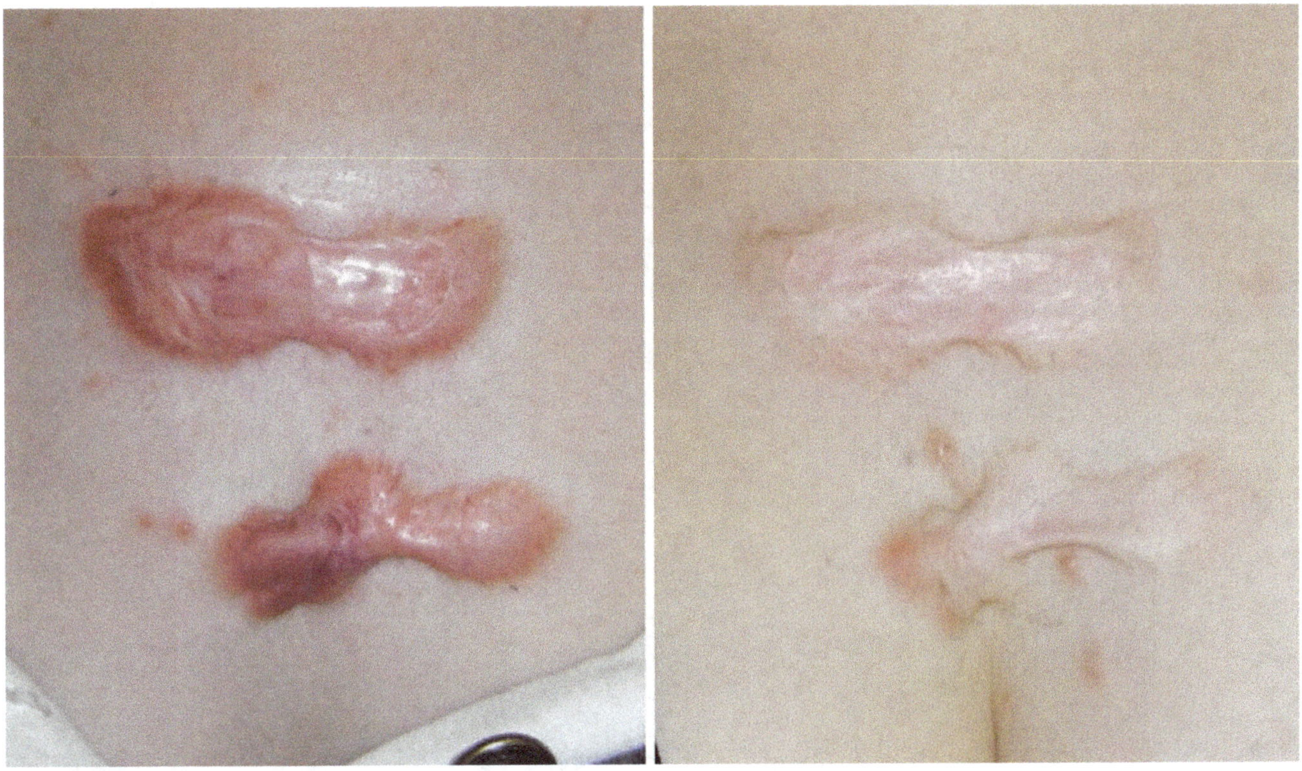

Fig. Anterior chest wall keloid. Left: before treatment. Right: 1 year after treatment. Eleven years before her referral to our clinic, a 29-year-old female developed butterfly-shaped keloids on her anterior chest. Treatment with steroid ointment and tape at other clinics did not improve these scars. Long-pulsed Nd:YAG laser was used at the following settings: 5 mm spot diameter, 65–75 J/cm^2, 25 ms, and 2 Hz. After 1 year of treatment, the textural differences and elevation had improved but there was remaining redness on some parts. (This figure is cited from Ref. [13] with approval from the publisher. © All rights reserved)

response to minor stimulation. Thus, these patients should be educated in the self-management of both their abnormal scars and new wounds. In particular, they should be encouraged to apply steroid tape/plasters during the early stages of scar development. This will rapidly reduce the inflammation in the scar and improve its appearance. Moreover, laser therapy, anti-allergy agents (including tranilast), anti-inflammatory agents, bleaching creams, and make-up therapies can be used on a case-by-case basis [3].

Conclusion

Long-pulsed 1064 nm Nd:YAG laser has been used to treat keloids and hypertrophic scars. This laser was developed for the treatment of vascular diseases, including inflammatory scars that exhibit neovascularization. The depth that is reached is determined by the spot size, the laser power, and the fluence: the larger the spot size, power, or fluence, the deeper the laser beam penetrates. The standard treatment setting is a spot diameter of 5 mm, an energy density of 75 J/cm^2, an exposure time per pulse of 25 ms, and a repetition rate of 2 Hz. Moreover, it is important that patients with keloids and hypertrophic scars who undergo sequential treatments are followed up over the long term and that they are appropriately educated about scar management.

Take-Home Messages

- It has been used long-pulsed 1064 nm Nd:YAG laser to treat keloids and hypertrophic scars.
- Long-pulsed 1064 nm Nd:YAG laser was developed for the treatment of vascular diseases, including inflammatory scars that exhibit neovascularization.
- The depth that is reached is determined by the spot size, the laser power, and the fluence: the larger the spot size, power, or fluence, the deeper the laser beam penetrates.
- The standard treatment setting is a spot diameter of 5 mm, an energy density of 75 J/cm^2, an exposure time per pulse of 25 ms, and a repetition rate of 2 Hz.

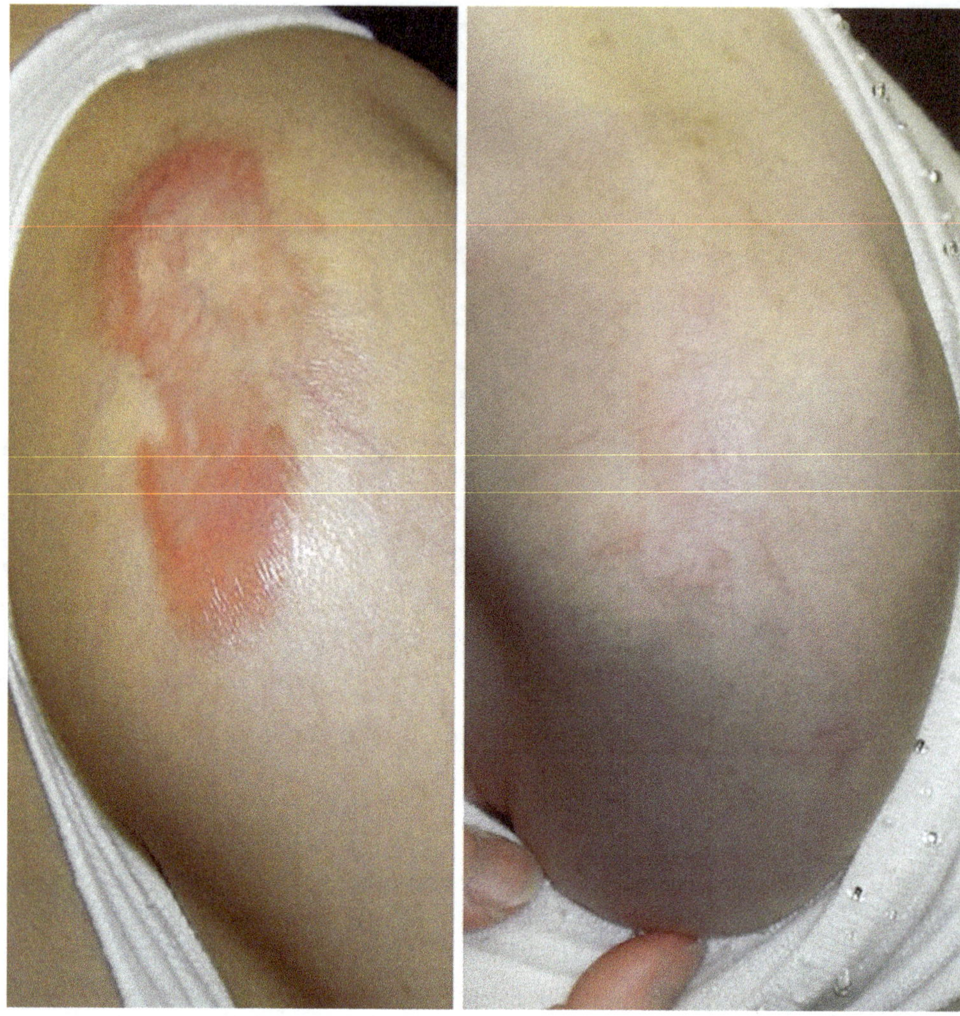

Fig. Shoulder keloid. Left: before treatment. Right: 30 months after treatment. About 20 years before her referral to our clinic, a 52-year-old female developed butterfly-shaped keloids on her upper arm and shoulder. Long-pulsed 1064 nm Nd:YAG laser was used at the following settings: 5 mm spot diameter, 70–75 J/cm^2, 25 ms, and 2 Hz. After 1 year of treatment, there were clear improvements in the textural differences and elevation but there was remaining redness on some parts. There was also some capillary dilation that was the result of steroid injections in the past. (This figure is cited from Ref. [13] with approval from the publisher)

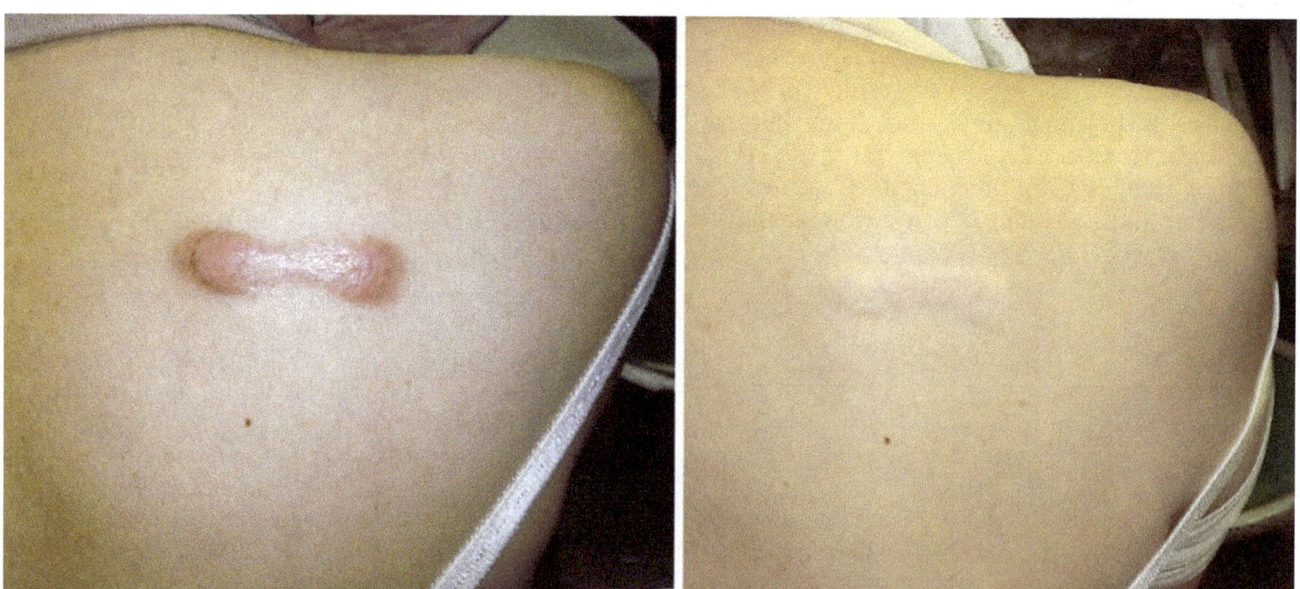

Fig. Scapular keloid. Left: before treatment. Right: 3 years after treatment. About 30 years before her referral to our clinic, a 52-year-old female developed a butterfly-shaped keloid on her scapula. Steroid injections and tape at other clinics yielded little improvement. Long-pulsed 1064 nm Nd:YAG laser was used at the following settings: 5 mm spot diameter, 70–75 J/cm^2, 25 ms, and 2 Hz. After 2 years of treatment, the texture, redness, induration, and elevation of the scar had clearly improved. (This figure is cited from Ref. [13] with approval from the publisher)

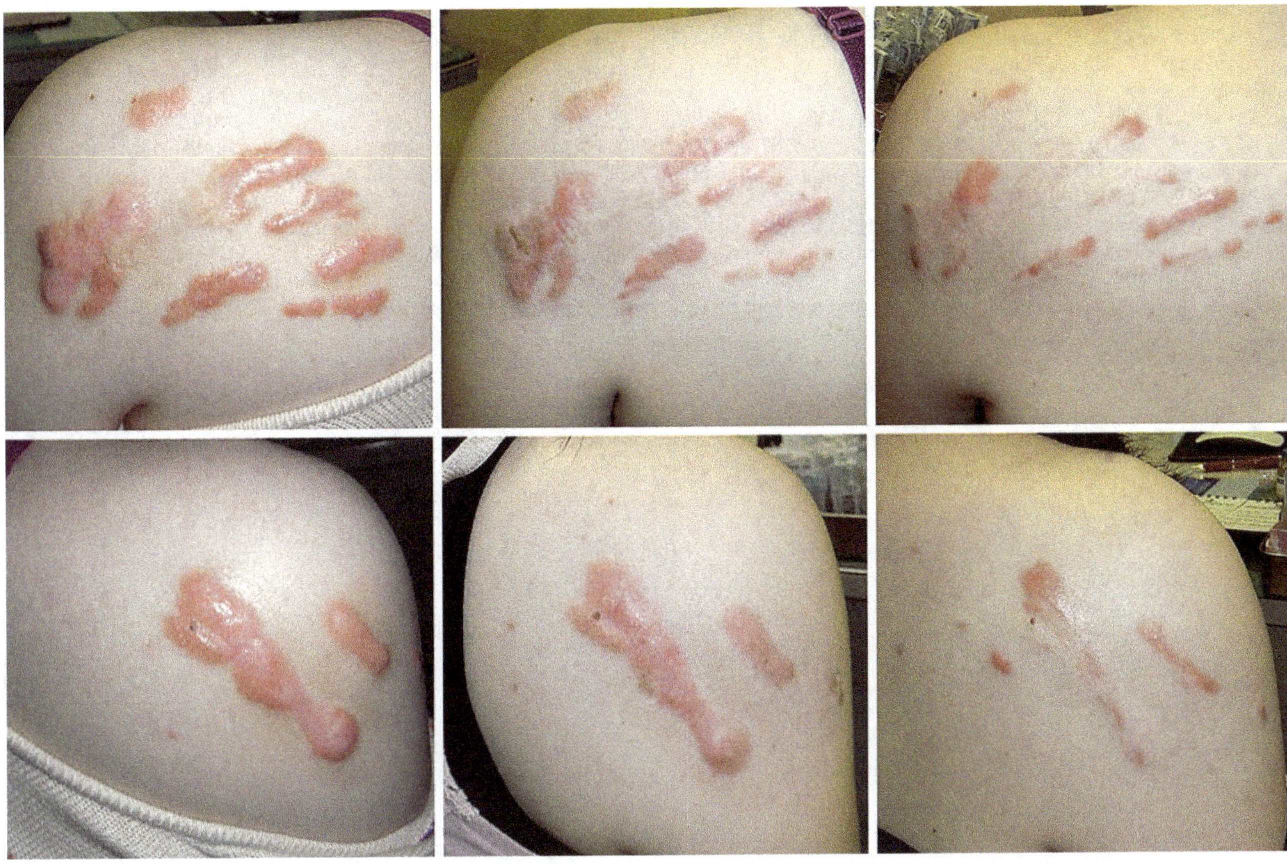

Fig. Scapular keloid. Left images: before treatment. Middle images: after 1 year of treatment. Right images: after 4 years of treatment. About 30 years before her referral to our clinic, a 42-year-old female developed multiple keloids on both the left (top images) and right (bottom images) scapular areas. The keloids had been slowly increasing in size. Steroid injections and tape treatment at other clinics yielded little improvement. Long-pulsed 1064 nm Nd:YAG laser was used at the following settings: 5 mm spot diameter, 75 J/cm^2, 25 ms, and 2 Hz. Moreover, a Chinese herb (Saireito) was administered every day. After 4 years of treatment, the texture, redness, induration, and elevation of the scars have improved. However, the scars are not yet completely cured

References

1. Tredget EE, Nedelec B, Scott PG, Ghahary A. Hypertrophic scars, keloids, and contractures. The cellular and molecular basis for therapy. Surg Clin North Am. 1997;77(3):701–30.
2. Huang C, Murphy GF, Akaishi S, Ogawa R. Keloids and hypertrophic scars: update and future directions. Plast Reconstr Surg Glob Open. 2013;1(4):e25.
3. Ogawa R, Akaishi S, Kuribayashi S, Miyashita T. Keloids and hypertrophic scars can now be cured completely: recent progress in our understanding of the pathogenesis of keloids and hypertrophic scars and the most promising current therapeutic strategy. J Nippon Med Sch. 2016;83(2):46–53.
4. Nakashima M, Chung S, Takahashi A, Kamatani N, Kawaguchi T, Tsunoda T, Hosono N, Kubo M, Nakamura Y, Zembutsu H. A genome-wide association study identifies four susceptibility loci for keloid in the Japanese population. Nat Genet. 2010;42(9):768–71.
5. Ogawa R, Watanabe A, Than Naing B, Sasaki M, Fujita A, Akaishi S, Hyakusoku H, Shimada T. Associations between keloid severity and single-nucleotide polymorphisms: importance of rs8032158 as a biomarker of keloid severity. J Invest Dermatol. 2014;134(7):2041–3.
6. Arima J, Huang C, Rosner B, Akaishi S, Ogawa R. Hypertension: a systemic key to understanding local keloid severity. Wound Repair Regen. 2015;23(2):213–21.
7. Huang C, Ogawa R. The link between hypertension and pathological scarring: does hypertension cause or promote keloid and hypertrophic scar pathogenesis? Wound Repair Regen. 2014;22(4):462–6.
8. Moustafa MF, Abdel-Fattah MA, Abdel-Fattah DC. Presumptive evidence of the effect of pregnancy estrogens on keloid growth. Case report. Plast Reconstr Surg. 1975;56(4):450–3.
9. Mendelsohn ME, Karas RH. Estrogen and the blood vessel wall. Curr Opin Cardiol. 1994;9(5):619–26.
10. Ogawa R, Okai K, Tokumura F, Mori K, Ohmori Y, Huang C, Hyakusoku H, Akaishi S. The relationship between skin stretching/contraction and pathologic scarring: the important role of mechanical forces in keloid generation. Wound Repair Regen. 2012;20(2):149–57.
11. Ogawa R, Akaishi S, Huang C, Dohi T, Aoki M, Omori Y, Koike S, Kobe K, Akimoto M, Hyakusoku H. Clinical applications of basic research that shows reducing skin tension could prevent and treat abnormal scarring: the importance of fascial/subcutaneous tensile reduction sutures and flap surgery for keloid and hypertrophic scar reconstruction. J Nippon Med Sch. 2011;78(2):68–76.

12. Akaishi S, Akimoto M, Ogawa R, Hyakusoku H. The relationship between keloid growth pattern and stretching tension: visual analysis using the finite element method. Ann Plast Surg. 2008;60(4):445–51.
13. Koike S, Akaishi S, Nagashima Y, Dohi T, Hyakusoku H, Ogawa R. Nd:YAG laser treatment for keloids and hypertrophic scars: an analysis of 102 cases. Plast Reconstr Surg Glob Open. 2015;2(12):e272.
14. Akaishi S, Koike S, Dohi T, Kobe K, Hyakusoku H, Ogawa R. Nd:YAG laser treatment of keloids and hypertrophic scars. Eplasty. 2012;12:e1.
15. Dover JS, Arndt KA. New approaches to the treatment of vascular lesions. Lasers Surg Med. 2000;26(2):158–63.
16. Alster TS, Williams C. Treatment of keloid sternotomy scars with 585 nm flashlamp-pumped pulsed-dye laser. Lancet. 1995;345:1198–200.
17. Paquet P, Hermanns JF, Pierard GE. Effect of the 585nm flash-pumped pulsed dye laser for the treatment of keloids. Dermatol Surg. 2001;27(2):171–4.
18. Dragoni F, Bassi A, Cannarozzo G, Bonan P, Moretti S, Campolmi P. Successful treatment of acne keloidalis nuchae resistant to conventional therapy with 1064-nm ND:YAG laser. G Ital Dermatol Venereol. 2013;148(2):231–2.
19. Rossi A, Lu R, Frey MK, Kubota T, Smith LA, Perez M. The use of the 300 microsecond 1064 nm Nd:YAG laser in the treatment of keloids. J Drugs Dermatol. 2013;12(11):1256–62.
20. Al-Mohamady AE, Ibrahim SM, Muhammad MM. Pulsed dye laser versus long-pulsed Nd:YAG laser in the treatment of hypertrophic scars and keloid: a comparative randomized split-scar trial. J Cosmet Laser Ther. 2016;8:1–5.
21. Tian WC. Savior of post-blepharoepicanthoplasty scarring: novel use of a low-fluence 1064-nm Q-switched Nd:YAG laser. J Cosmet Laser Ther. 2016;18(2):69–71.
22. Goutos I, Ogawa R. Steroid tape: a promising adjunct to scar management. Scars Burn Heal. 2017;3:2059513117690937.
23. Tsai CH, Kao HK, Akaishi S, An-Jou Lin J, Ogawa R. Combination of 1,064-nm Neodymium-doped Yttrium Aluminum Garnet Laser and Steroid Tape. Decreases the Total Treatment Time of Hypertrophic Scars: An Analysis of 40 Cases of Cesarean-Section Scars [published online ahead of print, 2019 Nov 5]. Dermatol Surg. 2019;10.1097/DSS.0000000000002235.

5

Scar Epidemiology and Consequences

M. El Kinani and F. Duteille

Contents

Introduction and Background

Cutaneous scarring is a dynamic process following a physical alteration of the cutaneous barrier. It is a slow process, taking place in three phases: debridement, granulation and epidermization, each of these phases bringing into play different cellular mediators. Then comes the maturation phase of the scar, which reaches its final appearance usually after two years of evolution.

It is important to distinguish between defective scars, which may result out of poor surgical technique, issuing to a dermal separation, keeping the epidermal layer in continuity. These scars are stable over time and do not belong to the same category than pathological scars, which are true evolutionary abnormalities of cutaneous scarring, linked to abnormal cell proliferation of myofibroblasts, with different scenarios depending on the degree of anarchy of the collagenic bundles.

Reminder of the Spectrum of Scars

Contractures

Located generally opposite the joints or when a wound is perpendicular to the lines of Langer, they can alter considerably the function according to their importance and their localization. They are particularly common in burned patients or after a thin or semi-thick skin graft.

Extended Scar

They are mainly observed from the first postoperative weeks. Most often pale, asymptomatic, they pose mostly aesthetic problems without functional discomfort. Stretch marks (often abdominal) are a type of enlarged scar and a consequence of a rupture of the dermis, without epidermal alteration. The absence of elevation or thickening differentiates them from hypertrophic scars.

Atrophic Scar

The plan of these scars lies under the plan of healthy peripheral skin. They are usually small. Frequent on the face, they are mostly consequences of acne or chicken pox.

Hypertrophic Scar

They are characterized clinically by an elevation of the plane of the scar which is thickened, inflammatory, but which remains limited to the cicatricial banks. They never invade the healthy peripheral skin. They are also distinguished from keloid scars by their spontaneous regression within two years of the onset of the wound. They are often itchy and even painful.

Keloid Scar

Unlike hypertrophic scars, keloid scars extend beyond the margins and also affect healthy skin around the scar. Functional symptoms (itching and pain) are very common and hinder quality of life. They have no tendency to regress. After excision, the rate of recurrence is major, making the management of these scars, which must be multimodal, complex.

Pathological (hypertrophic or keloid) healing is a complex process, resulting from many factors. During normal healing, the myofibroblasts participating in the cutaneous contraction enter apoptosis. A lack of apoptosis of these myofibroblasts, and consequently their excessive accumulation, explains the occurrence of raised and inflammatory scars [1]. Another factor contributing to the pathogenesis of these scars is an accumulation of immature collagen [2].

Hypertrophic Scars

Hypertrophic scars are the result of excessive proliferation of myofibroblasts and increased deposition of collagen within the scar [1, 2]. The scar then exceeds to the surface of the healthy peripheral skin, can be inflammatory and itchy, and even painful. They differ from keloid scars due to their tendency to regress within two years and because they never exceed the scarred margins [3, 4, 5]. However, diagnostic errors are still common in practice.

Basic Epidemiology

The frequent confusion between hypertrophic scars and keloids (despite the above definitions) means that there is little data on their epidemiology. The studies found are often of low level of evidence, centered on a given geographic population. Mahdavian Belavary et al [5] studied the rate of hypertrophic scars after breast reduction or median sternotomy. At three months, 60% of patients developed hypertrophic scars. At one year, there was persistent hypertrophy in 32% of patients included. These figures are consistent with previous studies, found between 38% and 68% postoperative hypertrophic scars [6]. An analysis of data over time would be interesting, in order to evaluate the average duration of evolution of these scars. No sex ratio was found in the literature, as men and women were similarly affected by the occurrence of hypertrophic scars.

Risk Factors

Many risk factors for the occurrence of scarring hypertrophy are admitted. There are many studies in the literature but many are of a low level of proof (levels IV–V). Butzelaar et al. [7] found as major risk factors the age, the existence of allergic terrain, the existence of bacterial colonization (with or without infection) within the wound, and cutaneous tension. Most of the hypertrophic scars are found between the ages of 11 and 30 years. This can be explained by the presence of sagging skin with age and a decrease in the inflammatory response [8]. It is often accepted that a dark phototype (African skin) is a risk factor for hypertrophic scars. Nevertheless, in the literature, the studies are of a low level of proof and the opinion of the authors is partaged, not allowing to bring a valid and reliable conclusion to this idea. Unlike keloid scars, there does not appear to be a genetic cause for the occurrence of hypertrophic scars [9]. Butzelaar et al [7] found a protective trend of smoking for the development of hypertrophic scars. Cancer chemotherapy also seems to be a protective factor; however, there are many confounding factors to consider in the studies in question (role of cancer itself, possible undernutrition).

Keloid Scars

The keloid scar is an abnormality of cutaneous healing specific to humans. The main problems, apart from their unattractive and annoying appearance, are their non-improvement in the time and frequency of recurrence despite the medical and surgical treatments undertaken. They can even be aggravated by surgical resection if it is not strictly intra-lesional.

Basic Epidemiology

Again, few studies have investigated the prevalence or incidence of keloid scars. Yet each year, it is estimated that about 100 million scars are developed, and among them 11 million would become keloids [10].

In the literature, the prevalence varies widely according to the population studied [3, 11].The estimations are as follows:

- 4.5 to 16% in black and Hispanic populations of American origin
- 16% in Zaire
- only 0.09% in England

They are responsible for pruritus or pain in 20–40% of cases [3].

Risk Factors

Keloid scars may be found on all localizations, but are more frequent in some areas [11, 12]:

- Ear lobe
- Pre-stern and deltoid region
- Under umbilical area (pubic area)

These are areas where skin tension is important, thus joining the frequent locations of hypertrophic scars. By definition, they do not touch the mucous membranes.

They can be observed at any age but peak frequency is between 10 and 30 years [13, 18]. Some authors explain this by the role of cutaneous tension which is more important in young subjects [3]. There also appears to be a hormonal factor, keloid scars being more frequent in the pubertal period [3]. The hormonal role is still discussed: if they are actually more common in pubertal period, keloids that appear at these ages also have a tendency to hyperpigmentation. During pregnancy, some authors have observed a more frequent appearance or enlargement of keloid scars [14].

It is also accepted that subjects with a dark phototype are more frequently affected, although we may experience keloid scars in all phototypes [15, 16].

The hypothesis of a genetic predisposition is beginning to be well anchored. It is estimated that 5 to 10% of cases have family keloids [17]. Marneros et al. [18] found that transmission is autosomal-dominant mode, the clinical penetrance is incomplete, and the expression is highly variable. There appears to be susceptibility to the development of keloids in Japanese and African-American families in relation to chromosomes 2 and 7 [19].

There are cases of spontaneous keloids in the literature, but these would ultimately be due to undetected microtrauma [20]

Specific Situation: The Burnt Patient Healing

Hypertrophic scarring after a burn (whether it has healed spontaneously or required skin grafting) is a common problem in clinical practice. In addition to being dysgraculous, these scars are generally itchy and even painful and can significantly alter function and quality of life, especially if they are responsible for skin retraction. Since this type of healing is quite specific to the burned patient, we chose to treat it in a separate chapter.

Scarred Hypertrophy in Burned Patients: Epidemiology

The data of the literature are very variable on this subject. In the majority of cases, the studies are small, and few distinctions are made between the different populations (adults vs. children, light phototype vs. dark phototype, spontaneously scarred burn vs. transplanted).

Deitch et al [21] found a prevalence of 15% (white patients) to 30% (black patients) in burn patients who healed spontaneously.

Mc Donald and Deitch [22] analyzed the prevalence of scar hypertrophy in patients treated with thin skin grafts. Of the children included, 75% had cicatricial hypertrophy. In adults, the prevalence was 50% in patients with black skin, compared to 7% in patients with fair skin.

Spurr and Shakespeare [23] followed 82 children and found 65% hypertrophic scars. Bombaro et al. [24] reported an average of 67% cicatricial hypertrophy (up to 100% in children with non-white skin). Finally, Delavary et al. [25] found a rate of 60% hypertrophic scars in burn patients, mainly in the first three months after the onset of the burn. According to them, young and non-smoking subjects are more likely to develop hypertrophic scars. In each of these studies, the number of patients remains low and the population monocentric. Further and larger studies would be needed to better identify populations at risk. The risk factors identified to date are young age, location of the upper limbs or neck, dark phototype, repetition of surgical procedures, initial severity of burn, and time to heal [25]. Lawrence et al [26] also find these risk factors in the literature, in addition to the female sex and skin grafts that required expansion (mesh-graft). Their review of the literature found a prevalence of hypertrophic scars ranging between 32 and 72%.

Retracted Scars

Retraction or contraction of the skin following a burn results from an excessive, hypertrophic scarring, of which we have just spoken. Functional consequences can be major and threaten the socio-professional future of patients. They are frequent and particularly disabling in the articular areas. The prevalence is very variable according to the studies, one finds on average between 38 and 54% of contraction in the years following the occurrence of the burn [27]. According to the authors, these would be more common in severely burned patients, children, women, and upper limb. Gangemi et al. [28] analyzed 703 burned patients and found on average 77% of pathological scars (44% hypertrophy, 5% contractures, 28% combining both). They also found as risk factors the female sex, the young age, localization of the burning of the upper limb or the neck, the repetition of the surgical procedures, and the expansion of the skin grafts when these are realized.

Impact of Scars

Although many studies concern the epidemiology and management of scars, very few have been interested in the consequences of these scars. However, it is estimated that more than one in two patients are not satisfied with the appearance of their scars, 20% of patients suffer from anxiety, and more than 50% feel that their privacy is affected by the presence of their scars [29].

Conclusion

Few studies have really focused on the epidemiology of scars and their consequences. When studies are conducted, they often concentrate around a given geographic population and report only a small number of patients. There are probably many lost sight, since many patients live surely with their scars (hypertrophic, keloids) without consulting. Larger scale studies should be carried out to determine the frequency of occurrence of these scarring abnormalities, in order to better identify them and, consequently, to better treat them.

Take Home Message

The epidemiology of pathologic scars is diverse. Sixty percent of scars located on the thorax may become hypertrophic, and a patient from Zaire has 100% more risks to develop a keloid than a patient native from England. Burns may issue up to 77% of pathologic scars, combining hypertrophic, retractile, and keloid scars. The role of hormonal status, nutrition, and many other factors has been suspected in keloids.

References

1. Sarrazy V, Billet F, Micallef L, Coulomb B, Desmoulière A. Mechanisms of pathological scarring: role of myofibroblasts and current developments. Wound Rep Reg. 2011;19:S10–5.
2. Ehrlich HP, Desmouliere A, Diegelmann RF, et al. Morphological and immunochemical differences between keloid and hypertrophic scar. Ann J Pathol. 1994;145:105.
3. Rockwell WB, Cohen IK, Ehrlich HP. Keloids and hypertrophic scars. A comprehensive review. Plast Reconstr Surg. 1989;84:827–37; Burd A, Huang I. Hypertrophic response and keloid diathe-

sis: two very different forms of scar. Plast Reconstr Surg. 2005;116:150e–7e.

4. Atiyeh BS, Costagliola M, Hayek SN. Keloid or hypertrophic scar, the controversy: review of the literature. Ann Plast Surg. 2005;54(6):676–80.d.
5. Mahdavian Delavary B, Van der Veer WM, Ferreira JA, Niessen FB. Formation of hypertrophic scars: evolution and susceptibility. J Plast Surg Hand Surg. 2012;46:95–101.
6. Elliot D, Cory-Pearce R, Rees GM. The behavior of presternal scars in a fair-skinned population. Ann R Coll Surg Engl. 1985;67:238–40.
7. Butzelaar, et al. Currently known risk factors for hypertrophic skin scarring: a review. J Plast Rec Aesth Surg. 2016;69:163–9.
8. Enoch S, Price PE. Cellular, molecular and biochemical differences in the pathophysiology of healing between acute wounds, chronic wounds and wounds in the aged. World Wild Wounds;2004;ISSN 1369–2607.
9. Brown JJ, Bayat A. Genetic susceptibility to raised dermal scarring. Br J Dermatol. 2009;161:8–18.
10. Bayat A, McGrouther DA, Ferguson MW. Skin scarring. BMJ. 2003;326:88–92.
11. Philandrianos C, et al. Keloid scars (part I): Clinical presentation, epidemiology, histology and pathogenesis. Ann Chir Plast Esthet. 2015;1181
12. Crockett DJ. Regional keloid susceptibility. Br J Plast Surg. 1964;17:245–53.
13. Bayat A, Arscott G, Ollier WE, McGrouther DA, Ferguson MW. Keloid disease: clinical relevance of single versus multiple site scars. Br J Plast Surg. 2005;58(1):28–37.
14. Moustafa MF, Abdel-Fattah MA, Abdel-Fattah DC. Presumptive evidence of the effect of pregnancy estrogens on keloid growth. Plast Reconstr Surg. 1975;56:450–3.
15. Allah KC, Yeo S, Kossoko H, Assi Dje Bi Dje V, Richard KM. Keloid scar on black skin: myth or reality. Ann Chir Plast Esthet. 2013;58(2):115–22.
16. Niessen FB, Spauwen PH, Schalkwijk J, Kon M. On the nature of hypertrophic scars and keloids: a review. Plast Reconstr Surg. 1999;104(5):1435–58.
17. Martinet L. La cicatrice chéloïde: étude retrospective sur quinze ans. [Thèse 2007]
18. Marneros AG, Norris JEC, Olsen BR, Reichenberger E. Clinical genetics of familial keloids. Arch Dermatol. 2001;131(11): 1429–34.
19. Marneros AG, Norris JEC, Watanabe S, Reichenberger E, Olsen BR. Genome scans provide evidence for keloid susceptibility loci on chromosomes 2q23 and 7p11. J Invest Dermatol. 2004;122:1126.
20. Pitche P. What is true in "spontaneous keloids"? Ann Dermatol Venerol. 2006;133:501.
21. Deitch EA, Wheelahan TM, Rose MO, Clothier J, Cotter J. Hypertrophic burn scars: analysis of variables. J Trauma. 1983;23:895–8.
22. McDonal WS, Deitch EA. Hypertrophic skin grafts in burned patients: a prospective analysis of variables. J Trauma. 1987;27:147–50.
23. Spurr ED, Shakespeare PG. Incidence of hypertrophic scarring in burn-injured children. Burns. 1990;16:179–81.
24. Bombaro KM, Engrav LH, Carrougher GJ, Wiechman SA, Faucher L, Costa BA, et al. What is the prevalence of hypertrophic scarring following burns ? Burns. 2003;29(4):299–302.
25. Delavary BM, Van der Veer WM, Ferreira JA, Niessen FB. Formation of hypertrophic scars: evolution and susceptibility. J Plast Surg Hand Surg. 2012;46:95–101.
26. Lawrence JW, Mason ST, Schomer K, Klein MB. Epidemiology and impact of scarring after burn injury: a systematic review of literature. J Burn Care Res. 2012;33:136–46.
27. Oosterwijk, et al. Prevalence of scar contractures after burn: a systematic review. Burns. 2017;43:41–9.
28. Gangemi EN, Gregori D, Berchialla P, et al. Epidemiology and risk factors for pathological scarring after burn wounds. Arch Facial Plast Surg. 2008;10:93–102.
29. Brown BC, McKenna SP, Siddhi K, McGrouther DA, Bayat A. The hidden cost of skin scars : quality of life after skin scarring. J Plast Recon Aesth Surg. 2008;61:1049–58.

6

International Scar Classification in 2019

Thomas A. Mustoe

Contents

There has been a wide variety of therapies proposed for the treatment of scars, most of them with a lack of firm randomized controlled clinical trials to support their efficacy, and among other deficiencies, there has been often a lack of appropriate labeling or classification of scars to allow optimal evaluation of existing literature. There is a real benefit to a consistent classification of different types of scars so that different clinicians use a consistent vocabulary allowing a systematic evaluation of treatments and outcomes. One problem has always been the changes in scars over time so that improvements may not necessarily be due to the treatment intervention but simply scar maturation.

Scar classifications have previously been published including notably the 2002 publication in PRS which gained widespread acceptance because it represented the consensus of 12 experts from an international group incorporating Europe, North America, and Australia. In subsequent publications, this classification has been found to sound and not needing further modification. We will use this classification again in this updated textbook.

Scarring is the inevitable consequence of tissue injury as opposed to tissue regeneration which is the true restoration of the normal architecture of the skin. True tissue regeneration after injury occurs only in the fetus during the first two trimesters and in amphibians who can even regenerate amputated limbs. In the optimal outcome of a thin flat thin linear scar, the sequence of tissue repair after injury is tightly regulated. After initial platelet aggegation, provisional matrix is deposited, followed by influx of inflammatory cells and subsequent cell proliferation including fibroplasia and angiogenesis. Wound healing overlap, and are followed by cellular apoptosis with resolution of inflammation. Permanent matrix deposition (collagen) begins within 3 days. Maximal collagen deposition occurs in the first few weeks with a combination of type 1 and type 3, followed by many months of collagen breakdown and synthesis with increasing type 1 collagen with increased organization and scar strength. These phases of inflammation, cell proliferation and collagen remodeling result in a fine line scar in the scenario of an incison ("normal" scar), and a wider flat scar in the scenario of an injury over a broader area.

Immature Scar

Even a normal scar goes through a period when it is immature, meaning it is pink, often with a healing ridge (edema plus collagen synthesis). Collagen accumulation typically peaks about 3 weeks after surgery and then goes through about 6 months of remodeling with steadily increasing collagen organization, conversion from a mix of type 1 and type 3 collagen to almost entirely type 1 collagen with increased cross-linking, and continued increase in tensile strength. The gains in scar strength are due to improvement in collagen organization and cross-linking rather than an increase in collagen. A useful analogy is to compare the difference between raw wool from a sheared sheep, versus the fine knit of a woolen coat. The amount of wool is the same, but the woven wool is far stronger. However, although the strength of a scar is maximal in approximately 6 months, complete scar maturation as measured by resolution of erythema typically takes a year or even longer. In a human volunteer study conducted by Renovo, superficial scars took longer than a year for the erythema to fully resolve in one-third of patients. In scars in thicker skin with more depth, or in a group of patients with more active scarring process, it probably takes even longer. In my own clinical practice with approximately 20,000 patients of all ages and ethnic backgrounds, my experience mirrors the study by Renovo (■ Table 9.1).

The resolution of erythema is a useful marker of scar maturity (■ Fig. 9.1). In all scars, erythema eventually resolves, but in a few percent of patients, I have seen it take longer than 2 years and in a rare hypertrophic scar as long as 10 years. In a study we conducted on burn patients, we found that the average scar elasticity (a measure of collagen remodeling), as measured by a device that applied a constant force to the skin and measured how much it stretched, continued to increase over 5 years (Bartell et al). Although the patients were not followed longitudinally, we simply correlated elasticity to the age of the scar, and it can be inferred that it can take a long time indeed for a scar to reach full maturity.

In an immature scar histologically, there are an increased number of inflammatory cells. After 2 weeks or so, the predominant inflammatory cells are macrophages with scattered lymphocytes and an occasional mast cell. There are increased numbers of fibroblasts including myofibroblasts, increased numbers of blood vessels, and for a period of up to a few months epidermal hyperplasia. The visual appearance is a scar that is erythematous and slightly raised due to increased fluid in the tissues and increased collagen as well as increased cellularity.

Mature Scar

In undergoing the transition from an immature scar to a mature scar, the key visual marker is resolution of erythema (■ Fig. 9.2). At this point, the inflammatory cells, endothelial cells, and most of the fibroblasts have undergone apoptosis, and the epithelium looks completely normal as compared to the adjacent unwounded

Table Scar Classification

Scar type	Description
Immature scar	Pink slightly raised
	Sometimes itchy
	Firm but not hard
	Begins soon after injury, months to resolve
	Peaks at a few weeks after injury
Mature flat scar	Flat scar without erythema, stable
	No symptoms
Hypertrophic linear scar	Ropy (elevated) and pink or red
	Evolves from immature scar within several weeks
	Progressive enlargement for months before slow decrease in activity
	Often itchy or slightly sore to touch
	Resolution results in a persistently elevated scar that is no longer pink
Hypertrophic wide scar	Elevated, pink or red
	Arises from widespread injury such as a burn
	Frequently with severe pruritis and can be tender
	Very stiff with limitation of mobility across joint surface
Minor keloid	Round or elevated, extends beyond scar
	Most often at site of pierced earring or surgical incision
	Strong genetic component which is different than hypertrophic scars
	Simple surgical excision with very high rate of recurrence
Major keloid	Elevated, large often irregular in shape (i.e., butterfly appearance)
	Frequently seen in multiple locations on person
	Initial injury can be very minor
	Often symptoms of pain and pruritis are debilitating
	Treatment options are limited

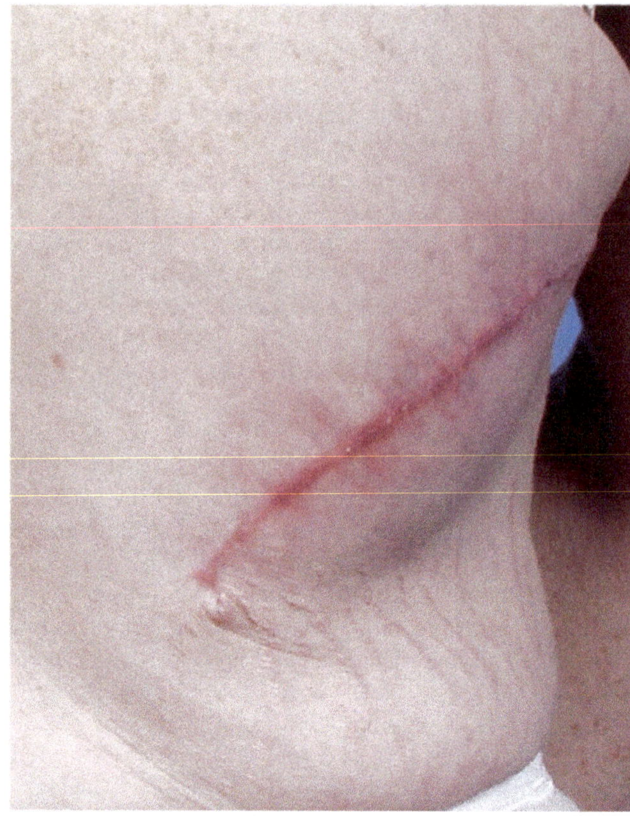

Fig. Immature scar

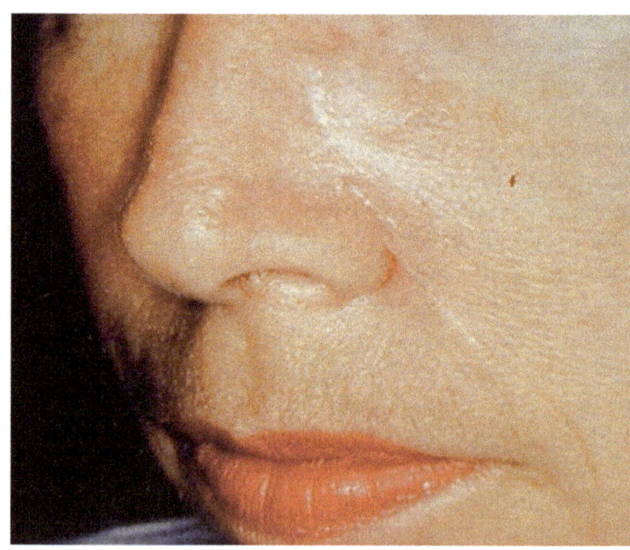

Fig. Mature scar

skin. What is left is a band of collagen fibers that are clearly demarcated from the surrounding dermis histologically lacking the completely ordered collagen organization characteristic of normal skin. The collagen fibers go in multiple directions giving the scar stiffer biomechanical properties and are of variable width depending on the genetics of the patient and the underlying tension placed on the healing immature scar. There is no longer any increased fluid in the tissues (edema) and so the scar is flat. The color of the scar ranges from white (absence of melanocytes) to hyperpigmented (often characteristic of ethnicities with increased melanocytes in the basal layer of the epidermis such as Asian, South Asian, Middle Eastern, Mediterranean, and Latin American or patients with brown skin).

Atrophic Scar

In some cases, a scar will become depressed or thinned as it transitions from an immature scar (◘ Fig. 9.3). This can occur when collagen synthesis is depressed and inflammation is less than usual. Examples of atrophic scars are the stretch marks or striae that can be a complication of systemic steroid excess either from exogenous steroids or Cushing's disease or in some scars after radiation therapy.

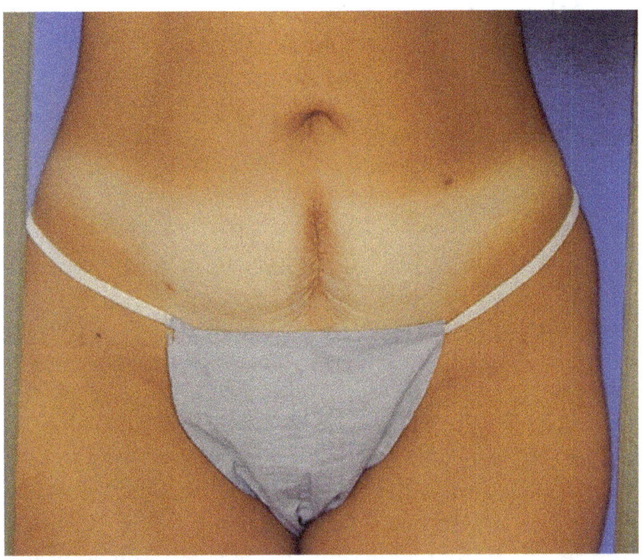

◘ **Fig.** Atrophic mature scar

Linear Hypertrophic Scar

In many cases, scars fail to transition normally from immature to mature with resolution of inflammation and an equilibrium of collagen synthesis and breakdown. Collagen continues to accumulate, and the scar widens and becomes elevated or ropy in appearance and the erythema fails to resolve. This active process of scar growth can continue for many months but eventually slowly resolves, with resolution of erythema that can take years. The collagen accumulation stabilizes but with a residual scar that is elevated and wider than a normal mature scar (◘ Fig. 9.4). During the period of active collagen accumulation and erythema, the scar can be itchy and/or painful. The residual scar is less elastic (stiffer) than normal skin and, if it crosses a joint, can limit motion. A key feature of hypertrophic scar (versus keloid) is that the scar tissue remains within the confines of the original scar (although it may be widened). Hypertrophic scars are more common in patients of color, particularly East Asians, and the susceptibility to hypertrophic scars is often inherited. Prolonged inflammation for any reason (delays in epithelization, blocked sebaceous glands, ingrown hairs, and tension) contributes significantly to the incidence of hypertrophic scars. Frequently portions of a scar will be hypertrophic in hair-bearing areas, while the adjacent scars evolve into normal mature scars.

Widespread Hypertrophic Scar

In many cases, most notably from burns, the initial injury is not linear but covers a larger area (◘ Fig. 9.5). In general, when epithelization (complete epithelial resurfacing) is not completed within 2 weeks, the risk of

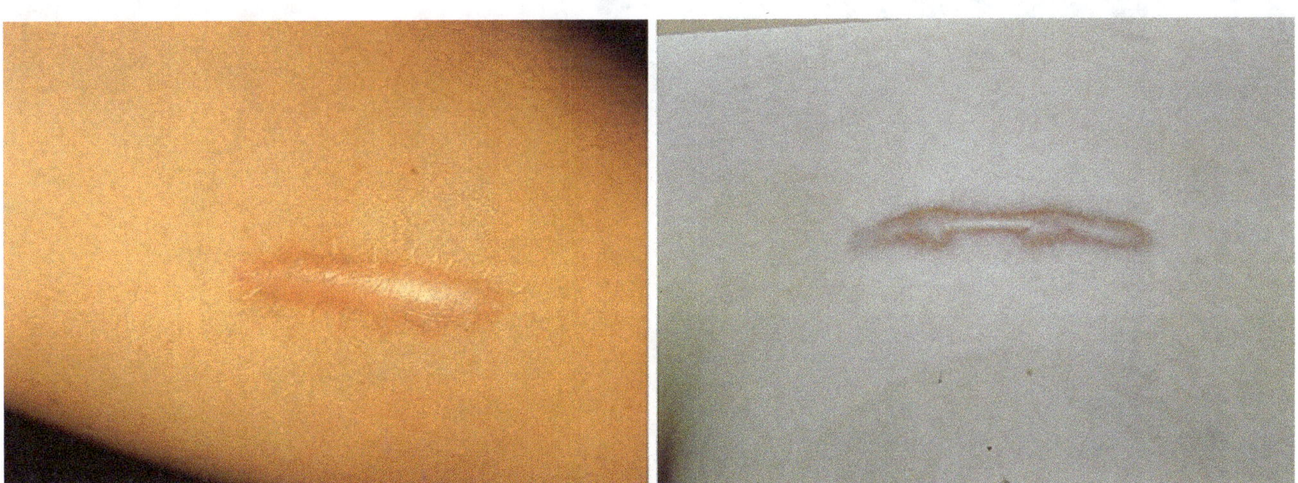

◘ **Fig.** Linear hypertrophic scar

hypertrophic scar increases, particularly in children and in adults under the age of 40. In a hypertrophic scar, the period of collagen accumulation is prolonged up to 6–12 months resulting in a scar that is elevated and thickened and is very stiff. Erythema will be prolonged and the scars are often intensely pruritic or even painful.

Keloid

A keloid unlike a hypertrophic scar behaves more like a tumor in that growth can occur even years after the original injury and extend far beyond the confines of the original scar. The keloid often has a mushroom or cauliflower type of appearance. Keloids are frequently symptomatic with pain or itch. The genetics of keloids are quite complex and beyond the scope of this chapter, but many are familial and are much more common among many African tribes and to a lesser degree among Asians. The central portion of a keloid is very dense fibers with a characteristic pattern histologically and relatively acellular, while the active spreading edge has a significant inflammatory and cellular component.

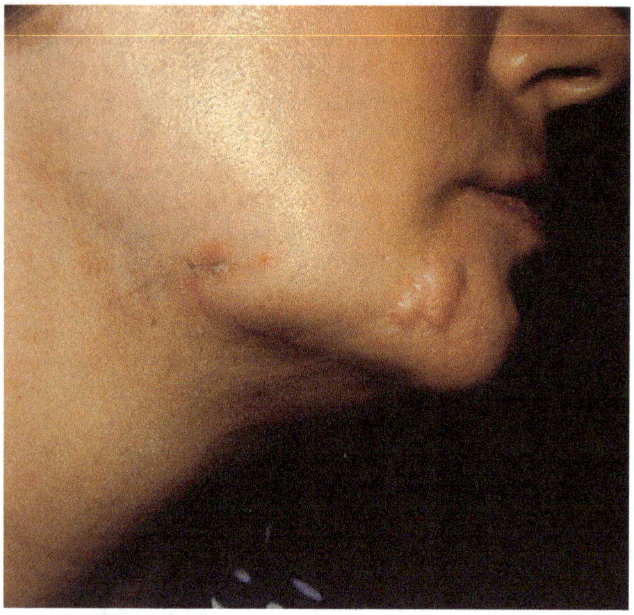

Fig. Hypertrophic broad scar

Minor Keloid

Most keloids arise from localized injuries such as a pierced ear (the most common location of minor keloid), and although they extend beyond the margins of the original scar, their growth stabilizes and allows more options for treatment including surgical excision combined with other modalities such as steroid injections or radiation therapy (Fig. 9.6).

Major Keloid

In extreme situations in patients with a very strong genetic predisposition, keloids can extend into large plagues with a very actively growing outer edge that in some areas has a characteristic butterfly pattern (Fig. 9.7a) due to forces on the keloid exerted by the surrounding skin. The peripheral edge of the keloid is active, while the central portion is less active with less cell proliferation. Often the original injury can be as minor as a scratch or seemingly spontaneous (Fig. 9.7b Keloid arising from small tracheotomy

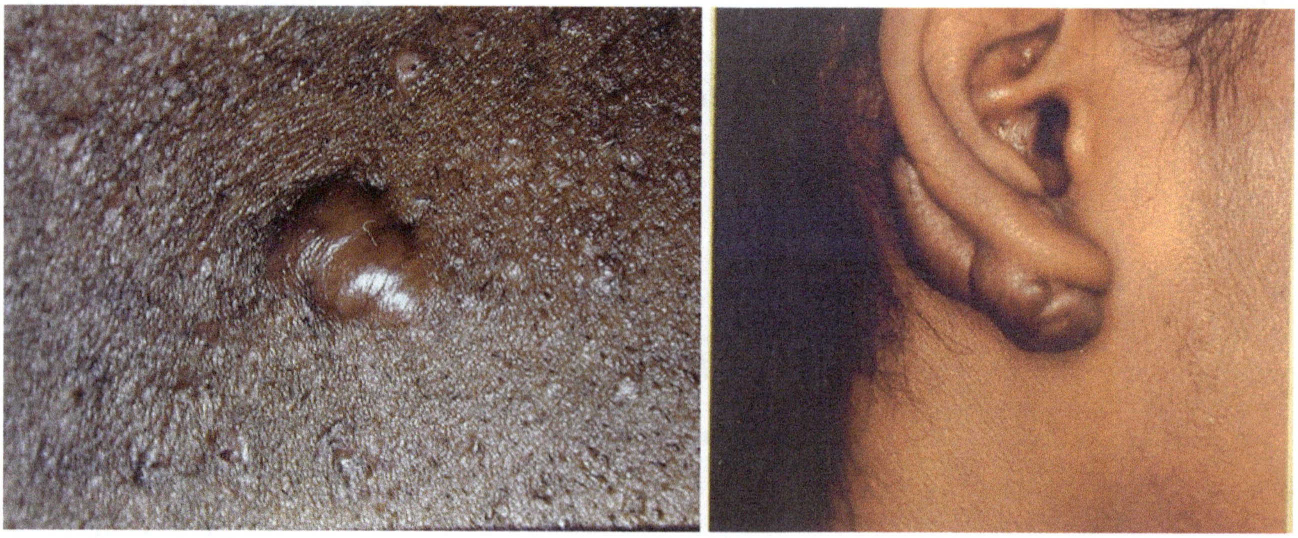

Fig. Minor keloid

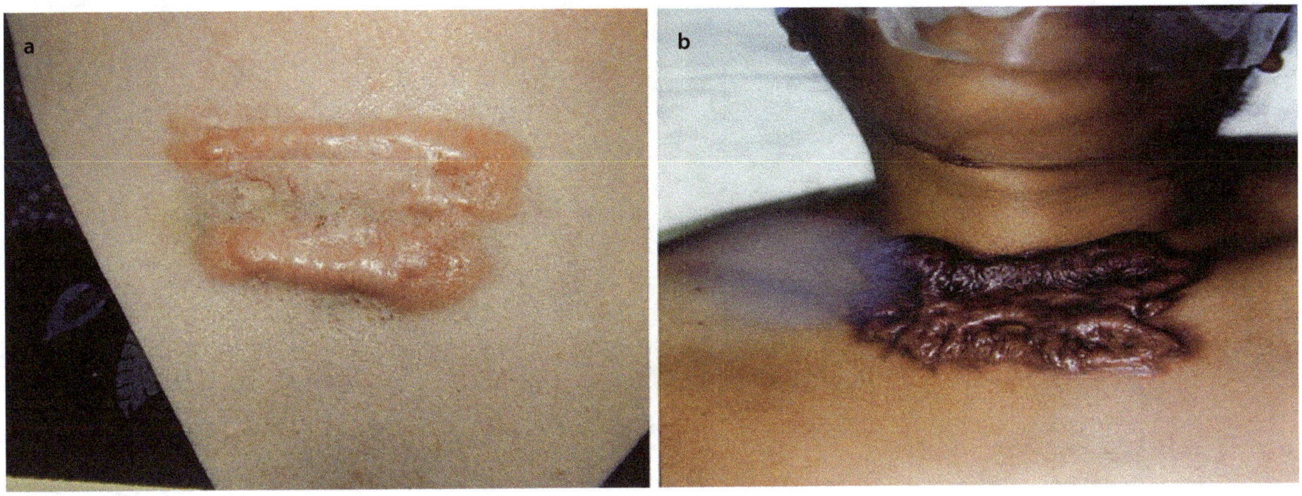

Fig. Major keloid. **a** Chest keloid with typical butterfly pattern. **b** Major keloid

scar), and the unfortunate patients with major keloids can form them all over their body. These are extraordinarily difficult to treat and are both deforming and debilitating. Intensive research on the defining genetic characteristics and pathogenesis of keloids continues, and in a few cases genetic loci have been identified, but the genetics are complex, as well as the pathogenesis.

Bibliography

1. Mustoe TA, Cooter R, Gold M, Hobbs R, Ramelet AA, Shakespeare P, Stella M, Teot L, Wood F, Ziegler U. International clinical guidelines for scar management. Plast Reconstr Surg. 2002;110:560–72.
2. Kim S, Choi TH, Liu W, Ogawa R, Mustoe TA. Update on scar management: guidelines for treating Aisian patients. Plast Reconstr Surg. 2013;132:1580–9.
3. Gold MH, Berman B, Clementoni MT, Gauglitz GG, Nahai F, McGuire M, Mustoe TA, Pusic A, Sachdev M, Teo L, Waibel J. International clinical recommendations on scar management: part 1 – evaluating the evidence and updated international clinical recommendations on scar management: part 2 – algorithms for scar prevention and treatment. Dermatol Surg. 2014;40(8):825–31.
4. Bartell TH, Monafo WW, Mustoe TA. Noninvasive in vivo quantification of elastic properties of hypertrophic scar: hand held elastometry. J Burn Care Rehabil. 1988;9:657–60.
5. Widgerow AD, Chait LA. Scar management practice and science: a comprehensive approach to controlling scar tissue and avoiding hypertrophic scarring. Adv Skin Wound Care. 2011;24(12):555–61. (meta-analysis).
6. Al-Attar A, Mess S, Thomassen JM, et al. Keloid pathogenesis and treatment. Plast Reconstr Surg. 2006;117(1):286–300.
7. Wolfram D, Tzankov A, Pulzi P, Piza-Katzer H. A review of hypertrophic scars and keloids-their pathophysiology, risk factors and management. Dermatol Surg. 2009;35:171–81.

7

Scar Symptoms: Pruritus and Pain

Osama Farrukh and Ioannis Goutos

Contents

Pain: Definition and Subtypes

Pain is defined as a distressing sensory experience associated with potential or actual tissue damage with cognitive, emotional, and social components [1]. Pain can be classified into acute and chronic, based on the duration of symptoms as well as nociceptive and non-nociceptive subtypes with regards to the neurophysiological processes involved.

Acute pain is the predicted physiological response to an adverse mechanical, thermal, or chemical stimulus and most frequently occurs after traumatic injury/surgery as part of the inflammatory response. Chronic pain is defined as pain lasting for three or more months showing no resolution to treatment [1].

Nociceptive pain can be defined as pain arising from the sensitization/activation of peripheral nociceptors and will only continue if the inciting stimulus is maintained [2]. Non-nociceptive pain can be classified into neuropathic and psychogenic pain. Neuropathic pain denotes a primary anatomical or biochemical abnormality arising within the CNS, resulting in persistent and chronic sensory disturbance following the initial injury [3]. It occurs as a result of damage to neural tissue in peripheral and central nervous system and relates to aberrant somatosensory processing. While a detailed account of psychogenic pain is outside the remit for this review, we will elaborate extensively on neuropathic phenomena since they are frequently observed in scar practice.

Pain Pathway

Peripheral Receptor Activation

Specialized sensory nociceptor fibers in peripheral tissues are activated by a broad spectrum of stimuli including mechanical, thermal as well as chemical with the most frequent being acetylcholine, bradykinin, adenosine triphosphate, and prostaglandins [4].

Ascending Pathway

First-order neuron pathways are responsible for carrying impulses to the dorsal column initially and then other parts of the CNS as part of the ascending pathway and comprise the following different subtypes [5].

A-beta fibers: These are low stimulation threshold, myelinated fibers, activated by vibration and touch; under normal conditions, they convey nonpainful stimuli; nevertheless, they play a crucial role in carrying painful sensations in chronic neuropathic pain.

A-delta fibers: These thinly myelinated fibers have a high threshold potential and are involved in the initiation of the reflex response associated with painful stimuli; they transmit pain faster than unmyelinated C fibers and contain the neurotransmitter L-glutamate.

C-fibers: These fibers are unmyelinated, have a high threshold for activation, and their stimulation causes delayed perception of pain that is often described as diffuse stabbing or burning. As well as glutamate, they contain other neurotransmitters like substance P (SP) and calcitonin gene-related peptide (CGRP).

Second-order neurons start from the dorsal horn and cross over to the contralateral side of the ascending spinothalamic tract to reach the thalamus and pons. The components of the dorsal horn involved in nociception express several receptors including α-amino-3-hydroxy-5-methyl-4-isoxazolepropionic acid (AMPA), voltage-gated calcium channels, N-methyl-D-aspartate (NMDA), as well as gamma-aminobutyric acid–alpha (GABA-A) receptors [4].

Third-order neurons start at the thalamus and end at a number of different cerebral loci.

Processing regarding the magnitude and spatial characteristics of painful stimuli is provided by the somatosensory cortex and the ventral posterior thalamic nuclei. At the same time affective and motivational aspects of pain are processed by the ventromedial posterior thalamic nucleus and its cortical connections [6].

Furthermore, positron emission tomography studies have proposed that pain-related activation of anterior cingulate cortex (ACC) has a direct relationship with an individual's emotional and behavioural reactions to pain [7]. Midbrain periaqueductal gray matter, the region responsible for fight or flight response has also been shown to have interconnections with the ACC [8].

Descending Pathway

The dorsal horn of the spinal cord receives input from higher centers, which can modulate the peripheral nociceptor input barrage by the descending pathway.

The descending pathway starts at the limbic system of the brain area, namely the periaqueductal gray/parabrachial area, rostral ventromedial medulla, and nucleus raphae magnus, whose stimulation, in turn, inhibit nociceptors in the laminae of the spinal cord. Key transmitters involved include noradrenaline, serotonin, as well as endogenous endorphins and encephalins [9].

Aside from descending signals, nociceptive impulses can also be modulated by segmental input from A-beta fibers under the gate control theory of pain. In other words, non-nociceptive fiber signals carried by the large diameter A fibers can interrupt the transmission of pain indirectly by inhibiting the effect of pain fibers ("closing the gate") [10].

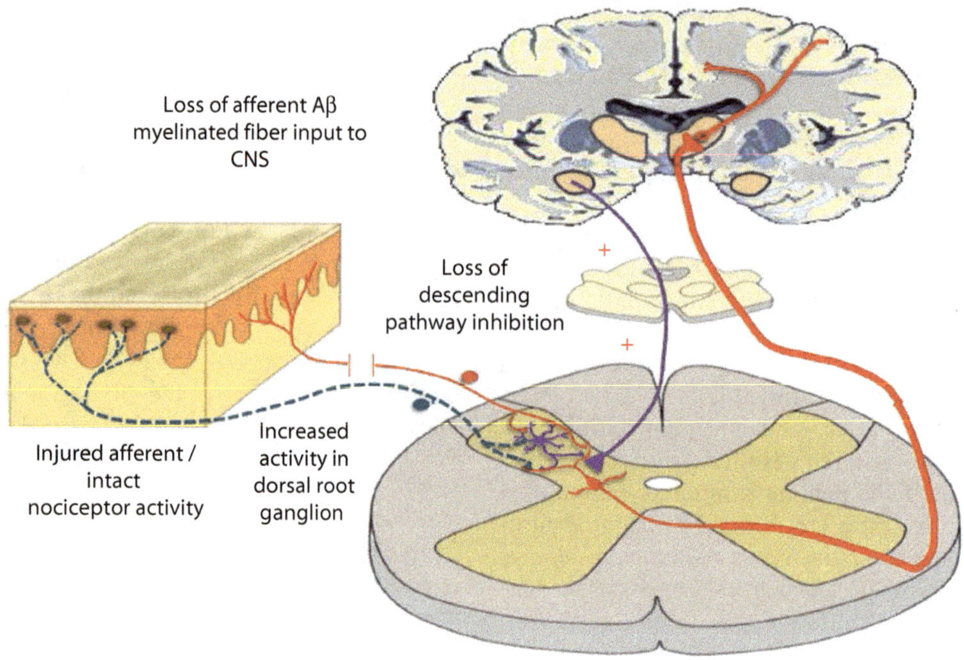

Fig. Schematic diagram of several mechanisms of periph-eral and central nervous system neuropathies. Peripheral sensitiza-tion include injured afferent hypothesis when a neuroma formed by injury to peripheral afferent fibres causes increased sesitvity to different stimuli resulting in abnormal excitability [11]; intact nocioceptor hypothesis in which spontaneous activity may develop in the nocioceptors that survived peripherally after injury innervating the region of the transected nerve secreting agents altering the activity of uninjured afferents [12] Central sensitization include increased activity in of the dorsal horn projection neurons in the dorsal root ganglion after a peripheral nerve injury causing the release of excitatory neurotransmitter glutamate [13]; loss of Aβ-myelinated fibers input causing loss of afferent inhibition resulting in more noxious stimuli reaching the CNS (Deafferentation theory) [14]; degenration of inhibitory CNS neurons (GABA interneurons) in the dorsal horn resulting in decreased inhibtion of nociceptive pathways causing chronic pain [15]; loss of anti-nociceptive descending pathways resulting in increased excitability to the CNS resulting in increased pain [16]; abnormal cotical input as a result of misdirected axonal growths at the site of injury causing reorganization of the somatosensory cortex with distorted skin mapping of the area innervated by the injured afferent [17]

Neuropathic pain refers to a type of non-nociceptive pain, which has many neurophysiological phenomena central to its genesis and symptom maintenance. These can involve the central nervous system primarily or secondarily due to changes to the peripheral nervous system components (sensitization). Figure 10.1 provides a pictorial representation of key processes involving the peripheral and central nervous system in neuropathic states.

Peripheral Sensitization

Different mechanisms have been proposed for the occurrence of abnormal signals in the peripheral nervous system capable of ultimately sensitizing the central system, including:

- Injured afferent hypothesis: According to this theory, a neuroma formed by injury to the peripheral afferent fibers causes growth of unmyelinated C fibers from damaged axons and results in abnormal excitability. This spontaneous activity occurs due to increased sensitivity to mechanical, chemical, and thermal stimuli [11, 12].
- Intact nociceptor hypothesis: This concept proposes that intact nociceptors (i.e., those surviving the original injury in the periphery and innervating the region affected by the transected nerve fibers) develop spontaneous activity [11]. Changes in ion channels, expression of receptors, and secretion of agents like prostaglandin, bradykinin, and tumor necrosis factor-alpha have the potential to sensitize nociceptors, thereby altering the properties of uninjured afferents [12].

Central Sensitization

The following mechanisms have been proposed to underlie central sensitization:

- Increased activity of dorsal horn projection neurons: There is an upregulation of $\alpha_2\delta$ subunit of calcium channels in the dorsal root ganglion and spinal cord after a peripheral nerve injury; this results in increased release of excitatory neurotransmitter glutamate [13].
- Deafferentation theory (loss of afferent inhibition): Tissue injury causes loss of Aβ-myelinated fibers input, which is the primary mechanism promoting hypoactivity of interneurons. These interneurons primarily inhibit nociceptive afferents resulting in more noxious stimuli reaching the CNS centers [14].
- Loss of CNS inhibitory neurons: γ-Aminobutyric acid (GABA) interneurons in the dorsal horn nerve fibers undergo degeneration, causing decreased inhibition of the nociceptive pathway contributing to chronic pain and hypersensitivity [15].
- Loss of descending inhibition: Inhibition of the anti-nociceptive descending pathways can result in increased excitability of the CNS, and this is thought to cause loss of sensory input following peripheral nerve injury [16].
- Synaptic reorganization: Acute deafferentation in the nervous system is thought to stem from peripheral nerve transection resulting in a misdirected axonal growth at the site of injury and cause abnormal cortical input. This mediates somatosensory cortex reorganization with distorted skin mapping originally innervated by the injured afferent [17].

The sensitization phenomena described above appear to play a key role in the generation and maintenance of chronic sensory phenomena in burn scars (see the following section) as well as keloid scars. It is interesting to note that the clinical profile of symptoms in keloids is such that pain in keloid is felt at the center while itch is mostly felt at the periphery raising the suspicion of a small fiber neuropathic state. Its severity has been suggested to correlate with pruritic intensity with a disproportionate number of regenerating unmyelinated C fibers at the periphery causing itch. Keloids with itch have also demonstrated an overall lower epidermal innervation density pointing toward mechanisms of peripheral nervous sensitization [18, 19]. Another study reporting a large number of thinner nerve fibers in deeper layers of keloidal skin has hypothesized the presence of the intensive fibrous compression (entrapment neuropathy) accounting for painful symptoms [20].

Pruritus: Definition and Subtypes

Pruritus is derived from the Latin word *prurio*, which means "to itch" and can be defined as the unpleasant sensation, which leads to the desire to scratch [21]. It can be divided into acute and chronic as well as into different subtypes based on the pathophysiological processes involved. In terms of chronicity, the acute itch has been proposed to last up to 6 months post-injury/insult to the skin in burns patients, corresponding to the early remodeling phase of wound healing [22]. Pruritic sensations in the healing wound could potentially be explained on the basis of histamine release as part of the inflammatory response and partly by virtue of abundant mast cell present in hypertrophic scars [23]. Nevertheless, the persistence of these symptoms beyond the wound healing and into scarring phase could not be solely explained on a histaminergic basis (see below).

Twycross et al. [24] has classified pruritus into the following four main subtypes:

- Pruritogenic: Arising in the skin because of injury/inflammation
- Neuropathic: Stemming from within the afferent neurologic pathway
- Neurogenic: Having a central nervous system origin in the absence of neurologic pathology
- Psychogenic: Associated with psychiatric conditions

While a number of non-skin pruritic disorders may appear to consistently fit in one discreet category, the scar-related itch is thought to have a number of non-pruritogenic origins.

Pruritic Pathway

Peripheral Receptor Activation

A wide variety of substances have been implicated in the generation and propagation of antegrade pruritic stimuli including:

Histamine

A number of histamine receptors have been described in the literature. The surface of sensory nerve endings have H1 and H2 receptors that are activated by histamine stored in the keratinocytes and mast cells [25]; H3 and H4 receptors are also found on peripheral and central neurons regulating neurotransmitter release and mast cells [26, 27]. As a by-product of collagen production, histamine synthesis is increased in the healing wound, and this can account for the generation of pruritic stimuli in the healing wound/freshly formed scar [28].

Acetylcholine

Human keratinocytes have been shown to synthesize, store, and release acetylcholine, which, through the activation of M3 muscarinic receptors in the skin, can produce an itch-associated response [29, 30].

Bradykinin

Histamine release can be caused by bradykinin secretion through mast cell degranulation [31]. It also stimulates the release of calcitonin gene-related peptide, substance P, and prostaglandin E2 at the site of tissue injury resulting in inflammation [32].

Proteinases

Dermal mast cells synthesize proteinases, including tryptase and chymase, which interact with proteinase-activated-receptor-2 located on C fibers neurons, contributing to impulse generation [33].

Peripheral Nerve Fibers (PNF)

A specific group of "unmyelinated C fibers" appears to be responsible for the transmission of itch; they start at the dermo-epidermal junction and reach the spinal cord via the dorsal root ganglion. These fibers have a characteristic slow conduction velocity (0.5 m/sec) with a prolonged histamine response and extensive terminal branching. The main transmitters released include substance P and calcitonin gene-related peptide [34].

Spinal Cord/Itch Specific Neurons

Andrew and Craig, in their experiments on cats, showed "itch-specific" neurons to be located in the superficial part of the dorsal lamina I of spinothalamic tract [35]. They are characterized by their lack of ongoing discharge and low conduction velocities and terminate at the thalamus before crossing over to the contralateral side in the spinal cord.

Thalamocortical Level

The exact parts of the brain activated by the pruritic pathway are still not fully characterized; lamina I of the spinothalamic tract was originally postulated to terminate in the medial dorsal and ventral medial nucleus of the thalamus in primates [36]. However, positron emission tomography studies have failed to show any subcortical activation in healthy individuals and instead show significant activation in contralateral somatosensory cortex and in both ipsilateral and contralateral motor areas (premotor cortex, primary motor cortex, and supplementary motor area). The cingulate gyrus and prefrontal cortex have also been implicated in neuronal transmission and this may potentially be the reason for the associated emotional component seen in scratching behaviour of patients suffering from pruritus [37].

The generation and maintenance of pruritic symptoms into a chronic state has been postulated to relate to a state of central nervous system sensitization, based on a combination of clinical, neurophysiological, as well as pharmacological data [38]. The salient observations supporting a neuropathic state in chronic pruritus in burns patients are summarized below.

(a) Emerging pharmacological evidence behind the effectiveness of antihistamines at different time-points during rehabilitation indicates that in the later phases of healing, wounds and scars become unresponsive to antihistamine therapy [39, 40, 41]. This may point toward the involvement of the central nervous system in the maintenance of these symptoms and is further supported by the superiority of centrally acting agents including gabapentin and pregabalin [34, 35, 42, 43] and transcutaneous electrical nerve stimulation modalities in symptom management [41, 44].

(b) Neurophysiological studies in burn scars show that phenomena similar to those occurring in chronic neuropathic pain exist in terms of the presence of increased sensitivity to stimuli (hyperalgesia/hyperkinesis) on the background of otherwise overall decreased sensibility. This finding provides some evidence of possible deafferentation as a mechanism for CNS sensitization [44, 45].

(c) Clinical presentation highlights a pattern of symptom exacerbation at night time, which is found typically in neuropathic states [46, 47].

(d) The neurological pathways of both symptoms share common features including the role of substance P and CGRP as well as similar areas of the central nervous system activated in the generation of symptoms as in neuropathic pain [48, 49].

(e) Neuropeptide expression data. Hypertrophic scar biopsies in patients with pain and itch demonstrated a higher density of neuropeptides (SP and CGRP) compared to controls, whereas these were absent in non-hypertrophic scars providing a link between neuropeptide expression and impulse transmission. Interestingly, SP immunoreactivity was present in the densely packed areas of scar hypertrophy [50].

Another study in grafted burn skin showed the coexistence of overall decrease in axonal population and a preferential increase in SP fibers correlating with pruritic symptoms; this provides a link between a state of SP hyperinnervation in a milieu of deafferentation possibly leading to a neuropathic state [32]. Furthermore, neuropeptides like SP are thought to play a key role in perpetuating fibroproliferative pathology establishing a cycle of nociception and scar hypertrophy [50, 51].

Other authors have proposed the role of opioids in the generation of pruritic impulses in hypertrophic burn scars [52].

Incidence/Prevalence of Pain and Itch in Scars

Pain is a major sensory disturbance and has been described as contributing to the "hidden cost" of cutaneous scars. According to a study based on semi-structured interviews in a UK scar specialist service, it has been identified that 26% and 44% of patients reported pain and itch in association with their scars, affecting their physical comfort and functioning [53].

In a corroborative study, pain and itch have been found to correlate with physical impairment ($P \leq 0.001$) in a study of 100 patients with keloid and hypertrophic scarring attending a German dermatology department using the Questionnaire on Experience with Skin Complaints. Similar work utilizing the Dermatology Life Quality Index (DLQI) tool confirmed that keloids have a statistically significant effect on the quality of life compared to physiologic scars ($p < 0.001$); additionally, they are associated with a statistically significant increase in pain and itch disturbances ($P < 0.01$ and 0.001 respectively) [54].

A cross-sectional health-related quality of life (HRQL) assessment study focused on indicators of the burden for 106 keloid patients using one disease-specific (Skindex-29) and two generic (SF-36 and EQ-5D-5L) HRQL measures; results indicated that pain and itch were the strongest predictors of impairment and related to low mental and emotional status [55].

A study evaluating chronic pain due to central sensitization in burn scars showed a 35% prevalence of pain in scarred tissue one or more years after injury [56, 57]. Additionally, work evaluating 98 burn survivors, reported 25% of patients having painful scars and 20% experiencing shooting pain more than 30 years post-injury [21]. A retrospective review involving 72 patients suggested that the first complaint of neuropathic pain presents on average at 4.3 months after injury and that there is a qualitative progression pattern; symptoms are initially reported as "pins and needles," then being predominantly stabbing or burning pain followed by "shooting" sensory qualities [58].

A multicenter cohort involving 510 patients was used to evaluate the incidence and prevalence of burns itch. In this long-term prospective study, 64% of individuals reported itch to be a significant problem over a 2-year period. At three months, 87% of individuals reported severe itching; this fell to 70% at 12 and 64% at 24 months respectively. Predictors of itch at three months post-burn included total burned surface area (TBSA), female gender, number of surgical procedures (deep dermal injury), and post-traumatic stress disorder (PTSD) symptoms at two weeks post-injury. Interestingly, at 24 months the only predictors for itch complaints were the latter two (PTSD at two weeks post-injury and the presence of deep dermal injury). The authors proposed that acute itch (up to 6 months) corresponding to the early remodeling phase of wound healing effects, both partial and full-thickness burn injuries. Chronic itch, on the other hand, affects patients with certain predisposing factors, providing a link between the chronicity of symptoms and markers of injury severity as well as psychological stress [59].

Another multicenter, large cohort study of adult burn survivors, reported high prevalence and severity of post-burn pruritus. Two cohorts of individual with burns were studied; the first included 637 patients followed prospectively over a 2-year period and identified that pruritus initially affected more than 90% of individuals and persisted in more than 40% of burn survivors in the long term. The second cohort comprised 336 patients who sustained burn injury 4–10 years before assessment using the 5-D itch scale. Pruritus was reported as severe in 76% patients within this group, moderate in 29%, and mild in 52% [60].

Schneider et al. [61] conducted a retrospective review of 430 pediatric burn survivors with a mean TBSA of 40.8%. Findings included that pruritus is present in most children (93%) and is of moderate intensity at discharge. The frequency and intensity of symptoms decreased over time; nevertheless continued to affect 63% of children at two years post-injury; furthermore, regression analysis showed significant correlations between pain and itch intensity at each time point. Most interestingly, no association was identified between pruritic intensity and burn etiology, age, gender, or burn size.

Management of Symptoms

Sensory symptoms in scars can be managed using a variety of approaches; undoubtedly, the most important initial step toward successful management relies on reliable and consistent monitoring of symptoms. A plethora of clinical measurement scales have been described in the literature; some of the most commonly utilized mono-dimensional scales include verbal, visual, as well as numerical analogue scales [62]. Other evaluation methods like the "itch man scale" incorporate a pictorial element, which makes them more suitable for pediatric patients or those unable to complete analogue scales [63]. Multidimensional tools including the 5-D Pruritus Scale have the advantage of incorporating components of the sensory experience other than intensity, including duration and disability, hence offering the opportunity to capture the degree of disturbance in a more comprehensive manner [64].

A variety of pharmacological and non-pharmacological adjuncts are available and frequently using a combination of modalities provides an optimal therapeutic approach.

Non-pharmacological Adjuncts

Psychological Support

A multidisciplinary approach toward treating sensory disturbances in scars is vital, and psychological support has been suggested as an integral part of the management plan [65]. This is particularly pertinent given the association between psychological stress and perseverance of sensory symptoms into a chronic state [38].

Cooling

The application of cooling agents as part of wound care and scar management can help temporarily relieve pruritic sensations. The beneficial effect of cooling can be explained by the temperature-sensitive activation of certain excitatory ion channels, including vanilloid receptor 1 as well as ascending pathway C fibers [34, 66].

Hydration/Moisturization

Two recent literature reviews have found that there is limited and low-level evidence behind the optimal choice of a moisturizing and hydrating product for burn scars [67], with a small number of studies investigating the value of different products available. The rationale for moisturization of a scar relates to addressing the increased rate of transepidermal water loss (TEWL) seen in scars and potentially inhibits the fibrogenic action of fibroblasts by virtue of the hydrating effect [68].

The ideal moisturizer should have both occlusive as well as humectant ingredients. Occlusive substances (e.g., oils) function to impede water loss, whereas humectants (e.g., glycerin, propylene glycol, etc.) attract water from the dermis into the stratum corneum. The presence of a defective barrier against transepidermal water loss in scarred skin implies that a humectant-only-based preparation would enhance fluid loss, hence should be avoided [69].

A small randomized study has indicated that mugwort lotion is a promising topical agent for the relief of an itch in burns hypertrophic scarring [70]; additionally, a nonprescription moisturizer containing a blend of protease enzymes (Provase) applied every 8 hours for four weeks has been shown to reduce itch severity parameters as well as the affective burden significantly [71].

A similar randomized controlled study among 52 patients with postburn itch found that a preparation of beeswax and herbal oil had a statistically significant better effect on itch compared to aqueous cream ($P = 0.001$); additionally, symptoms recurred later comparatively ($P \leq 0.001$), and the use of antipruritic medications was lower ($P = 0.023$) [72].

A different literature report compared the effects of hydrocolloid dressing versus moisturizer in 20 patients with keloid and hypertrophic scars over a 2-month period in a randomized controlled prospective manner. Results indicate that both products achieved a similar reduction in itch ($P < 0.03$) and pain ($P < 0.08$) presumably by virtue of scar hydration [73].

One of the most interesting reports in the literature focused on the comparison between a hydrating gel-cream and three fluid silicones in a group of healthy volunteers. The moisturizer Alhydran (BAP Medical, Belgium) has been found to have an equivalent effect on hydration and occlusion suggesting that these may be the most important in topical scar care preparations as opposed to active substances like silicone, which have become extremely popular in recent decades [74].

Massage

Massage has been shown to be effective for the management of pain, itch, and anxiety associated with scars in a number of studies [75–77]. The first randomized study included 20 patients in the remodeling phase of scar formation; these were divided into either a 30-minute massage with cocoa butter to a moderate-sized scar tissue area twice a week for five weeks or standard therapy (cocoa butter application to scars applied by physical therapists without massage motions). The massage therapy group showed reduced pain, itch (both measured using visual analogue scales), as well as anxiety scores consistently throughout the study period [75]. Similar results were obtained in a study with a comparable design with regards to pain, itch, and anxiety in adolescent burn victims [78].

A Korean group investigated the effects of skin rehabilitation massage for three months in a group of 18 burn survivors; this involved the combination of light stroking movements followed by acupressure using oil as a medium applied for 30 minutes once a week for three months. Results indicated a statistically significant improvement of pruritus in the massage group ($t = -2.942$, $p = 0.006$) as well as depression ($t = -2.920$, $p = 0.007$) [76]. The underlying mechanisms of action of massage include the principles of the "gate theory" of pain modulation as well as the increased vagal activity, reducing stress hormone levels in the recipient [10, 79, 80].

Silicone Gels/Sheets

Silicone is widely used for the treatment of symptomatic hypertrophic scars. The proposed beneficial mechanisms involved include increased skin hydration (by virtue of occlusion) and a decrease in fibroblastic activity [81, 82].

The literature contains a number of high-quality studies regarding the role of silicone for the prevention of hypertrophy including a randomized placebo-controlled, double-blind prospective trial on sternotomy wounds showing a statistically significant effect on pain and itch symptoms [83].

Topical application of silicone gel versus placebo gel has been investigated in a randomized within-subject comparative clinical trial. Results suggested that silicone gel promoted maturation of early burn scars (mean age of scars in the study 4 months) and a decrease in itch symptoms in a statistically significant manner [84]. Similar beneficial effects were reproduced in a different study employing silicone gel application to burns hypertrophic scarring showing a significant difference in terms of scar vascularity starting at the first month of application [85].

Another study utilized silicone gel sheets in the conservative management of six keloid patients for 24 weeks. Symptoms of pain and itch showed a decrease after four weeks of the gel sheeting application and disappeared after 12 weeks. After 24 weeks, a histological decrease in the number of mast cells was observed, which may explain the therapeutic benefit seen by virtue of a decreased concentration of mast cells derived mediators [86].

A number of comparative studies exist in the literature, which aimed to elucidate the role of silicone products in the scar care arena.

A randomized clinical trial of 45 post-traumatic hypertrophic scars found that silicone gel sheeting applied 24 hours/day for six months was superior to 15-minute-long daily massage in reducing scar thickness in a statistically significant manner ($p < 0.001$); of particular note is that pain and itch reduction did not reach statistical significance in this study [87].

A separate prospective single-blinded study compared the efficacy of 585 nm flashlamp-pumped pulsed dye laser and silicone gel sheeting and control in the management of 20 patients with hypertrophic scars; results showed an overall reduction of blood flow, volume, and pruritus for all the study subgroups but failed to show any statistically significant difference between treatment and control groups [88].

A prospective split sternotomy scar study [89] involving 14 patients randomized to treat one-half of the scar with triamcinolone acetonide (TAC) and the other with silicone gel sheeting worn for 12 hours for 12 weeks. The primary outcome of patient preference was analyzed, and recruitment was terminated after 11 patients had completed the study, 10 of whom favoured silicone gel treatment. The average time for the symptomatic improvement of silicone-treated patients was 3.9 days as compared to triamcinolone acetonide, which was 6.8 days ($p < 0.05$). The authors proposed that the enhanced compliance to silicone-based treatments relates to the painless and noninvasive nature of silicone-based adjuncts.

Transcutaneous Electrical Nerve Stimulation (TENS)

TENS involves the application of low-voltage electrical impulses to the nervous system by means of electrodes placed on the skin [90]. The underlying mechanism of action involves the stimulation of rapidly conducting A-fibers, which inhibit the transmission of noxious stimuli carried by the slower C fibers according to the "gate theory of pain" [10].

A pilot study involving 20 patients with healed burns complaining of severe itch following burns demonstrated a statistically significant change in the reported visual analogue scale compared with placebo over a 3-week period [90].

Pharmacological Adjuncts

Capsaicin

This is a naturally occurring alkaloid compound, which interacts with the transient receptor potential V1 receptor resulting in the depletion of neuropeptides from peripheral nerves. Despite the fact that capsaicin forms one of the mainstay topical agents in many chronic pain services, a double-blind placebo-controlled randomized trial using 0.025% capsaicin cream on 30 patients with pruritic wounds revealed no significant effects on pruritic symptom relief [91, 92, 93]. Further work is warranted involving preparations with different concentrations of this agent in order to elucidate its exact role in the management of symptomatic scars.

Antihistamines

Antihistamines have traditionally been used as first-line agents for the management of pruritus. First-generation compounds (diphenhydramine, hydroxyzine, cyproheptadine, and chlorphenamine) act on histaminic, serotonergic, muscarinic, and alpha-adrenergic receptors. Second-generation compounds, like cetirizine, have minimal activity on non-histaminic receptors and hence have a more favourable side effect profile as well as a longer duration of action [94, 95]. The pharmacological action of antihistamine relates primarily to a reverse agonist action at histaminic receptors as well a central nervous system sedative effect (the latter action refers to first-generation compounds).

One of the initial studies involving 35 burns patient complaining of severe itching after discharge assessed the efficacy of three first-generation antihistamines, namely chlorpheniramine, hydroxyzine, and diphenhydramine. The results of the study pointed toward no significant difference in therapeutic efficacy between the three compounds and only a 20% complete relief of symptoms in the cohort [96].

Gabapentin/Pregabalin

Gabapentin is a useful agent for the management of neuropathic pain associated with a variety of conditions, including post-herpetic neuralgia [97].

The mechanism of action of gabapentin involves a number of mechanisms, including:

1. Blockade of the $\alpha_2\delta$ subunits of voltage-gated Ca channels resulting in a reduced release of excitatory neurotransmitters [98].
2. Increased synthesis and release of γ-aminobutyric acid in the CNS [99].

A comparative study appraised two different therapeutic protocols for the management of burns pruritus in patients with healing and healed burns in a UK burn center incorporating a mixture of antihistamines and gabapentin; the authors concluded that gabapentin as monotherapy as well as in combination with another two antihistamines was more efficacious compared to chlorpheniramine alone and in combination with another two antihistamines ($t = 3.70$, df = 89, $P < 0.001$ for monotherapy and $x^2 = 12.2$, df = 1, $P = 0.001$ for polytherapy). Additionally, patients with higher initial pruritus scores needed a combination of pharmacological agents for effective symptomatic relief. This study raised the value of centrally acting agents in itch management and proposed the combination of peripherally and centrally acting agents in the treatment for burns pruritus [41].

Another landmark study comprised a four-arm, double-blind, randomized and placebo-controlled study of pregabalin in the management of postburn pruritus. Pregabalin is a newer analogue of gabapentin with comparatively better anxiolytic and pharmacokinetic properties. The study compared the following four groups: pregabalin; cetirizine and pheniramine maleate; the combination of pregabalin, cetirizine, and pheniramine maleate; and placebo. Results indicated that for moderate to severe pruritus (VAS 6-10) a centrally acting agent like pregabalin is indicated to significantly decrease itch; patients with milder itch (VAS 4-5) are best served with the addition of pregabalin even if massage and antihistamines can provide some control because of quicker, predictable response with the added benefit of anxiolysis [77].

Steroids

Steroid delivery to hypertrophic and keloidal scars is a well-established modality for the alleviation of scar-related symptoms, including pain and itch, and their beneficial effects were first recorded in literature in the 1950s [100]. The international advisory panel in 2002 recommended triamcinolone acetonide (TAC) as the first-line treatment modality for keloid and second-line treatment for linear hypertrophic scar in reducing subjective symptoms associated with keloid and hypertrophic scar like pain and pruritus [101].

In 2014, a protocol re-evaluation was undertaken, which reinforced the prominent position of steroids in scar management albeit supported a combined approach incorporating the use of other agents including 5 fluorouracil, cryotherapy, laser, and silicone products [102].

Darvi evaluated the use of intralesional triamcinolone acetonide in treating hypertrophic and keloid scars in 65 patients with a 10-year follow-up. The dosage of TAC for 1–2 cm^2 of scar surface area was determined to be 20–40 mg, 40–80 mg for 2–3 cm^2, and 60–120 mg for scar surface area of 4–6 cm^2. In this study four injections of TAC were given for the total dose delivered to the scar at 1–2-week intervals with an ensuing symptomatic relief seen in 71% of patients; furthermore, a dramatic improvement of symptoms with full flattening of hypertrophic scars was seen in 50% and 71% in patients with keloid scars [103].

Manuskiatti [104] and colleagues performed a randomized controlled trial comparing the effects of intralesional triamcinolone acetonide with 5-fluorouracil or alone with 585 nm pulse dye laser. TAC-treated scars had better improvements in clinical symptoms (pain, itching) and scar induration, although the results were not statistically significant. Intralesional triamcinolone acetonide treatment, however, did produce side effects, including skin atrophy, telangiectasia, and hypopigmentation in 50% of the TAC-treated group. Boutli-Kasapidou and colleagues [105] evaluated a polytherapy protocol, including three triamcinolone acetonide intralesional injections every month combined with 12 monthly cycles of cryotherapy and 12-hour silicone dressing for 12 months. Patient satisfaction scale was used to grade the appearance cosmetically and subjective symptoms (pain, burning, and tension post 12 months). Similarly, an investigator satisfaction scale was used as well. The results showed that compared to monotherapy, polytherapy group had a major improvement in control of symptoms and appearance, reported by the patient and observed by the physician ($P < 0.01$). They concluded the beneficial effects of each treatment acting synergistically: Steroids downregulating the excessive collagen expression in keloids and making it softer, ischemic destruction and subsequent necrosis of keloids with cryotherapy, and silicon downregulating mastocytes.

Tan and colleagues [106] conducted a patient-controlled prospective study for 12 weeks with patients receiving intralesional triamcinolone acetonide (40 mg/mL), silicone gel sheeting, or no treatment (control).

The dose of triamcinolone acetonide varied between 0.1 ml to 0.5 ml of 40 mg/mL of TAC depending upon the size of the lesion. In this trial, 12% of silicone-treated keloids showed a significant reduction (>50%) in size compared with 94% of triamcinolone acetonide group (RR: 33.00, 95% CI: 2.14–509.33). There was also a significant improvement in erythema (RR: 21.00, 95% CI: 1.33–332.06). The improvement in itch and pain was not statistically significant when compared to control.

Martin et al. studied the combination of carbon dioxide fractional laser (10,600 nm), a pulsed dye laser (585 nm), and triamcinolone acetonide (40 mg/ml) injections monthly for seven sessions in a cohort of keloid scars; they reported favourable results in regards to pruritic relief [107].

Steroids can also be delivered to scars in the form of tape application. Advantages of this modality include the noninvasive nature and the ability to maintain a continuous level of steroid concentration to the symptomatic scar, which can ameliorate the inflammatory milieu responsible for the bulk as well as sensory symptoms [108].

Botulinum Toxin

Botulinum toxin is a protein neurotoxin produced by the spore-forming bacteria Clostridium Botulinum; it works by preventing the release of acetylcholine at the neuromuscular junction and causing chemoimmobilization as well as affecting a variety of cell types including fibroblasts [109]. It is an established adjunct in a variety of medical and aesthetic interventions and over the last number of years has been trialed in the scar management arena. The rationale for its use rests on the ability to decrease muscular tension underlying a scar as well as the ability to alter a host of fibroblast related pathways, including their proliferation and cell cycle [110].

A randomized, double-blind comparative trial [111] involving 24 females with idiopathic or post-traumatic keloids employed the use of either intralesional triamcinolone (10 mg/cc), given every four weeks for six sessions or 5 IU/cm^3 intralesional botulinum toxin every eight weeks for three sessions; in both groups, therapy was continued until complete improvement of keloid was noted. The authors concluded that the effects of intralesional botulinum toxin A comparable to that of intralesional steroids with a significant reduction in volume height and redness of scar in both groups ($p < 0.01$). In the 7-month follow up both treated groups had a statistically significant reduction in subjective symptoms of pain and itching with a statistically significant difference in favour of the botulinum toxin A treated group with the added advantage of no side effects which were typically seen in steroid-treated patients.

Another blind study compared the effect of triamcinolone acetonide (maximum of 40 mg dose) plus placebo versus triamcinolone acetonide and botulinum toxin (20IU) for keloid scars injected every four weeks for a total of 12 weeks. Although the difference in height, vascularization, and the pliability were not significant between the two groups, there was a significant difference in favour of the botulinum group in terms of pain and pruritus control (($p < 0.001$) at the end of the study [112].

Similar results in terms of the superior alleviating effect of botulinum toxin have been reached in another randomized, single-blind study in 32 keloid patients [113].

The use of botulinum toxin has been reported in the burns literature as part of a pilot study involving nine patients, eight of which had skin grafts for deep partial-thickness to full-thickness burns, with an average TBSA of 24%. At the beginning of the study, 87.5% of patients rated their burns itch as being severe (>7/10), which fell to 0 at four weeks following the administration of toxin [114].

Further studies are warranted to delineate the exact role of botulinum toxin in scar symptom management.

Emerging Modalities

Autologous Fat Grafting

Autologous fat grafting has been widely used for the treatment of contour deformities and increasingly employed to remodel and regenerate tissue by virtue of mesenchymal stem cells present in adipose tissue [115, 116].

The proposed mechanism supporting the alleviation of scar symptoms is suggested to relate to the mechanical release of adhesions, neovascularization, and remodeling of scar tissue architecture [117]. Other mechanisms proposed for controlling neuropathic pain symptoms include blockade of nociceptive impulses and an overall reduction of the signal input to the central nervous system [118].

Fredman et al. [119] in a retrospective case review evaluated the effectiveness of fat grafting in neuropathic burn scars using the patient-reported outcome measurement information system (PROMIS) to assess pain following two fat-grafting sessions eight weeks apart. Results showed a statistically significant improvement in subjective outcomes at 1-year follow-up.

Huang et al. [120] evaluated autologous fat grafting in 13 patients with neuropathic scar pain. Pain evaluations were undertaken using the Visual Analogue Scale (VAS) and Neuropathic Pain Symptom Inventory (NPSI) preoperatively and at 1, 4, and 24 weeks postoperatively. Both VAS and NPSI scores showed a significant decrease starting at one week, alleviating neuropathic scar pain in the short term, which were statistically significant ($P = 0.009$ and $P = 0.007$

respectively). The NPSI score continued to decrease at four weeks ($P = 0.0009$) till 24 weeks ($P = 0.0008$) with the most significant improvement in paresthesia, dysesthesia and evoked pain ($P < 0.001$). They concluded the autologous fat provides insulation and acts as a cushion to block abnormal sensations and prevent stimulation.

Two systematic reviews of the literature pertaining to the use of fat grafting and adipose-derived stem cells in scarring have shown improvements in scar characteristics including texture and size, improved pain profiles, increased angiogenesis, and an earlier return to function [121, 122]. It is clear that the use of fat-derived cells will play an important role in the future of scar treatments in the field of regenerative medicine.

Lasers

Laser stands for "Light Amplification by Stimulated Emission of Radiation" and exerts its effect on the tissue through photochemical/thermal/mechanical mechanisms [123].

The photothermal effect or photothermolysis is the most relevant mechanism in scar treatment with the main target being either blood vessels (pulsed dye laser) or water (CO_2 and Er:YAG laser). Lasers can be further subdivided into ablative and non-ablative based on whether the epidermis is affected or not and fractional and non-fractional: based on whether intact columns of skin are left behind or not after the treatment [124].

Pulsed Dye Laser is a vascular specific laser with haemoglobin being the target chromophore. Selective photothermolysis [125] with a short pulse duration leads to selective absorption of heat by haemoglobin, leading to thrombosis and vasculitis [126].

Ebid et al. [127] in a double-blind, randomized, placebo-controlled trial, compared the effects of pulsed high-intensity laser in the treatment of post-burn pruritus. They showed that a combination of a long period of high-intensity pulsed laser, antihistamine, and massage could effectively control moderate to severe burn pruritus, raising the value of incorporating laser modalities in antipruritic protocols.

Vasheghani and colleagues [128] showed that low-level laser therapy in second-degree cutaneous burns decreases the total number of mast cells in the remodeling phase while increasing the number of mast cells in the proliferative and inflammatory phases. Increased level of growth factors and anti-inflammatory cytokines and decreased level of pro-inflammatory cytokines like interleukin alpha and beta have been shown after treatment with laser therapy [129] elucidating potential mechanisms for the action of laser on pruritic pathways. Other proposed mechanisms include the direct action on reactive oxygen species, inhibition of cyclooxygenase (COX) and prostaglandin E2 [130], as well as the fast axonal flow and microtubule disruption of Aδ and C fibers transmission [131].

Alster and Williams [132], in an investigator-blinded split scar study of patients with keloid scarring, performed two sessions of flash pump 585 nm pulse-dyed laser treatment to half of the scar at 6–8-week intervals. They reported a significant improvement in the texture of the skin surface, scar height, erythema, pruritus with coarse, loose collagen, and increase number of mast cells seen histologically in the laser-treated side.

A prospective randomized controlled trial investigated the outcomes following ablative fractional CO_2 laser on 19 patients with burn scars (minimum age of scars for inclusion six months). Results demonstrated that three treatments of ablative fractional CO_2 laser (Deep FX setting on UltraPulse®, Lumenis; treatment parameters: single pass of 300 Hz, 5% density, and 50 mJ energy) significantly improved scar pain, itch based on Patient and Observer Scar Assessment Scale (POSAS) scores ($p = 0.047$ and <0.01 respectively). Additional findings included an improved dermal architecture at six weeks post-treatment [133].

Conclusion

Pain and itch represent the most common sensory symptoms accompanying scars and can have a significant impact on patients' quality of life. Over the last number of decades, our understanding of the pertinent pathophysiological mechanisms has improved considerably, especially with regards to the contribution of the central nervous system in the generation and maintenance of nociceptive and pruritic stimuli. Consistent and reliable monitoring of symptoms combined with a multimodal approach to treatment should be integral parts of holistic scar management.

Take-Home Messages

- Itch and pain can have a significant impact on individuals with scars.
- The contribution of the central nervous system in the generation and maintenance of symptoms is paramount.
- Accurate assessment and monitoring of symptoms are central to successful scar management.
- Multimodal approaches which target both peripheral and central nervous system components and incorporate non-pharmacological adjuncts are recommended.

References

1. Anwar K. Pathophysiology of pain. Dis Mon. 2016;62(9):324–9.
2. Woolf CJ, Bennett GJ, Doherty M, Dubner R, Kidd B, Koltzenburg M, et al. Towards a mechanism-based classification of pain? Pain. 1998;77(3):227–9.
3. Yosipovitch G, Samuel LS. Neuropathic and psychogenic itch. Dermatol Ther. 2008;21(1):32–41.
4. Schug SA, Daly HCS, Stannard KJD. Pathophysiology of pain. Mechanisms of vascular disease: a reference book for vascular specialists. Adelaide: University of Adelaide Press; 2011.
5. Woolf CJ. American College of Physicians, American Physiological Society. Pain: moving from symptom control toward mechanism-specific pharmacologic management. Ann Intern Med. 2004;140(6):441–51.
6. Mackey SC, Maeda F. Functional imaging and the neural systems of chronic pain. Neurosurg Clin N Am. 2004;15(3):269–88.
7. Rainville P, Duncan GH, Price DD, Carrier B, Bushnell MC. Pain affect encoded in human anterior cingulate but not somatosensory cortex. Science. 1997;277(5328):968–71.
8. Buhle JT, Kober H, Ochsner KN, Mende-Siedlecki P, Weber J, Hughes BL, et al. Common representation of pain and negative emotion in the midbrain periaqueductal gray. Soc Cogn Affect Neurosci. 2013;8(6):609–16.
9. Stamford JA. Descending control of pain. Br J Anaesth. 1995;75(2):217–27.
10. Melzack R, Wall PD. Pain mechanisms: a new theory. Science. 1965;150(3699):971–8.
11. Campbell JN, Meyer RA. Mechanisms of neuropathic pain. Neuron. 2006;52(1):77–92.
12. Truini A, Cruccu G. Pathophysiological mechanisms of neuropathic pain. Neurol Sci. 2006;27(S2):s179–82.
13. Kusuyama K, Tachibana T, Yamanaka H, Okubo M, Yoshiya S, Noguchi K. Upregulation of calcium channel alpha-2-delta-1 subunit in dorsal horn contributes to spinal cord injury-induced tactile allodynia. Spine J. 2018;18(6):1062–9. https://doi.org/10.1016/j.spinee.2018.01.010.
14. Zimmermann M. Pathobiology of neuropathic pain. Eur J Pharmacol. 2001;429(1–3):23–37.
15. Scholz J, Broom DC, Youn D-H, Mills CD, Kohno T, Suter MR, et al. Blocking caspase activity prevents transsynaptic neuronal apoptosis and the loss of inhibition in lamina II of the dorsal horn after peripheral nerve injury. J Neurosci. 2005;25(32):7317–23.
16. Porreca F, Ossipov MH, Gebhart GF. Chronic pain and medullary descending facilitation. Trends Neurosci. 2002;25(6):319–25.
17. Oaklander AL. Mechanisms of pain and itch caused by herpes zoster (shingles). J Pain. 2008;9(1):10–8.
18. Tey HL, Maddison B, Wang H, Ishiju Y, McMichael A, Marks M, et al. Cutaneous innervation and itch in keloids. Acta Derm Venereol. 2012;92(5):529–31.
19. Lee S-S, Yosipovitch G, Chan Y-H, Goh C-L. Pruritus, pain, and small nerve fiber function in keloids: a controlled study. J Am Acad Dermatol. 2004;51(6):1002–6.
20. Hochman B, Nahas FX, Sobral CS, Arias V, Locali RF, Juliano Y, Ferreira LM. Nerve fibres: a possible role in keloid pathogenesis. Br J Dermatol. 2008;158:651–2.
21. Holavanahalli RK, Helm PA, Kowalske KJ. Long-term outcomes in patients surviving large burns: the skin. J Burn Care Res. 2010;31(4):631–9.
22. Pereira MP, Ständer S. Chronic pruritus: current and emerging treatment options. Drugs. 2017;77(9):999–1007.
23. Wulff BC, Wilgus TA. Mast cell activity in the healing wound: more than meets the eye? Exp Dermatol. 2013;22(8):507–10.
24. Twycross R, Greaves MW, Handwerker H, Jones EA, Libretto SE, Szepietowski JC, et al. Itch: scratching more than the surface. QJM. 2003;96(1):7–26.
25. Hill SJ. Distribution, properties, and functional characteristics of three classes of histamine receptor. Pharmacol Rev. 1990;42(1):45–83.
26. Lippert U, Artuc M, Grützkau A, Babina M, Guhl S, Haase I, et al. Human skin mast cells express H2 and H4, but not H3 receptors. J Investig Dermatol. 2004;123(1):116–23.
27. Ohkubo T, Shibata M, Inoue M, Kaya H, Takahashi H. Regulation of substance P release mediated via prejunctional histamine H3 receptors. Eur J Pharmacol. 1995;273:83–8.
28. Ahuja R, Chatterjee P. Postburn pruritus: a practical review. Indian J Burns. 2014;22(1):13.
29. Miyamoto T, Nojima H, Kuraishi Y. Intradermal cholinergic agonists induce itch-associated response via M3 muscarinic acetylcholine receptors in mice. Jpn J Pharmacol. 2002;88(3):351–4.
30. Grando SA, Kist DA, Qi M, Dahl MV. Human keratinocytes synthesize, secrete, and degrade acetylcholine. J Invest Dermatol. 1993;101(1):32–6.
31. Walker K, Perkins M, Dray A. Kinins and kinin receptors in the nervous system. Neurochem Int. 1995;26(1):1–16; discussion 17–26.
32. Averbeck B, Reeh PW. Interactions of inflammatory mediators stimulating release of calcitonin gene-related peptide, substance P and prostaglandin E(2) from isolated rat skin. Neuropharmacology. 2001;40(3):416–23.
33. Cocchiara R, Lampiasi N, Albeggiani G, Bongiovanni A, Azzolina A, Geraci D. Mast cell production of TNF-alpha induced by substance P evidence for a modulatory role of substance P-antagonists. J Neuroimmunol. 1999;101(2):128–36.
34. Schmelz M, Schmidt R, Bickel A, Handwerker HO, Torebjörk HE. Specific C-receptors for itch in human skin. J Neurosci. 1997;17:8003–8.
35. Andrew D, Craig AD. Spinothalamic lamina I neurones selectively responsive to cutaneous warming in cats. J Physiol. 2001;537:489–95.
36 Jinks SL, Carstens E. Superficial dorsal horn neurons identified by intracutaneous histamine: chemonociceptive responses and modulation by morphine. J Neurophysiol. 2000;84(2):616–27.
37. Drzezga A, Darsow U, Treede RD, Siebner H, Frisch M, Munz F, Weilke F, Ring J, Schwaiger M, Bartenstein P. Central activation by histamine-induced itch: analogies to pain processing: a correlational analysis of O-15 H2O positron emission tomography studies. Pain. 2001;92:295–305.
38. Goutos I. Neuropathic mechanisms in the pathophysiology of burns pruritus: redefining directions for therapy and research. J Burn Care Res. 2013;34(1):82–93. https://doi.org/10.1097/BCR.0b013e3182644c44.
39. Vitale M, Fields-Blache C, Luterman A. Severe itching in the patient with burns. J Burn Care Rehabil. 1991;12(4):330–3.
40. Ahuja RB, Gupta R, Gupta G, Shrivastava P. A comparative analysis of cetirizine, gabapentin and their combination in the relief of post-burn pruritus. Burns. 2011;37(2):203–7.
41. Goutos I, Eldardiri M, Khan AA, Dziewulski P, Richardson PM. Comparative evaluation of antipruritic protocols in acute burns. The emerging value of gabapentin in the treatment of burns pruritus. J Burn Care Res. 31(1):57–63.
42. Jinks SL, Carstens E. Superficial dorsal horn neurons identified by intracutaneous histamine: chemonociceptive responses and modulation by morphine. J Neurophysiol. 2000;84:616–27.
43. Drzezga A, Darsow U, Treede R-D, Siebner H, Frisch M, Munz F, Weilke F, Ring J, Schwaiger M, Bartenstein P. Central activation by histamine-induced itch: analogies to pain processing: a correlational analysis of O-15 H2O positron emission tomography studies. Pain. 92(1):295–305.

44. Malenfant A, Forget R, Amsel R, Papillon J, Frigon JY, Choinière M. Tactile, thermal and pain sensibility in burned patients with and without chronic pain and paresthesia problems. Pain. 1998;77(3):241–51.
45. Shlash SOA, Madani JOA, Deib JIE, Alsubhi FS, Saifi SSA, Helmi AMA, et al. Demographic characteristics and outcome of burn patients requiring skin grafts: a tertiary hospital experience. Int J Burns Trauma. 2016;6(2):30–6.
46. Goutos I. Burns pruritus—a study of current practices in the UK. Burns. 2010;36(1):42–8.
47. Bell L, McAdams T, Morgan R, Parshley PF, Pike RC, Riggs P, et al. Pruritus in burns: a descriptive study. J Burn Care Rehabil. 1998;9(3):305–8.
48. Scholzen T, Armstrong CA, Bunnett NW, Luger TA, Olerud JE, Ansel JC. Neuropeptides in the skin: interactions between the neuroendocrine and the skin immune systems. Exp Dermatol. 1998;7(2–3):81–96.
49. Ständer S, Schmelz M. Chronic itch and pain-Similarities and differences. Eur J Pain. 2006;10:473.
50. Crowe R, Parkhouse N, McGrouther D, Burnstock G. Neuropeptide-containing nerves in painful hypertrophic human scar tissue. Br J Dermatol. 1994;130(4):444–52.
51. Scott JR, Muangman PR, Tamura RN, Zhu KQ, Liang Z, Anthony J, et al. Substance P levels and neutral endopeptidase activity in acute burn wounds and hypertrophic scar. Plast Reconstr Surg. 2005;115(4):1095–102.
52. Cheng B, Liu H-W, Fu X-B. Update on pruritic mechanisms of hypertrophic scars in postburn patients: the potential role of opioids and their receptors. J Burn Care Res. 2011;32(4):e118–5.
53. Brown BC, McKenna SP, Siddhi K, McGrouther DA, Bayat A. The hidden cost of skin scars: quality of life after skin scarring. J Plast Reconstr Aesthet Surg. 2008;61(9):1049–58.
54. Reinholz M, Poetschke J, Schwaiger H, Epple A, Ruzicka T, Gauglitz GG. The dermatology life quality index as a means to assess life quality in patients with different scar types. J Eur Acad Dermatol Venereol. 2015;29(11):2112–9.
55. Bijlard E, Kouwenberg C, Timman R, Hovius S, Busschbach J, Mureau M. Burden of Keloid disease: a cross-sectional health-related quality of life assessment. Acta Dermato Venereologica. 2017;97(2):225–9.
56. Bock O, Schmid-Ott G, Malewski P, Mrowietz U. Quality of life of patients with keloid and hypertrophic scarring. Arch Dermatol Res. 2006;297(10):433–8.
57. Choinière M, Melzack R, Papillon J. Pain and paresthesia in patients with healed burns: an exploratory study. J Pain Symptom Manag. 1991;6(7):437–44.
58. Schneider JC, Harris NL, El Shami A, Sheridan RL, Schulz JT, Bilodeau M-L, et al. A descriptive review of neuropathic-like pain after burn injury. J Burn Care Res. 2006;27(4):524–8.
59. Van Loey NEE, Bremer M, Faber AW, Middelkoop E, Nieuwenhuis MK. Itching following burns: epidemiology and predictors. Br J Dermatol.2007;071106220718003.
60. Carrougher GJ, Martinez EM, McMullen KS, Fauerbach JA, Holavanahalli RK, Herndon DN, Wiechman SA, Engrav LH, Gibran NS. Pruritus in adult burn survivors. J Burn Care Res. 34(1):94–101.
61. Schneider JC, Nadler DL, Herndon DN, Kowalske K, Matthews K, Wiechman SA, Carrougher GJ, Gibran NS, Meyer WJ, Sheridan RL, Ryan CM. Pruritus in pediatric burn survivors. J Burn Care Res. 36(1):151–8.
62. Phan NQ, et al. J der Deutschen Dermatologischen Gesellschaft. 2011;9:148–9.
63. Blankers K, Dankerlui N, van Loey N, Pursad M, Rode H, van Dijk M. Cross-cultural validation of the itch man scale in pediatric burn survivors in a South African setting. Burns. 2019;45(3):725–31.
64. Reich A, Heisig M, Phan N, Taneda K, Takamori K, Takeuchi S, et al. Visual analogue scale: evaluation of the instrument for the assessment of pruritus. Acta Dermato Venereologica. 2012;92(5):497–501.
65. Bell PL, Gabriel V. Evidence based review for the treatment of post-burn pruritus. J Burn Care Res. 2009;30(1):55–61.
66. McKemy DD, Neuhausser WM, Julius D. Identification of a cold receptor reveals a general role for TRP channels in thermosensation. Nature. 2002;416(6876):52–8.
67. Anthonissen M, Daly D, Janssens T, Van den Kerckhove E. The effects of conservative treatments on burn scars: a systematic review. Burns. 2016;42(3):508–18.
68. Klotz T, Kurmis R, Munn Z, Heath K, Greenwood J. Moisturisers in scar management following burn: a survey report. Burns. 2017;43(5):965–72.
69. Harte D, Gordon J, Shaw M, Stinson M, Porter-Armstrong A. The use of pressure and silicone in hypertrophic scar management in burns patients: a pilot randomized controlled trial. J Burn Care Res. 2009;30(4):632–42.
70. Ogawa R, Hyakusoku H, Ogawa K, Nakao C. Effectiveness of mugwort lotion for the treatment of post-burn hypertrophic scars. J Plast Reconstr Aesthet Surg. 2008;61(2):210–2.
71. Nedelec B, Rachelska G, Parnell LKS, LaSalle L. Double-blind, randomized, pilot study assessing the resolution of postburn pruritus. J Burn Care Res. 2012;33(3):398–406.
72. Lewis PA, Wright K, Webster A, Steer M, Rudd M, Doubrovsky A, Gardner G. A randomized controlled pilot study comparing aqueous cream with a beeswax and herbal oil cream in the provision of relief from postburn pruritis. J Burn Care Res. 33(4):e195–200.
73. Phillips TJ, Gerstein AD, Lordan V. A randomized controlled trial of hydrocolloid dressing in the treatment of hypertrophic scars and keloids. Dermatol Surg. 1996;22(9):775–8.
74. Hoeksema H, De Vos M, Verbelen J, Pirayesh A, Monstrey S. Scar management by means of occlusion and hydration: a comparative study of silicones versus a hydrating gel-cream. Burns. 2013;39(7):1437–48.
75. Field T, Peck M, et al. Postburn itching, pain, and psychological symptoms are reduced with massage therapy. J Burn Care Rehabil. 2000;21(3):189–93.
76. Roh YS, Cho H, Oh JO, Yoon CJ. Effects of skin rehabilitation massage therapy on pruritus, skin status, and depression in burn survivors. Taehan Kanho Hakhoe Chi. 2007;37(2):221–6.
77. Ahuja RB, Gupta GK. A four arm, double blind, randomized and placebo controlled study of pregabalin in the management of post-burn pruritus. Burns. 2013;39(1):24–9.
78. Gürol AP, Polat S, Akçay MN. Itching, pain, and anxiety levels are reduced with massage therapy in burned adolescents. J Burn Care Res. 31(3):429–32.
79. Schachner L, Field T, Hernandez-Reif M, Duarte AM, Krasnegor J. Atopic dermatitis symptoms decreased in children following massage therapy. Pediatr Dermatol. 2009;15(5):390–5.
80. Field T, Peck M, Krugman S, Tuchel T, Schanberg S, Kuhn C, et al. Burn injuries benefit from massage therapy. J Burn Care Rehabil. 1998;19(3):241–4.
81. Musgrave MA, Umraw N, Fish JS, Gomez M, Cartotto RC The effect of silicone gel sheets on perfusion of hypertrophic burn scars. J Burn Care Rehabil 23:208–1481
82. Quinn KJ, Evans JH, Courtney JM, Gaylor JDS, Reid WH. Non-pressure treatment of hypertrophic scars. Burns. 1985;12:102–8.
83. Chan KY, Lau CL, Adeeb SM, Somasundaram S, Nasir-Zahari M. A randomized, placebo-controlled, double-blind, prospective clinical trial of silicone gel in prevention of hypertrophic scar development in median sternotomy wound. Plast Reconstr Surg. 2005;116(4):1013–20; discussion 1021–2.

84. van der Wal MBA, van Zuijlen PP, van de Ven P, Middelkoop E. Topical silicone gel versus placebo in promoting the maturation of burn scars: a randomized controlled trial. Plast Reconstr Surg. 2010;126(2):524–31.
85. Momeni M, Hafezi F, Rahbar H, Karimi H. Effects of silicone gel on burn scars. Burns. 2009;35(1):70–4.
86. Eishi K, Bae S, Ogawa F, Hamasaki Y, Shimizu K, Katayama I. Silicone gel sheets relieve pain and pruritus with clinical improvement of keloid: possible target of mast cells. J Dermatol Treat. 2003;14(4):248–52.
87. Li-Tsang CWP, Lau JCM, Choi J, Chan CCC, Jianan L. A prospective randomized clinical trial to investigate the effect of silicone gel sheeting (Cica-Care) on post-traumatic hypertrophic scar among the Chinese population. Burns. 2006;32(6): 678–83.
88. Wittenberg GP, Fabian BG, Bogomilsky JL, Schultz LR, Rudner EJ, Chaffins ML, et al. Prospective, single-blind, randomized, controlled study to assess the efficacy of the 585-nm flashlamp-pumped pulsed-dye laser and silicone gel sheeting in hypertrophic scar treatment. Arch Dermatol. 1999;135(9):1049–55.
89. Sproat JE, Dalcin A, Weitauer N, Roberts RS. Hypertrophic sternal scars: silicone gel sheet versus Kenalog injection treatment. Plast Reconstr Surg. 1992;90(6):988–92.
90. Hettrick HH, O'Brien K, Laznick H, Sanchez J, Gorga D, Nagler W, et al. Effect of transcutaneous electrical nerve stimulation for the management of burn pruritus: a pilot study. J Burn Care Rehabil. 2004;25(3):236–40.
91. Choiniere M, Papillon J. Topical capsaicin treatment for post-burn pruritus: a double blind study. In: Abstract: 9th Congress of the International Society for Burn Injuries; 2001.
92. Hercogová J. Topical anti-itch therapy. Dermatol Ther. 18(4):341–3.
93. Staňder S, Steinhoff M, Schmelz M, et al. Neurophysiology of pruritus: cutaneous elicitation of itch. Arch Dermatol. 2003;139:1463–70.
94. Simons FER. Advances in H_1-antihistamines. N Engl J Med. 2004;351(21):2203–17.
95. Simons FER. H1-antihistamines: more relevant than ever in the treatment of allergic disorders. J Allergy Clin Immunol. 2003;112(4 Suppl):S42–52.
96. Vitale M, Fields-Blache C, Luterman A. Severe itching in the patient with burns. J Burn Care Rehabil. 1991;12(4):330–3. https://doi.org/10.1097/00004630-199107000-00008.
97. Rowbotham M, Harden N, Stacey B, Bernstein P, Magnus-Miller L. Gabapentin for the treatment of postherpetic neuralgia: a randomized controlled trial. JAMA. 1998;280(21):1837–42.
98. Gee NS, Brown JP, Dissanayake VU, Offord J, Thurlow R, Woodruff GN. The novel anticonvulsant drug, gabapentin (Neurontin), binds to the alpha2delta subunit of a calcium channel. J Biol Chem. 1996;271(10):5768–76.
99. Kuzniecky R, Ho S, Pan J, Martin R, Gilliam F, Faught E, et al. Modulation of cerebral GABA by topiramate, lamotrigine, and gabapentin in healthy adults. Neurology. 2002;58(3):368–72.
100. Conway H, Stark RB. ACTH in plastic surgery. Plast Reconstr Surg (1946). 1951;8(5):354–77.
101. Mustoe TA, Cooter RD, Gold MH, et al. International clinical recommendations on scar management. Plast Reconstr Surg. 2002;110(2):560–71. https://doi.org/10.1097/00006534-200208000-00031.
102. Gold MH, Berman B, Clementoni MT, Gauglitz GG, Nahai F, Murcia C. Updated international clinical recommendations on scar management: part 1–evaluating the evidence. Dermatol Surg. 2014;40(8):817–24.
103. Darzi MA, Chowdri NA, Kaul SK, Khan M, Wood M, Rollins C. Evaluation of various methods of treating keloids and hypertrophic scars: a 10-year follow-up study. Br J Plast Surg. 1992;45(5):374–9.
104. Manuskiatti W, Fitzpatrick RE. Treatment response of keloidal and hypertrophic sternotomy scars comparison among intralesional corticosteroid, 5-fluorouracil, and 585-nm flashlamp-pumped pulsed-dye laser treatments. Arch Dermatol. 2002;138(9):1149–55.
105. Boutli-Kasapidou F, Tsakiri A, Anagnostou E, Mourellou O. Hypertrophic and keloidal scars: an approach to polytherapy. Int J Dermatol. 2005;44(4):324–7.
106. Tan E, Chua S, Lim J. Topical silicone gel sheet versus intralesional injections of triamcinolone acetonide in the treatment of keloids — a patient-controlled comparative clinical trial. J Dermatol Treat. 1999;10(4):251–4.
107. Martin MS, Collawn SS. Combination treatment of CO_2 fractional laser, pulsed dye laser, and triamcinolone acetonide injection for refractory keloid scars on the upper back. J Cosmet Laser Ther. 2013;15(3):166–70.
108. Goutos I, Ogawa R. Steroid tape: a promising adjunct to scar management. Scars Burns Healing. 2017;3:2059513117690937.
109. Wright G, Lax A, Mehta SB. A review of the longevity of effect of botulinum toxin in wrinkle treatments. Br Dent J. 2018;224(4):255–60.
110. Sohrabi C, Goutos I. The use of botulinum toxin in keloid scar management: a literature review [Internet]. National Plastic Surgery Research Forum; 2019 [cited 2019 Aug 1]. Available from: https://nationalplasticsurgeryresearchforum.org/the-use-of-botulinum-toxin-in-keloid-scar-management-a-literature-review.
111. Shaarawy E, Hegazy RA, Abdel Hay RM. Intralesional botulinum toxin type A equally effective and better tolerated than intralesional steroid in the treatment of keloids: a randomized controlled trial. J Cosmet Dermatol. 2015;14(2):161–6.
112. Rasaii S, Sohrabian N, Gianfaldoni S, Hadibarhaghtalab M, Pazyar N, Bakhshaeekia A, et al. Intralesional triamcinolone alone or in combination with botulinium toxin A is ineffective for the treatment of formed keloid scar: a double blind controlled pilot study. Dermatol Ther. 2019;32(2):e12781.
113. Li J, Wu X-Y, Chen X-D. Observation on clinical efficacy of intralesional injection of glucocorticoid combined with botulinum toxin type A for treatment of keloid | J Li. J Clin Dermatol. 2017;46(9):629–32.
114. Akhtar N, Brooks P. The use of botulinum toxin in the management of burns itching: preliminary results. Burns. 2012;38(8):1119–23.
115. Gregoire FM, Smas CM, Sul HS. Understanding adipocyte differentiation. Physiol Rev. 1998;78:783–809 103.
116. Conde-Green A, Baptista LS, de Amorin NFG, de Oliveira ED, da Silva KR, Pedrosa CDSG, Borojevic R, Pitanguy I. Effects of centrifugation on cell composition and viability of aspirated adipose tissue processed for transplantation. Aesthet Surg J. 2010;30(2):249–55.
117. Klinger M, Lisa A, Klinger F, Giannasi S, Veronesi A, Banzatti B, et al. Regenerative approach to scars, ulcers and related problems with fat grafting. Clin Plast Surg. 2015;42(3): 345–52.
118. Cheville AL, Sloan JA, Northfelt DW, Jillella AP, Wong GY, Bearden JD III, et al. Use of a lidocaine patch in the management of postsurgical neuropathic pain in patients with cancer: a phase III double-blind crossover study (N01CB). Support Care Cancer. 2009;17(4):451–60.
119. Fredman R, Edkins RE, Hultman CS. Fat grafting for neuropathic pain after severe burns. Ann Plast Surg. 2016;76:S298–303.
120. Huang S-H, Wu S-H, Chang K-P, Lin C-H, Chang C-H, Wu Y-C, et al. Alleviation of neuropathic scar pain using autologous fat grafting. Ann Plast Surg. 2015;74:S99–104.

121. Condé-Green A, Marano AA, Lee ES, Reisler T, Price LA, Milner SM, Granick MS. Fat grafting and adipose-derived regenerative cells in burn wound healing and scarring. Plast Reconstr Surg. 2016;137:302–312 116.
122. Negenborn VL, Groen J-W, Smit JM, Niessen FB, Mullender MG. The use of autologous fat grafting for treatment of scar tissue and scar-related conditions. Plast Reconstr Surg. 2016;137:31e–43e.
123. Elsaie ML, Choudhary S. Lasers for scars: a review and evidence-based appraisal. J Drugs Dermatol. 2010;9:1355–62.
124. Chrastil B, Glaich AS, Goldberg LH, Friedman PM. Second-generation 1,550-nm fractional photothermolysis for the treatment of acne scars. Dermatol Surg. 2008;34(10):1327–32.
125. Anderson RR, Parrish JA. Selective photothermolysis: precise microsurgery by selective absorption of pulsed radiation. Science. 1983;220(4596):524–7.
126. Nakagawa H, Tan OT, Parrish JA. Ultrastructural changes in human skin after exposure to a pulsed laser. J Invest Dermatol. 1985;84(5):396–400.
127. Ebid AA, Ibrahim AR, Omar MT, El Baky AMA. Long-term effects of pulsed high-intensity laser therapy in the treatment of post-burn pruritus: a double-blind, placebo-controlled, randomized study. Lasers Med Sci. 2017;32(3):693–701.
128. Vasheghani MM, Bayat M, Rezaei F, Bayat A, Karimipour M. Effect of low-level laser therapy on mast cells in second-degree burns in rats. Photomed Laser Surg. 2008;26(1):1–5.
129. Peplow PV, Chung T-Y, Baxter GD. Application of low level laser technologies for pain relief and wound healing: overview of scientific bases. Phys Ther Rev. 2010;15(4):253–85.
130. Lim W, Lee S, Kim I, Chung M, Kim M, Lim H, et al. The anti-inflammatory mechanism of 635 nm light-emitting-diode irradiation compared with existing COX inhibitors. Lasers Surg Med. 2007;39(7):614–21.
131. Chow R, Armati P, Laakso E-L, Bjordal JM, Baxter GD. Inhibitory effects of laser irradiation on peripheral mammalian nerves and relevance to analgesic effects: a systematic review. Photomed Laser Surg. 2011;29:365–81.
132. Alster TS, Williams CM. Treatment of keloid sternotomy scars with 585 nm flashlamp-pumped pulsed-dye laser. Lancet. 1995;345(8959):1198–200.
133. Douglas H, Lynch J, Harms K-A, Krop T, Kunath L, van Vreeswijk C, McGarry S, Fear MW, Wood FM, Murray A, Rea S. Carbon dioxide laser treatment in burn-related scarring: a prospective randomised controlled trial. J Plastic Reconst Aesthet Surg. 2019;72(6):863–70.

8

The Epidemiology of Keloids

Chenyu Huang, Zhaozhao Wu, Yanan Du, and Rei Ogawa

Contents

Take-Home Messages

- Despite the fact that keloids are common throughout the world, their epidemiology has not been adequately investigated.
- The demographic distribution of keloids, mainly on the geographical regions and ethnic racies.
- Genetic risk factors can shape keloid rates, in particular certain diseases appear to amplify or suppress keloid formations.
- Environmental factors also contribute to keloid development and progression and therefore shape keloid rates, such as local mechanical stimuli.

Background

Keloids are pathological scars that are characterized histologically by an overwhelming aggregation of fibroblasts and collagen type I within the inflammatory reticular dermis [1]. Their clinical characteristics include continuous growth and invasion into the neighboring healthy skin beyond the original wound boundary via an erythematous and pruritic leading edge. They also show a strong tendency to recur when they are surgically excised in the absence of adjuvant therapies. Despite the fact that keloids are common throughout the world, their epidemiology has not been adequately investigated.

In this chapter, we will summarize the limited epidemiological data on keloids that exists to date. Most of these data are from English language papers that are listed in PubMed. Below, we will describe what is known about (1) the demographic distribution of keloids, mainly on the geographical regions and ethnic races; (2) the internal genetic factors that shape keloid rates; and (3) the external environmental factors that influence keloid epidemiology. The aim of the chapter is to facilitate a greater understanding of the complexity and diversity of keloids from an epidemiological perspective, thereby potentiating further and deeper explorations into individualized strategies that prevent and treat keloids.

Demographic Risk Factors That Shape Keloid Rates

The studies on the demographic distribution of keloids in the world are sparse and occasionally contradictory. However, keloid rates can be affected by geography and ethnicity.

In terms of geographical distribution, it has long been cited that the incidence of keloids ranges widely from 0.09% in England to 16% in Zaire [2, 3]. While these reviews did not indicate how these incidences were determined, they are somewhat supported by the few large-scale studies on geographical incidence that have been performed. One of these was a review of the 5735 patients who underwent surgery in the 33 surgical facilities in Zambia between 1993 and 2008: the study showed that of the 5774 surgical diagnoses, 514 are related to keloids. Thus, keloids accounted for nearly 9% of all those surgical cases in Zambia during the study period [4]. Moreover in Kenya, the keloid prevalence is 8.5% among people with normally pigmented skins [5]. By contrast, the keloid incidence in Japan is around 0.1% [6] (◘ Table 4.1). Considering that the keloid incidence data is limited and scattered, which can hardly be comparable in a strictly defined background covering key factors such as statistical period/cycle, population size/composition, and diagnostic criteria on scar type/severity, it is still difficult to depict an accurate keloid distribution map at this time. And the average keloid incidence can only be estimated as 5–10% in African, 0–0.1% in Asian, and <0.1% in other countries, as seen in ◘ Fig. 4.1.

◘ Table The incidences of keloid reported in different countries

Country	Keloid incidence (%)	Reference
England	0.09%	[2, 3]
Japan	0.10%	[6]
Kenya	8.50%	[5]
Zambia	9%	[4]
Zaire	16%	[2, 3]

It is suspected that this large geographical variation in keloid rate may reflect racial differences in skin pigmentation (◘ Fig. 4.2). However, the data on keloid prevalence in various races is conflicting. First, Louw states that both Blacks and Asians are more susceptible to keloid formation than Caucasians [3]. Indeed, the Black/Caucasian ratio was reported varying from 14:1 to 2:1 [7]. However, the above reports may suggest that Asians could have similarly low incidences of keloid as Caucasians (0.1% in Japan versus 0.09% in England) [2, 3, 6]. Two studies also suggest that at least one specific type of keloid, acne keloidalis nuchae (AKN), is much more common in Blacks than in Asians. Na et al. showed that of 254,785 patients who attended the dermatology department of a Korean hospital in 2005–2017, 17 had AKN (0.007%) [8]. By contrast, another study showed that of 13,422 new patients who visited a large university hospital in Benin in 1993–2002, 0.7% (90 cases) had AKN, and the prevalence was reported as 0.37% (90

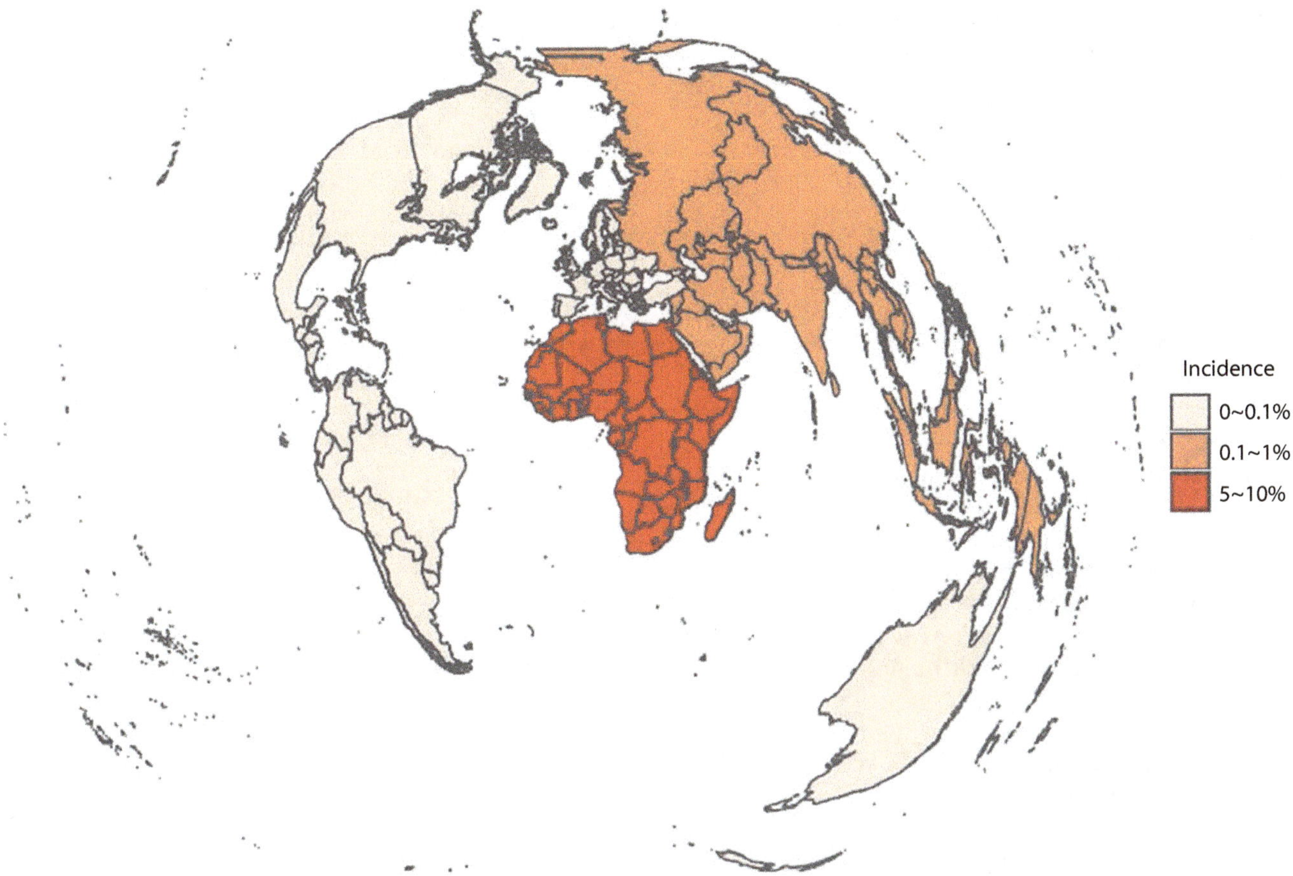

Fig. Heatmap of keloid epidemiology in the world. The average keloid incidence can only be estimated as 5–10% in African, 0–0.1% in Asian, and <0.1% in other countries

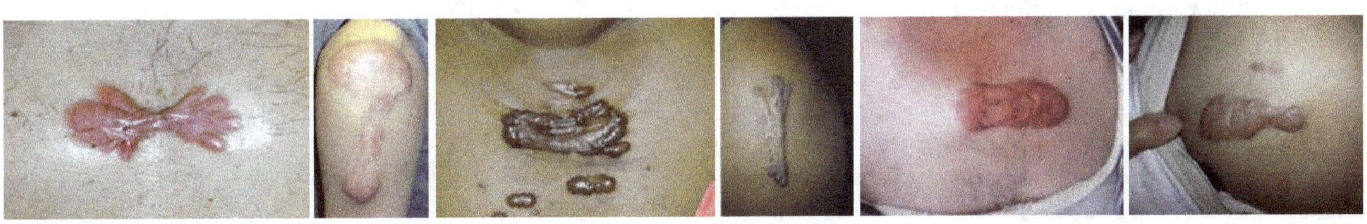

Fig. Chest and shoulder keloids in different racial groups of Asians, Africans, and Caucasians. 4.2.1 The images are from Huang et al. with permission (Huang et al. [11]). 4. 2.2 The images are from Bayat et al. with permission (Bayat et al. [12]). 4. 2.3 The images are from Shaheen et al. with permission (Shaheen et al. [13]. © All rights reserved)

cases out of 26,522 patients overall) [9]. The latter study is supported by several other studies that show that AKN is common in Blacks. For example, as high as 4.7% of Black boys in the last year of high school in South Africa can develop AKN [10]. Moreover, the postulated relationship between high skin pigmentation and greater susceptibility to keloid formation is not borne out by two studies. One is a cross-sectional study on randomly selected villages in Kenya and people with albinism who were recruited via an albino association in Kenya and dermatology training center clinics and special schools in Tanzania. Of the 1416 African people who were recruited, 1185 had normally pigmented skin, and 231 had albinism. And 954 among the 1416 people have scars on their body. For them, the total prevalence of keloid was 8.3%. The subjects with normal pigmentation did not differ significantly from the subjects with albinism in terms of keloid prevalence (8.5% versus 7.8%; $P = 0.599$) [5]. The second study described the 175 keloid patients who visited the General Hospital in Kuala Lumpur in West Malaysia in 1959–1967. West Malaysia has a multiracial population. An analysis of the ethnicities of the keloid patient cohort showed that keloid was more common in the relatively fair-skinned Chinese: while 56% of the keloid patients were Chinese, this ethnicity accounted for only 47.47% of the population. By contrast, 22.86% and 17.14% of the keloid patients were darker-skinned Indians and Malays, respectively; these ethnicities accounted for 19.52% and 29.58% of the population, respectively [7].

Genetic Risk Factors That Shape Keloid Rates

The effect of ethnicity on keloidogenesis suggests that keloid formation is somewhat underpinned by genetic variation. This is borne out by multiple genetic studies that show that keloidogenesis associates with certain gene mutations or polymorphism [14]. Keloids also show a familial tendency [15]. Here, we will discuss less well-known genetic associations with keloids, namely, certain diseases that appear to amplify or, conversely, suppress keloid rates.

The diseases that associate with an increased risk of keloid include the Rubinstein-Taybi syndrome (RSTS), the Ehlers-Danlos syndrome, the Lowe syndrome, and the novel X-linked syndrome, and others (◘ Table 4.2). RSTS is also called broad thumb-hallux syndrome. It is characterized by broad thumbs and toes, facial abnormalities, and short stature [16]. The etiological mutation lies in gene encoding the cyclic AMP response element-binding protein (CBP) on chromosome 16p13.3 [17] and E1A-binding protein (EP300) gene which encodes p300 protein (a cAMP response element-binding protein homologue) [18]. Keloid is reported to occur in 24% (15/62) of RSTS patients, either spontaneously or secondary to minor trauma [19]. The Ehlers-Danlos syndrome type IV (the vascular subtype) is an inherited disorder of connective tissue that is characterized by acrogeria, translucent skin, propensity to bruising, and significant arterial, digestive, and uterine complications [20]. The causative mutation is in COL3A1 gene, which encodes the pro-α1(III) chain of collagen type III [21]. Several case reports show that this syndrome can paradoxically associate with extensive keloid formation [22]. The Lowe syndrome (also called the oculocerebrorenal syndrome of Lowe [OCRL]) affects the eyes, nervous system, and kidneys [23]. It is caused by a mutation in the OCRL gene that reduces the amount of the OCRL-1 protein [24]. The formation of corneal keloids in patients with Lowe syndrome is relatively common. It is generally provoked by corneal contact lens use or after intraocular lens implantation [25]. Novel X-linked syndrome is characterized by symptoms of cardiac valvular disease, spontaneous keloid scarring, and reduced joint mobility. The causal mutation is filamin A (FLNA) substitution G1576R [26]. Other syndromes that may associate with spontaneous keloid formation include the Dubowitz syndrome [27], the Noonan syndrome [28], and the Goeminne syndrome [29], which are inherited in autosomal recessive, autosomal dominant, and sex-linked incomplete dominant ways, respectively, though the actual gene mutation remained unclear.

The diseases that associate with protection from severe pathological scarring are Hansen's disease and von Recklinghausen's disease. Hansen's disease (also known as leprosy) is a chronic disease that arises after infection with *Mycobacterium leprae* and *Mycobacterium lepromatosis*. It is characterized by granulomas of the nerves, respiratory tract, skin, and eyes and the gradual destruction of the intraepidermal innervation. Extensive scarring is extremely rare in patients with Hansen's disease [30, 31]. von Recklinghausen's disease is also known as neurofibromatosis type I (NF-I). It is characterized by the growth of tumors on the nerves. A study of 30 Nigerian patients with neurofibromatosis who underwent surgery showed that none of them developed keloid or hypertrophic scars after surgery, even though their wound healing was poor and some of their wounds were closed under tension [32]. Similarly, a worldwide multicenter study on 57 patients with von Recklinghausen's disease showed that none of the patients developed hypertrophic scar or keloid after surgery: in general, their wounds healed remarkably well. The main complications were the development of hematoma and wide white scar in six patients. By contrast, two of the 35 patients with a solitary neurofibroma who were included in the study developed hypertrophic scars after surgery [33].

Environmental Risk Factors That Shape Keloid Rates

Environmental factors also contribute to keloid development and progression and therefore shape keloid rates. One such factor is local mechanical stimulus. An interesting feature of keloids is that they show a distinct site specificity. When we analyzed 1500 keloids in 483 Japanese patients (the keloids generated from artificially created wounds, namely, those created by surgery and piercing, were excluded), we found they tended to occur on the anterior chest region (48.9%), scapular regions (26.9%), lower jaw/neck region (12.1%), upper arm (4.8%), dorsal regions (2.5%), lower abdomen (1.9%), femoral regions (1.7%), knee (0.5%) and upper abdomen (0.5%) [34]. All of these regions are characterized by high skin tension/friction. That skin tension promotes keloid development is also shown by the fact

Table The syndromes associated with keloidogenesis

Syndrome	Other names	Characteristic features	Keloid lesions	Genes or inheritance concerned	Reference
Rubinstein-Taybi syndrome (RSTS)	Broad thumb-hallux syndrome	Broad thumbs and toes, facial abnormalities, short stature	24%	CBP on chromosome 16p13.3; EP300	[16–19]
Ehlers-Danlos syndrome type IV (vascular type)		Acrogeria, translucent skin, propensity to bruising, and significant arterial, digestive, and uterine complications	Extensive keloid formation	COL3A1 gene that encodes the pro-α1(III) chain of collagen type III	[20–22]
Lowe syndrome	Oculocerebrorenal syndrome of Lowe (OCRL)	Affects the eyes, nervous system, and kidneys	Corneal keloids	OCRL gene that reduces the amount of the OCRL-1 protein	[23–25]
Novel X-linked syndrome		Cardiac valvular disease, spontaneous keloid scarring, and reduced joint mobility	Spontaneous keloid scarring	A G1576R mutation in filamin A (FLNA)	[26]
Dubowitz syndrome		Intrauterine growth retardation, low neonatal weight, short stature, characteristic facies, atopic dermatitis, and mental retardation	Spontaneous keloidal lesions	Autosomal recessive transmission	[27]
Noonan syndrome		Craniofacial appearance, congenital cardiac defects, orthopedic abnormalities, psychomotor and growth retardation, and some skin changes including keloidal tissue formation	Keloidal tissue formation	Autosomal dominant inheritance	[28]
Goeminne syndrome		Congenital muscular torticollis, multiple keloids, cryptorchidism, and renal dysplasia	Multiple spontaneous keloids	Sex-linked incomplete dominant inheritance	[29]

that the keloids on certain regions grow into specific shapes. Thus, anterior chest keloids form symmetrical butterfly shapes that reflect the predominant stretching directions of the chest skin that are caused by the upper arm movements. By contrast, keloids on the scapula form dumbbell shapes that run down the long axis of the arm and are caused by the skin stretching caused by the hanging upper arm. Moreover, earlobe keloids often grow into balls that reflect the circular nocturnal friction on the earlobe from the head moving on the pillow [34]. This role of mechanical tension in keloid growth is further supported by the recent case of a patient in our center whose symmetrically distributed butterfly keloid on the chest was accidentally split in half at the midline. The patient was right-handed. In the subsequent 2 years, the right half butterfly of the keloid continued to progress as usual. By contrast, the left half butterfly grew much less strongly and indeed exhibited signs of amelioration [11].

Conclusion

Regardless of whether keloids occur spontaneously or after trauma, these lesions are clearly the result of both internal genetic and external environmental factors. These factors underlie the association between keloids and various demographic risk factors, namely, geographical region and ethnicity. However, our understanding of these demographic factors is limited by the paucity of and inconsistencies in the epidemiological research on keloids. To identify the respective contributions of genetic and environment factors to keloid formation, it will be necessary to conduct large-scale investigations with specific study designs, such as studies on twin cohorts or cross-sectional studies on the members of families that show a predilection toward keloidogenesis. Such explorations will help to orient further keloid research, thereby aiding the development of effective therapeutic approaches.

References

1. Ogawa R. Keloid and hypertrophic scars are the result of chronic inflammation in the reticular dermis. Int J Mol Sci. 2017;18:606.
2. Kelly AP. Keloids. Dermatol Clin. 1988;6(3):413–24.
3. Louw L. Keloids in rural black south Africans. Part 1: general overview and essential fatty acid hypotheses for keloid formation and prevention. Prostaglandins Leukot Essent Fatty Acids. 2000;63(5):237–45.
4. Jovic G, Corlew DS, Bowman KG. Plastic and reconstructive surgery in Zambia: epidemiology of 16 years of practice. World J Surg. 2012;36(2):241–6.
5. Kiprono SK, Chaula BM, Masenga JE, Muchunu JW, Mavura DR, Moehrle M. Epidemiology of keloids in normally pigmented Africans and African people with albinism: population-based cross-sectional survey. Br J Dermatol. 2015;173(3):852–4.
6. Ogawa R. Importance of epidemiologic investigation on keloids. Scar Management. 2009;3:62–64.
7. Alhady SM, Sivanantharajah K. Keloids in various races. A review of 175 cases. Plast Reconstr Surg. 1969;44(6):564–6.
8. Na K, Oh SH, Kim SK. Acne keloidalis nuchae in Asian: a single institutional experience. PLoS One. 2017;12(12):e0189790.
9. Adegbidi H, Atadokpede F, do Ango-Padonou F, Yedomon H. Keloid acne of the neck: epidemiological studies over 10 years. Int J Dermatol. 2005;44(Suppl 1):49–50.
10. Khumalo NP, Jessop S, Gumedze F, Ehrlich R. Hairdressing is associated with scalp disease in African schoolchildren. Br J Dermatol. 2007;157(1):106–10.
11. Huang C, Liu L, You Z, Wang B, Du Y, Ogawa R. Keloid progression: a stiffness gap hypothesis. Int Wound J. 2017;14(5):764–71.
12. Bayat A, Arscott G, Ollier WE, Ferguson MW, Mc Grouther DA. Description of site-specific morphology of keloid phenotypes in an Afrocaribbean population. Br J Plast Surg. 2004;57(2):122–33.
13. Shaheen A, Khaddam J, Kesh F. Risk factors of keloids in Syrians. BMC Dermatol. 2016;16(1):13.
14. Shih B, Bayat A. Genetics of keloid scarring. Arch Dermatol Res. 2010;302(5):319–39.
15. Santos-Cortez RLP, Hu Y, Sun F, Benahmed-Miniuk F, Tao J, Kanaujiya JK, Ademola S, Fadiora S, Odesina V, Nickerson DA, Bamshad MJ, Olaitan PB, Oluwatosin OM, Leal SM, Reichenberger EJ. Identification of ASAH1 as a susceptibility gene for familial keloids. Eur J Hum Genet. 2017;25(10):1155–61.
16. Rubinstein JH, Taybi H. Broad thumbs and toes and facial abnormalities. A possible mental retardation syndrome. Am J Dis Child. 1963;105:588–608.
17. Petrij F, Giles RH, Dauwerse HG, Saris JJ, Hennekam RC, Masuno M, Tommerup N, van Ommen GJ, Goodman RH, Peters DJ, et al. Rubinstein-Taybi syndrome caused by mutations in the transcriptional co-activator CBP. Nature. 1995;376(6538):348–51.
18. Roelfsema JH, White SJ, Ariyürek Y, Bartholdi D, Niedrist D, Papadia F, Bacino CA, den Dunnen JT, van Ommen GJ, Breuning MH, Hennekam RC, Peters DJ. Genetic heterogeneity in Rubinstein-Taybi syndrome: mutations in both the CBP and EP300 genes cause disease. Am J Hum Genet. 2005;76(4):572–80.
19. van de Kar AL, Houge G, Shaw AC, de Jong D, van Belzen MJ, Peters DJ, Hennekam RC. Keloids in Rubinstein-Taybi syndrome: a clinical study. Br J Dermatol. 2014;171(3):615–21.
20. Germain DP. Ehlers-Danlos syndrome type IV. Orphanet J Rare Dis. 2007;2:32.
21. Smith LT, Schwarze U, Goldstein J, Byers PH. Mutations in the COL3A1 gene result in the Ehlers-Danlos syndrome type IV and alterations in the size and distribution of the major collagen fibrils of the dermis. J Invest Dermatol. 1997;108(3):241–7.
22. Burk CJ, Aber C, Connelly EA. Ehlers-Danlos syndrome type IV: keloidal plaques of the lower extremities, amniotic band limb deformity, and a new mutation. J Am Acad Dermatol. 2007;56(2 Suppl):S53–4.
23. Lowe CU, Terrey M, MacLachlan EA. Organic-aciduria, decreased renal ammonia production, hydrophthalmos, and mental retardation; a clinical entity. AMA Am J Dis Child. 1952;83(2):164–84.
24. Rendu J, Montjean R, Coutton C, Suri M, Chicanne G, Petiot A, Brocard J, Grunwald D, Pietri Rouxel F, Payrastre B, Lunardi J, Dorseuil O, Marty I, Fauré J. Functional characterization and

Rescue of a Deep Intronic Mutation in OCRL gene responsible for Lowe syndrome. Hum Mutat. 2017;38(2):152–9.
25. Esquenazi S, Eustis HS, Bazan HE, Leon A, He J. Corneal keloid in Lowe syndrome. J Pediatr Ophthalmol Strabismus. 2005;42(5):308–10.
26. Atwal PS, Blease S, Braxton A, Graves J, He W, Person R, Slattery L, Bernstein JA, Hudgins L. Novel X-linked syndrome of cardiac valvulopathy, keloid scarring, and reduced joint mobility due to filamin a substitution G1576R. Am J Med Genet A. 2016;170A(4):891–5.
27. Paradisi M, Angelo C, Conti G, Mostaccioli S, Cianchini G, Atzori F, Puddu P. Dubowitz syndrome with keloidal lesions. Clin Exp Dermatol. 1994;19(5):425–7.
28. Güleç AT, Karaduman A, Seçkin D. Noonan syndrome: a case with recurrent keloid formation. Cutis. 2001;67(4):315–6.
29. Goeminne L. A new probably X-linked inherited syndrome: congenital muscular torticollis, multiple keloids cryptorchidism and renal dysplasia. Acta Genet Med Gemellol. 1968;17(3): 439–67.
30. Facer P, Mann D, Mathur R, Pandya S, Ladiwala U, Singhal B, Hongo J, Sinicropi DV, Terenghi G, Anand P. Do nerve growth factor-related mechanisms contribute to loss of cutaneous nociception in leprosy? Pain. 2000;85(1-2):231–8.
31. Ogawa R, Hsu CK. Mechanobiological dysregulation of the epidermis and dermis in skin disorders and in degeneration. J Cell Mol Med. 2013;17(7):817–22.
32. Ademiluyi SA, Sowemimo GO, Oyeneyin JO. Surgical experience in the management of multiple neurofibromatosis in Nigerians. West Afr J Med. 1989;8(1):59–65.
33. Miyawaki T, Billings B, Har-Shai Y, Agbenorku P, Kokuba E, Moreira-Gonzalez A, Tsukuno M, Kurihara K, Jackson IT. Multicenter study of wound healing in neurofibromatosis and neurofibroma. J Craniofac Surg. 2007;18(5):1008–11.
34. Ogawa R, Okai K, Tokumura F, Mori K, Ohmori Y, Huang C, Hyakusoku H, Akaishi S. The relationship between skin stretching/contraction and pathologic scarring: the important role of mechanical forces in keloid generation. Wound Repair Regen. 2012;20(2):149–57.

9

Compression Therapy and Conservative Strategies in Scar Management After Burn Injury

Eric Van den Kerckhove and Mieke Anthonissen

Contents

Background
Since a few decades, the focus of treatment of burn patients has shifted from survival to optimizing the rehabilitation outcome of patients with severe scars. This outcome can influence both physical as well as psychological well-being and quality of life of the patient. Therefore, the interest in the field of conservative scar management of these patients has risen drastically. In this regard, the golden standard in all medical or paramedical treatments is aiming for evidence-based interventions. Also in this rather new domain of scar rehabilitation, caregivers strive to use the most efficient therapies. Unfortunately, for most of the daily used interventions, the number of proper scientific clinical trials is still limited and therefore the evidence-based level of many of them is often low. As a consequence, the recommended therapies are often based on recommendations or guidelines written by a group of specialists based on their expertise and available literature. This chapter focuses on the most relevant noninvasive strategies in the aftercare of patients with severe scarring after burn injury with special attention to compression therapy.

ferent conservative therapeutic strategies that are mostly used in the rehabilitation of patients with severe scars after burn injury. These strategies include pressure therapy, the use of silicones as a contact medium, massage, the use of moisturizers, splinting and positioning, exercise, and mobilizations. The relevance of the conservative therapeutic strategies will be situated within the field of the available scientific literature or guidelines.

According to the World Health Organization (WHO), annually nearly 11 million people worldwide are burned severely enough to require medical attention. Aesthetic and functional outcomes have become increasingly important, as overall mortality from burn injury has decreased. Hypertrophic scar formation is a common and bothersome complication after a severe burn injury or even after minor burns, due to its functional and aesthetic consequences. These scars, which usually develop after 6–8 weeks of wound closure, are typified by the following characteristics. The red to deep purple color of the scar reflects an enhanced microcirculation. The hypertrophic scar becomes more elevated, firm, warm to touch, hypersensitive, and itchy but the lesion remains within the confines of the original scar. The elevation, firmness, and retraction of the scar is probably due to an overabundant collagen deposition as a cellular response of the fibroblast during the proliferation phase of wound healing. The contraction of the scar has been linked to the presence of fibroblasts with contractile properties, called the "myofibroblasts." Generally, a period of at least 6–18 months is required for maturation of burn scars at which time the redness (erythema) of the scar subsides, the scar no longer appears inflamed, and the scar contraction diminishes.

Many factors can influence the presence or severity of hypertrophic scarring after a burn injury. Genetic predisposition, race, anatomical location of the burn, age, and depth of the burn are some of the factors that are known as "uncontrollable or extrinsic factors," whereas infection, type of wound healing (surgical intervention or not), and tension are factors that can be considered as "extrinsic or controllable" factors. The prevalence of hypertrophic scarring ranges from 32% to 72%. Female gender, young age, race or ethnicity, burn site (on face, neck, and upper limb), multiple surgical procedures, meshed skin grafts, time to heal longer than 2–3 weeks, more than 20% total body surface area (TBSA), and burn severity are some of the identified risk factors.

The scar management treatments in patients with burns have gained a lot of interest recently. This increase in interest is entirely correct, as the quality of life of these patients can be significantly influenced if one can improve the clinical parameters of scars. Burn scar-related symptoms show a proximal impact on health-related quality of life. Therefore, the scar management interventions have high interest in the improvement of quality of life of burn patients, especially those with visible scars and severe burns. Scar management in the treatment of burn patients includes a wide variety of aftercare methods and physio- and occupational therapeutic techniques such as pressure therapy, silicone therapy, massage, moisturizers, splinting and positioning, exercise, and mobilizations.

Of all the noninvasive therapeutic treatments, pressure therapy is one of the most successful, widely used, and evidence-based techniques in the prevention and treatment of hypertrophic (burn-related) scars [1]. In the late 1960s, Dr. Silverstein at Brooke Army Hospital in San Antonio observed that in a patient with burns, vascular support garments for the treatment of a postphlebitic syndrome decreased scarring after a burn injury and Larson noted the same effect with pressure-exerting splints on scar tissue. The use of compression in the prevention of burn scar hypertrophy was then further popularized at Shriners' Burns Institute in Galveston at the beginning of the 1970s.

Furthermore, silicone therapy is also a popular and evidence-supported conservative treatment to prevent or treat hypertrophic scars [2]. The first silicone applications were individually made as a pressure device or pad to solve concavity problems under pressure garments. The pressure pads are individually made using elastomer (medical grade with catalyst), putty, or foam, and fitted directly on the patient. They are usually worn in combination with classical pressure garments, masks, and splints. Silicone applications can also be applied directly to the scar without any intention to augment or establish pressure on the scar. In the 1980s, silicone gel sheets were effectively used for the first time in the treatment of burn-related scars, however without clear standardized treatment protocols. Since the beginning of the 1990s, publications and protocols about the use of silicone sheets and gels as contact media in the prevention of hypertrophic scarring and contractures started to appear. They remain very popular as a conservative strategy ever since.

Concerning the other noninvasive treatment modalities, such as massage, the use of moisturizers, positioning and splinting, exercise, and mobilizations, the number of published controlled trials (randomized controlled trials [RCTs] of controlled clinical trial [CCTs]) for each category is rather low and within each category, different techniques or types of applications and products are used. In the field of rehabilitation, especially in burn rehabilitation, controlled randomized double-blind trials are practically and ethically extremely difficult to perform. Due to this shortcoming, except for the effect of pressure on the thickness of a scar, there is no real scientific consensus on the actual effect of the various treatment modalities. Therefore, most recommendations are mostly made based on guidelines and consensus meetings of experts [3–8].

Pressure therapy is indicated to prevent and treat skin grafts and wounds that take longer than 14–21 days to heal, because of the higher risk of hypertrophic scar formation. As soon as the healing skin tolerates compression and shear forces, pressure therapy is recommended for 23 hours per day until scar maturation. Continuous pressure on scars can be exerted by means of custom-fitted pressure garments, orthoses or transparent face masks, casts, or splints, measured by trained technicians or therapists. The optimal amount of pressure required remains controversial. Theoretically, pressures that exceed 24 mmHg pressure to overcome capillary pressure are required. However, good clinical results have been reported with levels as low as 5–15 mmHg pressure. Many authors however state or show that 15 mmHg or even higher, 20 mmHg to 30 mmHg, is necessary to accelerate the maturation process and that the effects of pressures below 10 mmHg pressure are minimal [1, 9]. Higher pressure increases the effect, but can also induce complications such as paresthesia, blistering, abnormal bone growth, limb necrosis, etc. The generated pressure plays a crucial role and needs to be monitored regularly (e.g., by using a simple pneumatic pressure sensor, such as for instance the Kikuhime pressure sensor). The Kikuhime pressure sensor has been tested in clinical circumstances and was found to be reliable and valid in the assessment of the efficiency of pressure garment therapy. The pressure of pressure garments needs to be checked every 2–3 months and, if necessary, they need to be replaced or modified to achieve optimal results [1]. Frequent washing and proper hygiene with a minimal use of ointments, lotions, or moisturizers that contain unsaturated lipid acids can help in reducing the aging and wearing of the garments.

There are mainly two different types of pressure garments that are used in the treatment and prevention of hypertrophic burn scars: elastic tricot and powernet structures. The first type of elastic tricot garments are mostly woven knit structures with a biaxial stretch and a multidimensional structure. These elastic tricot garments usually tend to be delivered with less tension (or pressure values on the scar) but maintain the pressure longer than powernet garments. The powernet structure garments have mostly one-axial stretch and a plenary open structure. The second type, the powernet garments are a bit more comfortable pertaining to water vapor permeability in summer or warm climates, but are more fragile due to their open structure. Also therefore elastic tricot garments offer a far better protection against UV rays, a property that cannot be underestimated since pigment changes are one of the most important sequelae after a severe burn injury with a higher risk for UV-induced malignant changes as result. Although the exact value for this protecting factor of the garments (UPF) is not defined, for textiles of common daily worn clothing this factor is set on a value of 50.

Pressure is strongly recommended to decrease scar height and scar erythema [1]. The working mechanism of pressure therapy is not completely understood. First, pressure can control collagen synthesis [9]. The realignment of collagen fibers and the reduction of development of whorled-typed collagen nodules might induce thinning of scars. Secondly, pressure might reduce the vascular flow to scar tissue, which leads to a decrease of nutrient and oxygen supply for cellular activities. It might diminish fibrotic activity (TGF-β reduction), accelerate cell apoptosis of fibroblasts, and reduce scar redness [9]. In addition, application of pressure commonly reduces pain and itching and alleviates edema associated with active hypertrophic scars [4, 9]. Based on the evidence framework of Sharp et al., pressure therapy is strongly recommended and found to be evidence based to decrease scar height and recommended to diminish scar erythema [1].

Silicone gel sheets or gels are also used in the prevention of scars after wound healing of more than 21 days and in the treatment of hypertrophic scars. Silicone gel sheets or gels can be used as soon as wounds are re-epithelialized and until complete maturation of scars [2]. The silicone gel sheets are typically worn 12–16 hours per day. The topical silicone gels are applied twice a day

[2]. Skin reactions such as allergy, dermatitis, itch, or skin breakdown may occur, but fewer when using silicone gels compared to gel sheets. Progressive building-up of wearing the silicone and hygienic precautions of both the product and the skin are important actions to reduce the risks of adverse effects, especially in warm weather or climates. Besides there are no clear benefits to using gels versus gel sheets or non-silicone versus silicone products with respect to the treatment effect [2]; the silicone-containing occlusive sheets have the most substantial amount of publications and references [3].

Silicones are recommended to improve scar erythema, thickness, and pliability [2, 3]. The universally accepted mechanism of action of silicone is hydration and occlusion of the stratum corneum [6, 10, 11]. Based on the guidelines of Meaume et al., silicone is the current gold standard and the first-line, noninvasive option for the prevention and treatment of hypertrophic scars [6].

In daily practice, silicone applications are worn in combination with pressure garments, masks, or splints to achieve the best outcomes. Silicone applications can be prefabricated sheets or individually made by specialized manufacturers as a pressure device or pad to solve concavity problems (chin, breast, clavicle, neck, and face) or in soft tissue parts of the face and neck.

Therapists routinely use *massage* in the treatment of (hypertrophic) scars, which can be applied manually or with the use of a vacuum device. Different manual massage techniques, such as the GAF techniques by Jaudoin D. and the "massage dermo-épidermique" by Godeau J., are described to limit fibrosis of scar tissue and to free adhesions. Depending on scar age and/or inflammatory status of scar tissue, the applied technique can vary between applying a mild pressure combined with a "translation" of the epidermis and a moderate pressure to create a skinfold combined with small rotations in different directions. Also a mechanical suction device can be used for mature scars. This therapy is called "vacuum therapy" or "depressomassage." Using this mechanical massage, a skinfold is created in a treatment head with negative pressure after which the skinfold can be manipulated.

Massage therapy is used in the treatment of hypertrophic scars and skin grafts to improve pliability and to reduce pain and itching [3]. The mechanical disruption of fibrotic scar tissue explains the improvements in pliability. The gate theory of Melzack and Wall support the reduction of pain and pruritus. Following the literature, the applied massage therapies differ in the type of manual techniques and mechanical settings, with or without moisturizer, duration, and frequency. However, to our knowledge, massage therapy is applied daily using progressive techniques to obtain the best outcomes. The manual or mechanical technique depends on the inflammation status of the scar (immature scar versus mature scar).

Moisturizers and lotions are used in the treatment of hypertrophic scars, which are typically dry skin and often itchy. Hypertrophic scars show increased transepidermal water loss compared to healthy skin [12, 13]. Hydration can restore the skin barrier function. Little is known about the ideal composition of moisturizers and frequency of application for burn scar treatment [13], but we believe in an application of a water-based, neutral lotion or cream at least thrice a day.

Positioning and splinting are indicated in each burn rehabilitation phase. In the acute phase, positioning and splints aim to control edema and to bring pressure relief. In the intermediate phase, positioning and splinting are indicated for soft tissue or skin graft protection and tissue elongation, whereof the last indication is also important in the long-term phase. Positioning after a burn injury corresponds with an anti-comfort position. There is no universal position, but burn depth and location must be considered when determining optimal anti-contracture positioning. Positioning may be active, which is ideal for cooperative patients, or passive, which requires the use of splints. Three different types of splints are commonly used, a static, a static progressive, and a dynamic splint. Indication for one or the other type can be to protect a skin graft after surgery, to prevent or to treat contractures, or to improve joint mobility. However there is no consensus on the ideal splint-wearing schedule. The longer a splint is worn, the greater the benefit for tissue lengthening. Some suggest a regime of 2-hours-on, 2-hours-off; others advocate active exercises during the day and splinting only at night. Schedules should be established and adjusted according to the changes in joint mobility and activity level of the patient [14].

Positioning and splinting protocols must be supervised regularly for effectiveness and require cooperation of both the patient and the burn team.

Exercising and mobilizations are important components of the daily treatment of patients after a burn injury. After a severe burn injury, patients have an increased catabolism that leads to loss of lean body mass and causes muscle weakness and decreased functional capacity. The prolonged bed rest and the lack of physical activity have an important impact on recovery after burn injuries in the rehabilitation process. Further, the hypertrophic scar formation leads to scar contractures and decreased range of motion. Therefore, the rehabilitation program starts with passive and active movements, strength training of upper and/or lower limb and progressively includes more challenging exercises such as bed cycling, sit-to-stand-transfers, and walking with or without assistance. Depending on the patient's cooperation, general condition, and cardiovascular and neurological status, mobilizations start already after 24–48 hours after admission to the burn unit or surgical procedure, but always in dialogue with the attending physician.

In the literature, little is known about the best rehabilitation schemes to follow for adult burn patients. However, the aim of exercising is to maintain and restore the physical capacity, muscle strength, and autonomy of patients [15]. Mobilizations are required for realignment and lengthening of scar tissue, preventing joint and ligament stiffening.

Among experts, compression therapy is considered a first-line intervention in the aftercare of patients with severe scars related to burn injury while the use of all the other mentioned techniques are considered to be at least "best practice."

Conclusion

Although strong evidence is lacking for many of the different noninvasive therapeutic approaches that are used in the rehabilitation of patients with severe scars, all the interventions discussed in this chapter, that is, pressure and silicone therapy, massage, hydration, positioning and splinting, exercise, and mobilizations, are recommended and considered useful by the authors in the aftercare of these patients.

Take-Home Messages

- Pressure and silicone therapy have the best evidence in topical scar management.
- Massage is useful to treat pruritus and stiffness of scars.
- Combination strategies are mandatory and need to be individualized to optimize results.
- Hydration of scars is useful, but cost-effectiveness of the product that is used is also important.
- Positioning and splinting protocols must be individualized and supervised regularly for effectiveness.
- Physical activity and exercise are crucial to maintain and restore the physical capacity and muscle strength of burn patients.
- Mobilizations are required for realignment and lengthening of scar tissue as well as preventing joint and ligament stiffening.

References

1. Sharp PA, Pan B, Yakuboff KP, Rothchild D. Development of a best evidence statement for the use of pressure therapy for management of hypertrophic scarring. J Burn Care Res. 2016;37(4):255–64.
2. Nedelec B, Carter A, Forbes L, Hsu SC, McMahon M, Parry I, Ryan CM, Serghiou MA, Schneider JC, Sharp PA, de Oliveira A, Boruff J. Practice guidelines for the application of nonsilicone or silicone gels and gel sheets after burn injury. J Burn Care Res. 2015;36(3):345–74.
3. Anthonissen M, Daly D, Janssens T, Van Den Kerckhove E. The effects of conservative treatments on burn scars: a systematic review. Burns. 2016;42:508–18.
4. Monstrey S, Middelkoop E, Vranckx JJ, Bassetto F, Ziegler UE, Meaume S, Téot L. Updated scar management practical guidelines: non-invasive and invasive measures. J Plast Reconstr Aesthet Surg. 2014;67(8):1017–25.
5. Del Toro D, Dedhia R, Tollefson TT. Advances in scar management. Curr Opin Otolaryngol Head Neck Surg. 2016;24(4): 322–9.
6. Meaume S, Le Pillouer-Prost A, Richert B, Roseeuw D, Vadoud J. Management of scars: updated practical guidelines and use of silicones. Eur J Dermatol. 2014;24(4):435–43.
7. Gold MH, Berman B, Clementoni MT, Gauglitz GG, Nahai F, Murcia C. Updated international clinical recommendations on scar management: part 1 - evaluating the evidence. Dermatol Surg. 2014;40(8):817–24.
8. Gold MH, McGuire M, Mustoe TA, et al. Updated international clinical recommendations on scar management: part 2 – algorithms for scar prevention and treatment. Dermatol Surg. 2014;40(8):825–31.
9. Ai JW, Liu J, Pei SD, Liu Y, Li DS, Lin HM, Pei B. The effectiveness of pressure therapy (15–25 mmHg) for hypertrophic burn scars: a systematic review and meta-analysis. Sci Rep. 2017; 7:40185.
10. Friedstat J, Hultman C. Hypertrophic burn scar management: what does the evidence show? A systematic review of randomized controlled trials. Ann Plast Surg. 2014;72:S198–201.
11. Li-Tsang CW, Lau JCM, Choi J, Chan CC, Jianan L. A prospective randomized clinical trial to investigate the effect of silicone gel sheeting (Cica-Care) on post-traumatic hypertrophic scar among the Chinese population. Burns. 2006;32:678–83.
12. Suetake T, Sasai S, Zhen Y, Tagami H. Effects of silicone gel sheet on the stratum corneum hydration. Br J Plast Surg. 2000;53(6):503–7.
13. Klotz T, Kurmis R, Munn Z, Heath K, Greenwood JE. The effectiveness of moisturizers for the management of burn scars following severe burn injury: a systematic review protocol. JBI Database Syst Rev Implement Rep. 2014;12(11):212–20.
14. Dewey WS, Richard RL, Parry IS. Positioning, splinting, and contracture management. Phys Med Rehabil. 2011;22:229–47.
15. Porter C, Hardee J, Herndon DN, Suman OE. The role of exercise in the rehabilitation of patients with severe burns. Exerc Sport Sci Rev. 2015;43(1):34–40.

10. Scott JR, Muangman P, Gibran NS. Making sense of hypertrophic scar: a role for nerves. Wound Repair Regen. 2007;15(Suppl 1):S27–31.
11. Huang C, Akaishi S, Hyakusoku H, Ogawa R. Are keloid and hypertrophic scar different forms of the same disorder? A fibroproliferative skin disorder hypothesis based on keloid findings. Int Wound J. 2014;11(5):517–22.
12. Ogawa R, Akaishi S, Kuribayashi S, Miyashita T. Keloids and hypertrophic scars can now be cured completely: recent progress in our understanding of the pathogenesis of keloids and hypertrophic scars and the most promising current therapeutic strategy. J Nippon Med Sch. 2016;83(2):46–53.
13. Aarabi S, Bhatt KA, Shi Y, Paterno J, Chang EI, Loh SA, Holmes JW, Longaker MT, Yee H, Gurtner GC. Mechanical load initiates hypertrophic scar formation through decreased cellular apoptosis. FASEB J. 2007;21(12):3250–61.
14. Ogawa R, Okai K, Tokumura F, Mori K, Ohmori Y, Huang C, Hyakusoku H, Akaishi S. The relationship between skin stretching/contraction and pathologic scarring: the important role of mechanical forces in keloid generation. Wound Repair Regen. 2012;20(2):149–57.
15. Akaishi S, Akimoto M, Ogawa R, Hyakusoku H. The relationship between keloid growth pattern and stretching tension: visual analysis using the finite element method. Ann Plast Surg. 2008;60(4):445–51.
16. Arima J, Huang C, Rosner B, Akaishi S, Ogawa R. Hypertension: a systemic key to understanding local keloid severity. Wound Repair Regen. 2015;23(2):213–21.
17. Akaishi S, Akimoto M, Hyakusoku H, Ogawa R. The tensile reduction effects of silicone gel sheeting. Plast Reconstr Surg. 2010;126(2):109e–11e.

10

Scar Symptom: Erythema and Thickness

Yating Yang, Xiaoli Wu, and Wei Liu

Contents

Definition

Erythema is derived from the Greek *erythros*, which refers to the redness of skin or mucous membrane. Erythema is common in pathological scars (hypertrophic scar and keloid) and premature physiological scars where inflammation-induced angiogenesis and capillary dilation are mostly responsible. Different from the temporary and self-relieving redness in normal skin caused by allergy or mechanical friction (such as massage), the existence and severity of erythema in scar tissues are consistent with their maturity and inflammation state inside, serving as a convenient monitor of scar quality and treatment response. Scar thickness indirectly reflects the extent of scar development by collagen deposition.

Mechanisms of Erythema in Scar

In general, the common causes of erythema can be roughly categorized into four groups: inflammation, mechanical stimulation (massage, waxing, and tweezing of hairs), radiation (sunburn, radiotherapy), allergies and other chemical agents. Despite the pervasive nature of erythema in both physiological and pathological scars, the development mechanisms remain to be relatively less explored and therefore limited effective treatment options are available. However, previous studies demonstrated that inflammation, vascularization, and sometimes epidermis defect are the three major mechanisms that contribute to the erythema in scars.

Inflammation-Induced Capillary Perfusion Is Crucial for Erythema Initiation

Accumulated studies have confirmed that the inflammation induced by various reasons (infection, foreign body, immune dysfunction, etc.) is greatly associated with the formation of scars, especially hypertrophic scars and keloids [1]. Stimulated by inflammatory cytokines, capillaries constrict to increase the local blood flow and vessel permeability, resulting in erythema and sometimes elevated skin temperature [2]. It was shown that significant increase of blood flow values was detected in erythematous scars when compared to healthy skin [3, 4]. Besides, erythema (measured by colorimetry) is often interpreted as an indirect measurement of the blood flow in clinical practice as it indicates the hyperemia in superficial capillaries. Bae-Harboe *et al.* first introduced the term "postinflammatory erythema" (PIE) in 2013 to describe erythema often seen after the resolution of inflammatory acne or other inflammatory skin conditions [5]. To be specific, the symptom of erythema persists all along the inflammatory stage of wound healing and plays multiple roles in this process.

Vascularization Dynamically Participates in the Erythema Development

The chronic inflammatory stimulation and hyperproliferation of scar tissues deteriorate the local hypoxia and promote the secretion of angiogenic factors, such as vascular endothelial growth factor (VEGF), basic fibroblast growth factor (BFGF), and hypoxia-induced factor 1 (HIF-1) [2, 6]. As reported by Amadeu *et al.*, hypertrophic scars contain an increased number of dilated vessels in papillary and reticular dermis compared to normal skin [7]. The increased capillary density and dilated vessel diameter then contribute to the formation of erythema, in line with the study of Fullerton, who stated that erythema is determined by the blood volume under a given area, and not by the product of erythrocyte velocity and concentration [8]. Clinically, erythema disappears on finger pressure (blanching), which also suggests that the vascular remodeling is involved.

Scar erythema, blood flow, microvessels, and redness are four features of scar that are often interchangeably used under the item "vascularization" or "vascularity." However, by directly measuring erythema with colorimetry, blood flow with laser Doppler imaging (LDI), vessels with immunohistochemistry, and subjective scale of redness with POSAS, respectively, Jaspers *et al.* found only significant relevance between erythema and subjective redness, but no correlations between the others. In contrast, Mermans *et al.* found that erythema was associated with blood flow, but this correlation was not consistent at different test moments [9]. Moreover, Kischer *et al.* reported that most microvessels were occluded in hypertrophic scars due to an excessive number of endothelial cells [10, 11]. And the higher hematocrit and the enlarged vessels would then result in a more sluggish blood velocity and lower blood flow values. Taken together, it is now understood that the term "vascularity" describes a dynamic process, and the four criteria mentioned above can attribute to the redness either independently or interact with each other at different stages of scar development. These exploration studies express well the complexity of erythema formation and enlighten us to view this process dynamically instead of simply putting them under the umbrella of "vascularization," especially in clinical practice.

Thinner Epidermis Is Directly Responsible for the Transparency in Erythematous Scars with Skin Barrier Defect

The epidermal thickness and collagen synthesis are directly associated with the transparency of skin. Oliveira *et al.* and Busch *et al.* identified a thinned-out skin texture in burn scar that makes the intense circulation of blood becoming more apparent [3, 12]. They argued that increased skin redness is not only considered as an inflammatory symptom but also the structural modification of subdermal components. And the induction of percutaneous collagen (IPC) and angiogenesis therapies (medical needling and fractional laser) has been proven to be effective to adjust the skin color after repetitive treatments [12].

Different from the thinner epidermis in physiological scars resulting from normal wound-healing process, keloids and hypertrophic scars are characterized by extra collagen deposition and increased epidermal thickness [13]. But recent studies also hypothesized a skin barrier defect in keloid scars, which may possibly alter the opacity of epidermis [14].

Contributions of Erythema to Scar Development and Associated Clinical Symptoms

The wound-healing process contains three chronological but partially overlapped phases: inflammatory stage (day 1–6), proliferation stage (day 4–week 3), and remodeling stage (week 3–1 year). Parallel with this process, Van Der Wal *et al.* reported that the erythema index scores of scars reduce significantly within 12 months [15] as a result of the common pathological mechanisms they shared. To be specific, the alleviation and deterioration of erythema are closely associated with the scar development since they indirectly reflect the inflammatory state and angiogenic activity beneath the skin. And since the redness of erythema (from pink to scarlet to purple) is the result of different proportion of hemoglobin (the red oxygenated state, absorbed at 660 nm) and deoxyhemoglobin (dark red, absorbed at 940 nm) in the capillaries of the dermis, the color of scarred skin can serve as a monitor of local hypoxia, angiogenesis, and microcirculation.

Although the most commonly used principles for measuring scar color are narrow-band reflectance spectrophotometry and tristimulus reflectance colorimetry [4], researchers found statistically significant correlation between erythema values (colorimetry) and subjective redness assessment (Patient and Observer Scar Assessment Scale, POSAS) (r = 0.403, p = 0.030) [4], proving the reliability of subjective erythema measurement in clinical practice.

Similarly, erythematous scars are more likely to suffer from pain or pruritus as a result of inflammatory stimulation and suspicious vulnerability of scar fibroblasts (previous studies detected an elevation of α-adrenoreceptors expression on keloid fibroblasts and predicted that it might be related to paresthesia in scar tissues [16]).

Elevated temperature is directly associated with overperfusion of vessels especially arteries in deeper layer of the skin [4] and is not common in thickened scar tissues, but the existence of which could be explained as a sign of infection or active inflammatory state.

Generally, erythema reflects the inflammation and angiogenesis activity, as well as structural remodeling of scar tissues to serve as a monitor of scar maturation and quality. Since patients and clinicians often determine the success of treatment by the visual appearance of a scar, erythema measured by POSAS could be an accessible method to evaluate the treatment response and help to set the endpoint for the course.

Scar Erythema and Scar Thickness

There is no direct relation between scar erythema and scar thickness, because the former reflects the level of inflammation and angiogenesis process, whereas the latter indicates the extent of cell proliferation and extracellular matrix production and deposition. Such phenomenon has been frequently observed in clinical practice that a highly inflamed scar with sever erythema might be thin and soft in texture, whereas a dark-colored keloid could be thick and abundant with collagen. However, enhanced erythema by strong angiogenesis provides nutrition for fibroblast proliferation and matrix production, and therefore reducing erythema also helps to prevent scar thickening.

Clinical Measurement of Scar Redness and Thickness

Colorimetric plate along with photography is the conventional methodology to semi-objectively measure the redness of scars. Doppler ultrasound can detect blood flow inside a scar, but it reflects activity in a relatively deep blood vessel. For superficial blood flow inside the surface capillaries, laser speckle might be the technique to quantitatively measure the erythema change.

Manual measurement is the conventional way to assess scar thickness. With advances in technology, ultrasound and nuclear magnetic resonance can quantitatively provide data of scar thickness. In addition, 3D scanner not only provides the gross view of a thick scar, but also provides quantitative data of scar thickness and volume.

Clinical Relevance

Clinical Treatment Strategies of Erythema in Scars

Traditional clinical treatments of erythema in scar tissues mainly target on anti-inflammation and anti-proliferation, such as topical glucocorticoid and compression garments. The spreading applications of laser treatments and medical needling provide therapists with powerful arms that can interfere with erythema formation from various perspectives. Besides, systematic elements including imbalanced diets, stressful lifestyles, and even genetic predisposition may also be responsible.

Anti-inflammation Strategies to Alleviate Erythema and Hinder Scars Development

Inflammation is one of the major risk factors of both scar development and erythema. Since corticoid can effectively reduce the production of pro-inflammatory mediators and inhibit inflammatory processes in the dermis, the intralesional triamcinolone acetonide (TCA) injection has been widely used alone or as an adjuvant therapy to treat hypertrophic scars and keloids [17]. Besides, although the application of triamcinolone tapes is limited by its penetrating ability, it can be stuck to the scar area and release the drug all day long. Moreover, clinical studies observed a better performance of triamcinolone when combined with 5-Fluorouracil [17]. Other topical anti-inflammation treatment such as silicone gel sheeting that increases the elasticity of burn scar tissue also showed a reduction in pruritus, erythema, and scar thickness [18]. Systematic glucocorticoid application is not recommended for risks of complications such as diabetes, infections, and Cushing's syndrome.

Laser Treatments to Interfere with Erythema from Multiple Perspective

Laser therapy is one of the most widely used methods to treat erythema in scars. Ablative fractional lasers that create columns of vaporized tissue with surrounding eschar and coagulated tissue can improve various features of burn scars including erythema. Kawecki *et al.* observed that 31% of hypertrophic burn scar patients had resolution of erythema with resulting normal skin tone after ablative fractional laser treatment [19]. Coagulating microvessels with the selective photothermolysis of wavelengths around 595 nm, pulsed dye laser (PDL) can decrease inflammation and edema in erythematous scars and shows satisfactory outcomes in color repair. Similarly, Q-switched Nd:YAG lasers with a wavelength of 1064 nm in very short pulses are promising solutions to superficial angiogenesis of erythematous skin, especially in decreasing the vascular prominence in PIE [17, 18, 20]. Studies have demonstrated minimal side effects including atrophic scarring (0.8%), hyperpigmentation (1%), hypopigmentation (2.6%), and dermatitis (2%), among 500 patients treated with PDL [21]. Notably, although PDL and Nd:YAG have shown good results in reducing the red color of scars, skin erythema itself is one common adverse effect of laser treatment, which suggests that the laser therapy should be carefully selected and be practiced with cautions especially in patients with a history of post-treatment erythema or scar constitution.

Compression Therapy

Compression therapy (or occlusive dressings) has been widely applied to hypertrophic scar patients as a first-line agent with good results in decreasing erythema, thickness, and hardness of burn scars [22, 23]. A total of 60% of patients treated with compression devices showed 75–100% enhancement in scar condition according to previous studies [17]. The anti-scar effects of occlusive garments are thought to be related to occlusion and hydration [7, 17]. Some literature reported that this change is likely because of the inhibition of transforming growth factor (TGF)-β1 release and ultimately decreased fibroblast activity [24].

Medical Needling

Although sounding contradictory, the bleeding process of medical needling can influence vascularization by stimulating angiogenesis in the post-wound healing cascade and improve the vital thickness of the epidermis (directly related to skin transparency) by inducing percutaneous collagen synthesis.

Based on the outcomes of objective measurements, medical needling achieves a normalization of the skin color and an adjustment to healthy skin after repetitive treatments [12], and it has clinically shown to improve the abnormal vascular proliferation that occurs in PIE. Similarly, fractional resurfacing lasers have been used to induce structural remodeling and skin regeneration.

Clinical Treatment for Thick Scar

Contracture and functional disability caused by hypertrophic scars need surgical interventions. As for thick keloids, surgical therapy is also preferred. In addition, intralesional injection with 5-fluorouracil and steroid, cryotherapy, pressure therapy, and radiotherapy are all potential therapeutic options for thick scars, and these will be introduced in various chapters of this book and thus will not be the focus of this chapter.

Conclusion

The scar erythema is a burden for patients, as it amplifies the cosmetic problems and is associated with other unpleasant feelings such as pain and itching. Moreover, the development of erythema parallels with the dynamic process of inflammation, angiogenesis, scar formation, and thickening. Although most studies consider erythema as a concomitant byproduct following wound healing, it also promotes scar development via enhancing angiogenesis to provide scar fibroblasts essential nutrition for collagen production and deposition, and thus it has become an important therapeutic target as well. Although many issues remain to be explored such as what determines erythema presence, persistence, and disappearance, the erythema/redness itself can serve as a visible symptom reflecting treatment response and thus help both patients and therapists to set a relevant endpoint.

Take-Home Messages

Both erythema and thickness are key characteristics of scar, which can be used to monitor scar development and therapy efficacy. Angiogenesis represented by scar redness is a key contributor to pathological scar development due to enhanced inflammation, which can also serve as an important therapeutic target.

References

1. Ogawa R. Keloid and hypertrophic scars are the result of chronic inflammation in the reticular dermis. Int J Mol Sci. 2017;18:606.
2. Colgan SP, Campbell EL, Kominsky DJ. Hypoxia and mucosal inflammation. Annu Rev Pathol. 2016;11:77–100.
3. Oliveira GV, Chinkes D, Mitchell C, Oliveras G, Hawkins HK, Herndon DN. Objective assessment of burn scar vascularity, erythema, pliability, thickness, and planimetry. Dermatol Surg. 2005;31:48–58.
4. Jaspers M, Stekelenburg CM, Simons JM, Brouwer KM, Vlig M, van den Kerckhove E, van Zuijlen P. Assessing blood flow, microvasculature, erythema and redness in hypertrophic scars: a cross sectional study showing different features that require precise definitions. Burns. 2017;43:1044–50.
5. Bae-Harboe YS, Graber EM. Easy as pie (postinflammatory erythema). J Clin Aesthet Dermatol. 2013;6:46–7.
6. Sorg H, Tilkorn DJ, Hager S, Hauser J, Mirastschijski U. Skin wound healing: an update on the current knowledge and concepts. Eur Surg Res. 2017;58:81–94.
7. Amadeu T, Braune A, Mandarim-de-Lacerda C, Porto LC, Desmouliere A, Costa A. Vascularization pattern in hypertrophic scars and keloids: a stereological analysis. Pathol Res Pract. 2003;199:469–73.
8. Fullerton A, Fischer T, Lahti A, Wilhelm KP, Takiwaki H, Serup J. Guidelines for measurement of skin colour and erythema. A report from the standardization group of the european society of contact dermatitis. Contact Dermatitis. 1996;35: 1–10.
9. Mermans JF, Peeters WJ, Dikmans R, Serroyen J, van der Hulst RR, Van den Kerckhove E. A comparative study of colour and perfusion between two different post surgical scars. Do the laser doppler imager and the colorimeter measure the same features of a scar? Skin Res Technol. 2013;19:107–14.
10. Kischer CW, Thies AC, Chvapil M. Perivascular myofibroblasts and microvascular occlusion in hypertrophic scars and keloids. Hum Pathol. 1982;13:819–24.
11. Kischer CW, Shetlar MR. Microvasculature in hypertrophic scars and the effects of pressure. J Trauma. 1979;19:757–64.
12. Busch KH, Aliu A, Walezko N, Aust M. Medical needling: effect on skin erythema of hypertrophic burn scars. Cureus. 2018;10:e3260.
13. Limandjaja GC, van den Broek LJ, Waaijman T, van Veen HA, Everts V, Monstrey S, Scheper RJ, Niessen FB, Gibbs S. Increased epidermal thickness and abnormal epidermal differentiation in keloid scars. Br J Dermatol. 2017;176:116–26.
14. Limandjaja GC, Belien JM, Scheper RJ, Niessen FB, Gibbs S. Hypertrophic and keloid scars fail to progress from the cd34(−) /alpha-smooth muscle actin (alpha-sma)(+) immature scar phenotype and show gradient differences in alpha-sma and p16 expression. Br J Dermatol. 2020;82(4):974–86. https://doi.org/10.1111/bjd.18219.
15. van der Wal MB, Vloemans JF, Tuinebreijer WE, van de Ven P, van Unen E, van Zuijlen PP, Middelkoop E. Outcome after burns: an observational study on burn scar maturation and predictors for severe scarring. Wound Repair Regen. 2012;20:676–87.
16. Drummond PD, Drummond ES, Dawson LF, Mitchell V, Finch PM, Vaughan CW, Phillips JK. Upregulation of alpha1-adrenoceptors on cutaneous nerve fibres after partial sciatic nerve ligation and in complex regional pain syndrome type ii. Pain. 2014;155:606–16.
17. Berman B, Maderal A, Raphael B. Keloids and hypertrophic scars: pathophysiology, classification, and treatment. Dermatol Surg. 2017;43(Suppl 1):S3–S18.
18. Sadick NS, Cardona A. Laser treatment for facial acne scars: a review. J Cosmet Laser Ther. 2018;20:424–35.
19. Kawecki M, Bernad-Wisniewska T, Sakiel S, Nowak MAndriessen A. Laser in the treatment of hypertrophic burn scars. Int Wound J. 2008;5:87–97.
20. Anderson RR, Farinelli W, Laubach H, Manstein D, Yaroslavsky AN, Gubeli J 3rd, Dylla HF. Selective photothermolysis of lipid-rich tissues: a free electron laser study. Lasers Surg Med. 2006;38:913–9.
21. Levine VJ, Geronemus RG. Adverse effects associated with the 577- and 585-nanometer pulsed dye laser in the treatment of cutaneous vascular lesions: a study of 500 patients. J Am Acad Dermatol. 1995;32:613–7.

22. Friedstat JS, Hultman CS. Hypertrophic burn scar management: what does the evidence show? A systematic review of randomized controlled trials. Ann Plast Surg. 2014;72:S198–201.
23. Anthonissen M, Daly D, Janssens T, Van den Kerckhove E. The effects of conservative treatments on burn scars: a systematic review. Burns. 2016;42:508–18.
24. Atiyeh BS, El Khatib A, MDibo SA. Pressure garment therapy (pgt) of burn scars: evidence-based efficacy. Ann Burns Fire Disasters. 2013;26:205–12.

11

Scar Symptoms: Pigmentation Disorders

A. Pijpe, K. L. M. Gardien, R. E. van Meijeren-Hoogendoorn, E. Middelkoop, and Paul P. M. van Zuijlen

Contents

Background
To a significant degree, vascularization and pigmentation determine the color of scars. Pigmentation problems are often even more persistent than deviations in vascularization. Pigmentation problems are a common consequence after partial and full-thickness burns, skin pathology such as vitiligo, other skin trauma, and surgical procedures. Almost all these patients experience at least some pigmentation problems. Both hypopigmentation and hyperpigmentation can cause esthetic and psychological issues which affect the quality of life of patients. Information on the role and pathways of melanocytes in pigmentation problems and the changes that occur during scar maturation is increasingly more understood. Different subjective and objective methods are available to determine scar color. Hypo- and hyperpigmentation management options include surgical and nonsurgical techniques.

Pathophysiology and Epidemiology

Altered skin pigmentation, or pigmentation disorders, can result from increased or decreased melanin, abnormal melanin distribution, decreased hemoglobin, or deposition of exogenous substances. Melanin is produced by melanocytes, specialized cells of neural crest origin that reside in the basal layer of the epidermis. The biosynthesis of melanin occurs in lysosome-like organelles called melanosomes, which are transported to the cell periphery and transferred from the dendritic tips of the melanocytes to the surrounding keratinocytes. Each melanocyte is associated with approximately 36 basal keratinocytes to form the so-called "epidermal melanin unit."

Hypopigmentation

Hypopigmentation is characterized by skin becoming lighter than the individuals own color, but not completely lacking pigment (◘ Fig. 12.1). This should not be confused with depigmentation, which is the absence of all pigment. Hypopigmentation is common and approximately 1 in 20 have at least one hypopigmented macule [1]. Common causes include vitiligo, postinflammatory hypopigmentation, pityriasis versicolor, pityriasis alba, and halo naevi. Hypopigmentation disorders may be congenital or acquired. Acquired hypopigmentation may be the result of inflammatory conditions or trauma like a burn injury. In burn scars, hypopigmentation is a frequent pathology. Although the condition often improves over time with scar maturation, lasting depigmented or hypopigmented lesions may remain.

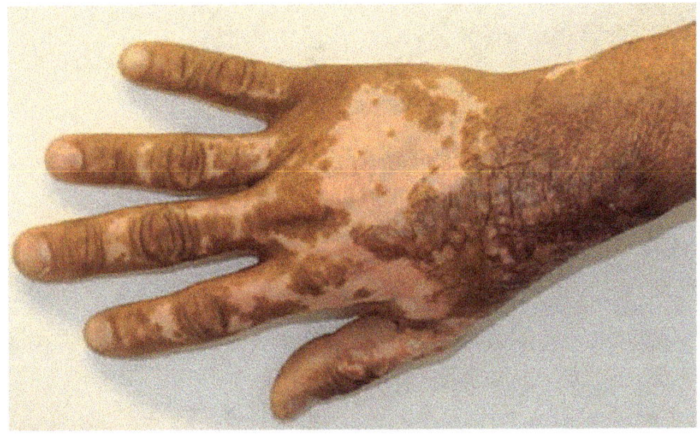

◘ **Fig.** Hypopigmentation in a hand after burn injury

Data on the prevalence of these conditions after burn injury are scarce.

Vitiligo is an autoimmune disease where melanocytes are affected. The condition affects approximately 0.5–1% of the population, occurs in patients of all ages, equally affects men and women, with an early onset in many cases (<20 years). There is no difference in prevalence with respect to skin type or race.

Hyperpigmentation

Hyperpigmentation is the darkening or increase in the natural color of the skin and results from overproduction or abnormal release of melanin in the epidermis and/or dermis in response to either endogenous or exogenous inflammatory conditions [2]. Superficial hyperpigmentation is located in the epidermis and causes a light- to dark-brown discoloration. As soon as the pigment lies deeper in the skin (dermal pigmentation), the hyperpigmentation acquires a gray-brown to gray-blue glow. Like hypopigmentation, hyperpigmentation disorders may be congenital or acquired.

Postinflammatory hyperpigmentation is a reactive hypermelanosis of the skin that occurs as a sequela of cutaneous inflammation. Common causes of include acne vulgaris, eczematous dermatoses, and burn injury. Postinflammatory hyperpigmentation may also occur as a complication of a chemical peeling.

Although this pigmentary change can be observed in all skin types, it more frequently affects individuals with higher degrees of skin pigmentation (meaning Fitzpatrick skin types IV–VI) due to increased reactivity of melanocytes within the skin. The modified Fitzpatrick skin type classification system contains six categories with types I–IV describing different types of white skin and type V "brown" and type VI "black" skin.

Severe burns significantly affect the process of pigmentation as it is tightly regulated by cell proliferation

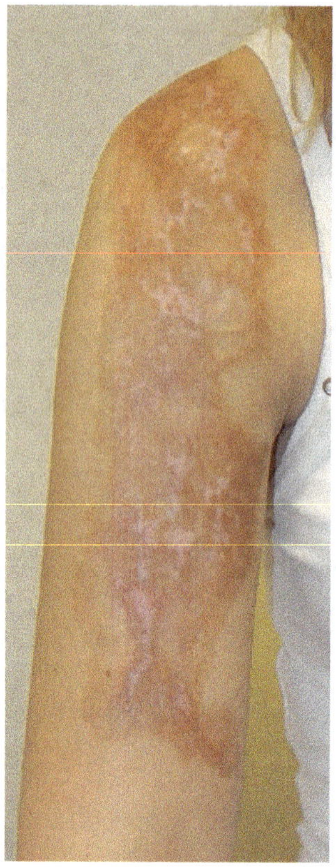

■ **Fig.** Burn scar with hyperpigmented and hypopigmented areas

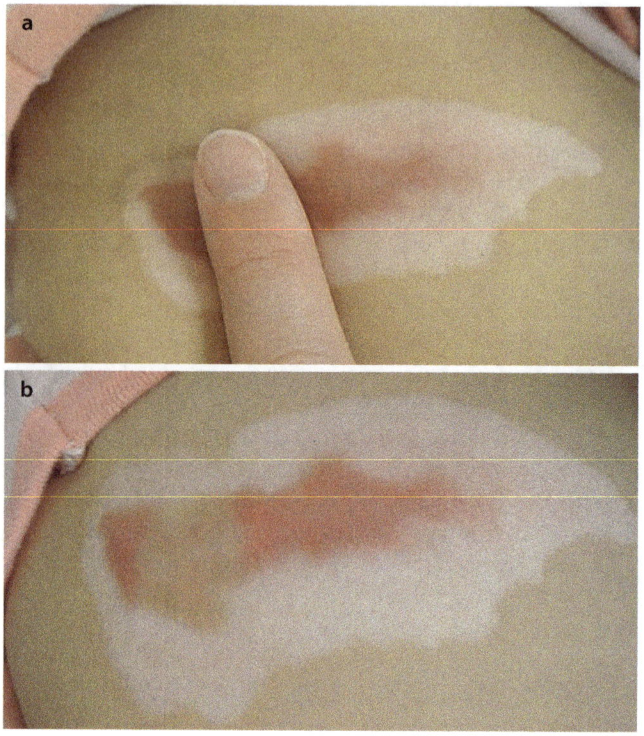

■ **Fig.** (**a**) Pressure on the scar with a finger reduces blood flow in the scar. (**b**) Immediately after release of the pressure, level of pigmentation of the scar is visible

and differentiation of melanocytes and melanocyte stem cells which are located in the epidermis and hair follicles of the skin. Almost all burn patients with deep partial-thickness wounds and full-thickness wounds experience at least some pigmentation problems (■ Fig. 12.2). Superficial burn wounds generally heal without pigmentation problems. Although scar-related hypo- and hyperpigmentation are not harmful, it can cause significant cosmetic problems and become a great psychological burden for patients which influences their quality of life.

Maturation

Maturation is the fourth and final stage of the wound healing process and is commonly referred to as remodeling. The cellular changes that occur during scar maturation are increasingly understood. They are associated with remodeling of the extracellular matrix as well as normalization of the ratio of type III to type I collagen. However, the process of scar maturation with regard to changes in clinical appearance over time is the least understood part of wound healing. Most studies suggest a mean maturation period of 1, 2, or several years. In this active stage it can be difficult to determine to what extent deviant skin color is caused by vascularization and/or pigmentation. By pressing the scar with a finger or transparent ruler like made from plexiglass, the blood flow is reduced and degree of pigmentation can be better established (■ Fig. 12.3).

Van der Wal et al. performed the first longitudinal study on the maturation pattern of individual scar characteristics and predictors of severe scarring in a representative burn population [3]. They conducted a detailed analysis on the clinical changes of burn scars in 474 patients following a longitudinal scar assessment protocol. The observations of the POSAS Observer Scale (see ► Sect. 2.2) showed that all scar parameters, except vascularization, become more apparent in the first 6 months after the injury. After 12 months, mean POSAS scores were significantly lower for vascularization, pigmentation, and pliability compared with the 6-month follow-up. Statistical significant improvement at 12 months was also found for the parameters vascularization and pigmentation compared with the 3-month evaluation.

Measurement Techniques

For the diagnosis, evaluation of progress of disease and/or therapy it is of major importance to be able to measure skin or scar color in a noninvasive, valid, and reliable way. Outcome measures receive more and more attention to evaluate therapies on an individual basis as well as at group level for efficacy studies. For this, validated techniques are a prerequisite.

To determine scar color, different subjective and objective methods are developed and available.

Objective Measurement Instruments

Several instruments are available to measure skin or scar color. The output is generally a combination of redness (erythema) and melanin (pigment). Most instruments use either narrow band spectrophotometry or reflectance colorimetry. The tristimulus reflectance colorimetry measures color through three broad wavelengths filters representing brightness, redness, and pigmentation. This system is suitable to measure any kind of color in the standard color space defined by Commission Internationale de l'Eclairage (CIE), where the output in L∗a∗b coordinates is defined as CIELAB color space values [4]. The LAB values express color as three values: L∗ for the lightness (black to white), a∗ from green to red, and b∗ from blue to yellow.

Narrow-band reflectance spectrophotometers measure erythema and melanin index, representing vascularization and pigmentation, based on differences in light absorption by hemoglobin and melanocytes, respectively, in selected bands of the light spectrum corresponding to hemoglobin and melanin absorption spectra.

Van der Wal et al. performed a study where the reliability, validity, and feasibility of narrow-band reflectance spectrophotometry and tristimulus reflectance colorimetry on normal skin and scar tissue were studied [5]. All three devices included in this study, Mexameter (narrow band spectrophotometer) and Colorimeter (tristimulus reflectance) (both from Courage & Khazaka Electronic GmbH, Cologne, Germany) and DSM II ColorMeter (narrow band spectrophotometer) (Cortex Technology, Hadsund, Denmark), obtained reliable results after a single measurement, performed by one observer.

Some aspects of these measurements need to be considered when using skin color data for therapeutic evaluation: Skin color is generally adapted to seasonal differences and is likely to be different on various anatomical regions of the body. Therefore, measurements of skin or scar lesions on specific locations need to be compared to the relevant normal skin of a nearby or contralateral comparative anatomical region. For narrow band spectrophotometric measurements, this needs to be performed by subtraction of the data of the normal skin from the lesional data. Furthermore, for the narrow band spectrophotometers, some caution is needed in interpretation of the data from highly pigmented skin: There is some influence on the erythema index by the melanin index, in that the erythema index apparently increases with increasing melanin index. Also, the melanin index is influenced by the oxygen saturation level of hemoglobin, since reduced hemoglobin absorbs more red light than oxyhemoglobin. For example, lowering the arm of a subject to be measured will lower the oxygenation, and give an increase in both erythema and melanin indices. Therefore, a standardized position for the measurements is recommended.

Scar Assessment Scales

Today, many scales exist to evaluate skin and scar characteristics [6]. One of the earliest and frequently reported is the Vancouver Scar Scale (VSS) [7]. Despite the fact that it is frequently used as a scale, especially the items "erythema" and "pigmentation" are nominal categories rather than ordinal ones. For the item "pigmentation" categories are normal, hypo, mixed, or hyper pigmentation; and for the item 'erythema' they are normal, pink, red, and purple. The VSS gives no intensity value of these parameters and therefore the numbers that are often attributed to these categories cannot be added to give a "severity score" for total scar characteristics. This is specifically important for pigmentation problems, since "hypopigmentation" cannot generally be considered to be less severe than "hyperpigmentation," which would be a consequence if the VSS categories would be used as a true scale.

To overcome these difficulties, the Patient and Observer Scar Assessment Scale (POSAS) was designed and validated [8]. The POSAS questionnaire represent the severity of burn scar quality including parameters that indicate skin color and pigmentation on a numerical 10-point rating scale. Furthermore, the categories "pale, pink, red, purple, mix" and "hypo, hyper, mix" are added for each assessment. Within these categories, the numerical data can be added to present an overall scar severity score.

Therapies

Hypopigmentation

Nonsurgical Techniques

Laser Therapy

Laser therapy can be used to treat pigment disorders in a scar. If there is hypopigmentation of a scar, it can be treated with the Excimer laser (308 nm) [9]. This laser produces a stimulation of melanocytes, thereby correcting hypopigmentation in the scar tissue.

Other pigment lasers mainly focus on the presence of hyperpigmentation and induce pigment reduction.

Dermatography

Dermatography, also known as medical tattooing, is an alternative method to improve the scar color, particularly in hypopigmented areas. Chemical-based pigments are injected into the dermis, as with other sorts of tattooing. Dermatography can be repeated if the color fades over time.

Camouflage Therapy

Camouflage therapy offers a temporary solution to hide a (hypopigmented) scar or make it less visible. Often a cream, spray, or powder that is close to the original skin color is used. Once the correct color has been determined, the application can be used independently in the home situation.

Surgical Techniques

Dermabrasion

Dermabrasion can help to treat the hypopigmentation of a scar.

By abrasion, the epidermis and a very small layer of the dermis are removed layer by layer, resulting in a superficial wound.

Normally, the abrasia is done until the whitish dermal layer is exposed with no more than fractional bleeding present.

Dermabrasion is performed as a single treatment modality or in combination with other treatments such as skin transplantation or cell spray. If it is used as a single treatment modality, the superficial wound has to recover by itself. In those cases abrasia must be carried out carefully to prevent wound-healing problems if the wound becomes too deep. This method is mainly used in case of hyperpigmentation where the excess pigment is shaved off and the new epidermis hopefully has a more balanced pigment and therefore color (see below).

In hypopigmentation the dermabrasion is mostly combined with a method to transplant melanocytes from healthy skin to the depigmented regions like skin grafting or cell therapy.

Skin Grafting

Skin-grafting techniques include split-thickness skin grafts, full-thickness skin grafts, punch-grafting, and epidermal grafts, such as grafts from suction blisters.

The split skin graft (SSG) contains the entire epidermis with only a thin layer of dermis. The skin is harvested with a dermatome preferably from a suitable, color-matching concealed donor site. A pigmented donor area with a thickness of 0.15 mm is identified to achieve optimal outcomes as the basal layer of the epidermis and a complement of melanocytes remain intact.

The full-thickness graft provides better functional and cosmetic outcomes in terms of scarring compared to the SSG. The entire epidermis and dermis are transplanted. For correction of pigment disorders, this is only indicated if the general quality of the scar is unacceptable/problematic and the scar area is limited.

In skin grafting, selecting a donor site of healthy skin with suitable normal pigmentation is key to ensure optimal outcomes.

Small full-thickness punch biopsies are harvested from healthy skin from a concealed body part, normally the upper arm or upper leg. The size of the biopsies can be 1–4 mm in diameter. Repigmentation occurs in 70% of the cases. Melanocytes migrate from the punch biopsies into the adjacent area in a centrifugal manner. A disadvantage of punch grafting is the cobblestone appearance that may remain in the long term.

Grafting of suction blisters is an interesting and successful technique for the treatment of hypopigmentation disorders. Negative pressure is exerted on healthy skin of the patient to create epidermal blisters. Devices such as a suction pump, vacuum bottle, hoses, or suction cups can be used for harvesting. This blister is harvested subsequently and transplanted to the depigmented area.

The donor site generally heals spontaneously with no or minimal scarring. Minor adverse effects such as donor site hyperpigmentation and color mismatching may be encountered.

Cell Therapy

An autologous epidermal cell suspension spray can be used to enhance repigmentation. The suspension can be sprayed on top of the wound after dermabrasion or injected in the hypopigmented area. This was studied by Falabella et al. already in 1971 and measured both by clinical score and by melanocyte counts, but the difference between the groups was not statistically significant in either case [10].

Later the RECELL® Autologous Cell Harvesting Device (AVITA Medical Europe Ltd., Melbourne, UK) became available, which uses an on-site device to isolate epidermal cells from a small piece of split skin graft.

Similar to the treatment of vitiligo, melanocytes are directly isolated and harvested from skin grafts prior to transplantation to the depigmented injured area. These cell-based treatments can be divided into (i) non-cultured cell suspension, (ii) cultured melanocyte suspension, (iii) cultured keratinocyte/melanocyte suspension, (iv) tissue-engineered melanocyte grafts. For current clinical practice mainly the non-cultured cell suspension is used. The other, more sophisticated options may be interesting but are rarely used as clinical therapy so far. These therapies are expensive and laborious and currently it has not been conclusively demonstrated that they are cost effective.

A limitation of cell transplantation is a potentially uneven cell dispersion across the recipient site. Furthermore, poor attachment of transplanted melanocytes to the recipient skin and unfavorable wound conditions may also affect cell survival and outcome.

Microneedling

Microneedling is a relatively new therapeutic modality in dermatology. It has shown promising results as an adjuvant therapy for enhanced drug delivery in the treatment of atrophic scars, alopecia, actinic keratoses, and disorders of pigmentation such as melisma [11]. The efficacy in treatment of vitiligo remains limited.

Excision

Excision of the hypopigmented area can be performed and needs to be combined with a technique for wound closure. For small areas direct wound closure is the first choice. For larger areas and in the case of considerable tension on the wound edges, additional closing techniques such as the skin stretching technique or tissue expansion can be performed.

The skin stretch technique is suitable for closing defects after excision of scars and wounds of limited size. The skin stretcher is a device that can stretch two widely spaced wound edges together. The force with which this goes can be set, but is usually in the order of 30 Newton. The best result is obtained when working in cycles of 4 minutes of stretch and 1 minute of rest. After a few cycles, the wound tension has dropped and the wound can be closed under acceptable tension. In a large study, the number of wound dehiscence was limited [12].

With the help of a tissue expander large areas of scar can be normally excised. The tissue expander technique is widespread and is frequently used for reconstruction of large scar areas such as alopecia areas of the hairy head. During the first operation, an expander is placed under flexible skin in the area of the scar area that needs to be reconstructed. This extension is a special balloon with a filling port. The filling port is also placed under the skin. The fill port can be triggered through the skin so the balloon can be filled in tempi until sufficient texture has been expanded for the scar reconstruction. However, despite good results, two interventions are needed, the total procedure may take several weeks to months with frequent visits to the clinic to fill the balloon.

Hyperpigmentation

Nonsurgical Treatment

Topical Treatments

Hydroquinone, either as monotherapy or in combination with alpha-hydroxy acid, ascorbic acid, retinoids, corticosteroids, and antioxidants, is a commonly used depigmenting agent [2]. Its working mechanism is thought to inhibit melanogenesis by acting as an alternative substrate for the enzyme tyrosinase. Hydroquinone may also result in inhibition of DNA/RNA synthesis, destruction of melanocytes, and degradation of melanosomes.

Topical retinoids, including tretinoin (all-trans-retinoic acid), tazarotene, and adapalene, are also used as monotherapy for treatment of hyperpigmented lesions. Retinoids are supposed to act by inhibition of tyrosinase, induction of melanocyte apoptosis, and acceleration of epidermal cell turnover.

Also azelaic acid is thought to inhibit tyrosinase and decrease melanogenesis.

Chemical Peels

A commonly used acid against hyperpigmentation is the use of lactic acid. Lactic acid is particularly known to prevent the formation of tyrosinase so that pigment cells can form less pigment. In addition, the accelerated exfoliation of the skin cells fades the pigment cells present. The mechanism of this effect might be due to epidermal remodeling and accelerated desquamation, which would result in quick pigment dispersion.

Laser Therapy

Hyperpigmentation can be treated with laser therapy, based on selective photothermolysis. Selecting the right wavelength can tackle pigment selectively. Selective photothermolysis suggests that laser therapy would allow discriminating destruction of pigment without injuring the surrounding tissue. Selective melanin photothermolysis can be obtained with any laser light having a wavelength in the absorption spectrum of melanin and sufficient energy levels to target melanosomes (mostly used: the Q-switched ruby laser (694 nm), Q-switched Nd:YAG laser (532 nm, 1064 nm), and the Q-switched alexandrite laser (755 nm)). Laser induces extreme heating of melanosomes with subsequent thermal expansion, local vaporization and generation of acoustic waves that damage the nucleus and eventually destroy the pigment-laden cells. The released melanin is then removed through transepidermal elimination or phagocytosis by dermal macrophages. To be effective and specific, wavelengths that avoid absorption by other skin chromophores and penetrate to the desired depth have to be used [13].

Surgical Treatment

Dermabrasion

As mentioned above, dermabrasion can help to reduce hypo- and hyperpigmentation of a scar. In the case of hyperpigmentation, dermabrasion is usually performed as a single treatment modality, that is, it is not combined with another treatment such as skin transplantation. The idea is to easily remove the epidermis including the melanocytes and the pigment and let it heal spontaneously resulting in an epidermis with a lower concentration of melanocytes. It is not recommended to go too deep because the regeneration capacity of the skin is limited in scars, due to lowered presence or even absence of hair follicles and sweat glands. If the wounds are too deep and stay open too long, problematic new scars can occur.

It is advisable to perform dermabrasion in the fall or winter season to anticipate low UV light exposure to reduce the risk of excessive new pigmentation. It is also recommended to start dermabrasion with a small test area, preferably in an area that can be easily evaluated by the patient.

Excision

Excision and closure is also a feasible therapeutic option for hyperpigmented lesions that are limited in size (see above under hypopigmentation). It should be taken into account that a (linear) scar will remain and that outcome may be more severe than the original situation.

Conclusion

Pigmentation problems are an important feature of scar quality and partly determine the visual characteristics of a scar. Both hypopigmentation and hyperpigmentation can cause aesthetic and psychological issues which influences quality of life. Pigmentation disorders are difficult to treat. Treatment options include camouflage therapy, topical treatments, chemical peels, laser therapy, dermatography, dermabrasion, microneedling, skin grafting, cell therapy, and excision. It is advised to first try the conservative options and to dose the treatment to prevent overshoot and complications.

Take-Home Messages

- Pigment abnormalities are divided into hyperpigmentation and hypopigmentation.
- Pigmentation disorders are difficult to treat.
- Nonsurgical and surgical options are available.
- Wait until the area has matured.
- First try the conservative options. If possible, first test the response to the therapy in a test area.
- Dose the treatment to prevent overshoot and complications.

References

1. Hill JP, Batchelor JM. An approach to hypopigmentation. BMJ. 2017;356:i6534.
2. Kaufman BP, Aman T, Alexis AF. Postinflammatory hyperpigmentation: epidemiology, clinical presentation, pathogenesis and treatment. Am J Clin Dermatol. 2018;19(4):489–503.
3. van der Wal MB, et al. Outcome after burns: an observational study on burn scar maturation and predictors for severe scarring. Wound Repair Regen. 2012;20(5):676–87.
4. Takiwaki H. Measurement of skin color: practical application and theoretical considerations. J Med Invest. 1998;44(3–4):121–6.
5. van der Wal M, et al. Objective color measurements: clinimetric performance of three devices on normal skin and scar tissue. J Burn Care Res. 2013;34(3):e187–94.
6. van der Wal MB, et al. A clinimetric overview of scar assessment scales. J Burn Care Res. 2012;33(2):e79–87.
7. Sullivan T, et al. Rating the burn scar. J Burn Care Rehabil. 1990;11(3):256–60.
8. Draaijers LJ, et al. The patient and observer scar assessment scale: a reliable and feasible tool for scar evaluation. Plast Reconstr Surg. 2004;113(7):1960–5; discussion 1966–7.
9. Alexiades-Armenakas MR, et al. The safety and efficacy of the 308-nm excimer laser for pigment correction of hypopigmented scars and striae alba. Arch Dermatol. 2004;140(8):955–60.
10. Falabella R. Epidermal grafting. An original technique and its application in achromic and granulating areas. Arch Dermatol. 1971;104(6):592–600.
11. Iriarte C, et al. Review of applications of microneedling in dermatology. Clin Cosmet Investig Dermatol. 2017;10:289–98.
12. Verhaegen PD, et al. Sustainable effect of skin stretching for burn scar excision: long-term results of a multicenter randomized controlled trial. Burns. 2011;37(7):1222–8.
13. Briganti S, Camera E, Picardo M. Chemical and instrumental approaches to treat hyperpigmentation. Pigment Cell Res. 2003;16(2):101–10.

12

Structural Assessment of Scars Using Optical Techniques

L. van Haasterecht, Paul P. M. van Zuijlen, and ML. Groot

Contents

Introduction

The skin, the largest organ of the body, consists of an epidermal layer and a dermal layer underneath. The thin epidermal layer functions as a barrier to the outer world. The dermis is much thicker, and its structural organization is responsible for the functional qualities of the human skin. It consists for almost 80% of collagen, elastin, and different types of cells, which render the skin strong and at the same time remarkably pliable. In scar tissue, visual aspects (discoloration and texture [1]), functional aspects (stiffness [1] and moisture retention [2]), and sensory functions [3] of the skin differ significantly from those of healthy skin.

In clinical practice, objective assessment of cutaneous scars remains a challenging task. The use of scar assessment tools has increased significantly in the last decade. The clinical follow-up of scar treatment necessitates precise measurement of thickness, surface area, and relief. Further, a better visualization of the precise 3D microstructural organization is crucial in understanding the etiology of pathological scarring. As most aspects of clinical scar assessment scales are based on the visual appearance, the potential for optical techniques as an objective assessment tool is high. With a so-called optical biopsy, it is possible to assess the microstructure below the surface of the skin with optical methods, negating invasive physical biopsies. Furthermore, a range of extensions for these techniques allow simultaneous structural, mechanical, and even chemical characterization.

This chapter aims to describe current progress in objective imaging techniques used in the clinical follow-up of scar progression on the one hand and some of the most powerful techniques for basic structural research of scar microstructures on the other hand. For the sake of brevity, we limit our discussion to techniques and devices that have been shown to be valid and reliable. For a complete overview of available devices, we refer the reader to an extensive review by Lee et al. [4].

Volumetric Analyses

The number of devices that measure scar volume has seen a rapid growth in the last decade, partly advanced by increased attention to wound and burn research.

Volumetric aspects of scars discussed here are surface area, thickness, and surface topology. Although there exists significant overlap between these aspects and some devices measure multiple aspects (surface roughness can be considered as fluctuations in scar height/thickness; newer analysis methods of surface area are often intrinsically three dimensional and therefore include information on surface topology), we discuss them separately as the reliability (the consistency of the measurements) and validity (whether the device measures what it intends to measure) of individual aspects of a device aren't necessarily similar.

Volumetric assessment has gone from manual paper tracing to high-tech 3D cameras.

Although manual tracing of scar surface area is reliable in the case of linear postoperative scars [5], for scars with irregular boundaries, the reliability decreases with scar size [6]. The LifeViz 3D camera (Quantificare SA, Valbonne, France) has been extensively tested in both the surface area and volumetric analysis mode by Stekelenburg et al., who reported it to be a reliable and valid tool [7, 8]. The LifeViz 3D works by comparing two photos from different angles, from a predefined distance. The Vectra 3D is a speckle pattern-based system that utilizes six cameras to construct a 3D image. Its interrater reliability was found to be excellent in a trial on raised scars [9]. A device with a similar working mechanism, MAVIS III (Photometrix, Pontypridd, United Kingdom), was assessed in a study on burn scars. The authors note that poorly delineated scars on curved surfaces pose a challenge in the boundary selection and subsequent analysis [10].

Rashaan et al. tested another stereophotogrammetry device, the Artec MHT (Artec 3D, San Diego, CA, USA), and found it to be highly reliable and valid in burn scars [11].

Other strategies that include laser scanning cameras and structured light scanners need additional clinical evaluation.

Surface Topology

Roughness, or surface irregularity, has a significant impact on a patient's perception of scars [12]. Furthermore, the predictive validity of long-term scar quality was found to be significantly influenced by the "relief" item on the POSAS observer scale [13] (see ► Chap. 16 for more on scar assessment scales). Most scar assessment scales include such a texture item, and even though subjective analysis isn't necessarily inferior to objective analysis, quantification of these aspect remains challenging.

Early attempts at quantitative evaluation of roughness entailed the casting of a positive or negative mold of the scar surface and its subsequent optical or mechanical analysis [14]. This process, although accurate, is overly cumbersome and time-consuming. Current contactless techniques use a combination of illumination and analysis of disturbance patterns. The most frequently used device, the Phaseshift Rapid In Vivo Measurement of the Skin (PRIMOS, Canfield Scienitifc, Inc., Parsippany, USA), has been shown to reliably measure scar topology [15, 16]. PRIMOS projects patterns of light onto the skin surface. Fluctuations in the surface profile cause disruptions in these patterns that are subsequently analyzed.

Antera 3D (Miravex, Dublin, Ireland) is based on photometric stereo, in which light from different angles produces shade based on surface topology. The reflected light is analyzed to form a surface reconstruction. Similarly, LifeViz Micro (Quantificare SA, Valbonne, France) is one of the devices in the LifeViz series mentioned earlier. Although they have been described in the context of clinical scar assessment [17, 18], their clinimetric properties have not been analyzed for the surface roughness aspect.

The Visioscan VC 98 uses software analysis of grayscale values in UVA-illuminated photographs (Visioscan VC 98). Reliability in healthy skin relies heavily on the chosen outcome measure of the "surface evaluation of living skin" method [16].

The analysis of relief can be considered a structural analysis of scar volume. Indeed, most devices offer some volumetric analysis. Furthermore, the Antera 3D offers additional colorimetric analysis. The abovementioned devices show great heterogeneity in measured parameters, resolution, and field of view, and thus, it is difficult to make a qualitative comparison. In the future, further cross-pollination between techniques can be expected. Askaruly et al. showed the potential of optical coherence tomography (OCT) to measure relief [19]. Although their study was not on scar tissue, the possibility of combining 3D surface analysis with structural analysis looks promising.

Thickness

Follow-up of scar thickness is especially important in both hypertrophic and keloid scars, where the aberrant deposition of ECM proteins leads to significant expansion. Therapies are mostly focused on reducing the scar's prominence over the surrounding tissue, and correctly analyzing the thickness of cutaneous scar is paramount.

Although not an optical technique, we discuss high-frequency ultrasound here as it's by far the most commonly used technique. Its inferior resolution compared to optical equivalents is mitigated by its superior penetration depth allowing thickness analysis, even in severe scar thickening. The working mechanism is based on reflection of sound waves of structures with different acoustic impedances and the analysis of the reflection time to determine the depth of the structure. The penetration depth ranges from the upper dermal layers to full-thickness skin and subcutaneous structures, depending on the employed frequency.

Numerous ultrasound systems exist that are marketed for dermatological applications; we succinctly limit our discussion to systems that have been applied to scars. The frequency used by these systems ranges from 5 to 50 MHz and forms the most important limitation in scars, as this limits the penetration depth. For example, the most frequently described device, the Dermascan C (Cortex Technology ApS), utilizes a frequency of 20 MHz which has a penetration depth described as inadequate in up to a third of burn scars in a study by Gankande et al. [20] (using the DermaLab Combo).

Reliability of these instruments has been tested in several studies and shows excellent inter-observer [20–23] and intra-observer reliability [20, 21, 23–25].

From a validity standpoint, it is of interest to note that a golden standard does not currently exist. Comparison with scar assessment scales has yielded inconsistent results, possibly due to heterogeneity in scar scales and ultrasound frequency [23, 26]. Histology has several drawbacks that include deformation during the biopsy process dependent on resting skin tension, manipulation during fixation, and slicing [27]. Agabalyan et al. found poor correlation between 20Mhz ultrasound analysis and histological analysis of skin graft scars in a small group of patients [26]. Andrew et al. found biopsies to be significantly thicker after excision, advising the use of pinning during formaldehyde fixation to mitigate this effect [27]. Li et al. compared ultrasound measurements with the use of a micrometer [24], theoretically bypassing the negative effects of sample preparation for histology. Although they achieve a high correlation, sonographic analysis was performed on porcine excised tissue in which it is conceivably easier to recognize the skin's boundaries.

Scar height can be measured using volumetric analyses like the 3D camera LifeViz 3D (Quantificare SA, Valbonne, France), although studies comparing this device with ultrasound measurements have favored the latter [23, 28]. It seems that the reliability is suboptimal due to the device having difficulty scanning over curved surfaces.

Experimental Techniques

Scarring involves the aberrant deposition of matrix molecules. The collagen content of scars, especially, differs from healthy skin in terms of amount, type, and, importantly, organization. In the past decades, quantification of the extracellular matrix (ECM) organization was mostly limited to two-dimensional images from fixated and stained tissue. Depending on the orientation of histological slices relative to the skin surface, analysis of orientation will yield different results. For example, Verhaegen et al. found significantly different supramolecular organization depending on which cross section was imaged (e.g., perpendicular to the surface or in the parallel plain) [29]. Gaining a better three-dimensional perspective of ECM organization is paramount in elucidating the etiology of pathological scars.

As the goal is not only to assess scar tissue based on texture, volume, and color but also to perform microstructural analysis, more advanced microscopic tools are required. An ideal optical scar assessment technique would have a resolution with which microstructural changes can be clearly identified, even in the deeper parts of the dermis. However, in optics, there exists a common trade-off between spatial resolution and penetration depth, and the marked thickening of hypertrophic and keloids scar complicates this trade-off. In this sense, a "perfect technique" does not exist. A technique's suitability depends merely on whether the application matches its strength. In the following, we will discuss several microscopic techniques and their applications in scar assessment and research.

Optical Coherence Tomography

Colloquially known as "Ultrasound based on light," OCT is a promising technique based on low-coherence interferometry. In short, light with a broad bandwidth is split into a sample arm and a reference arm. The interference pattern that arises from the combination of the reference arm and the sample arm, containing reflected light from different depth layers of the sample, creates a depth profile of the sample. Combining a lateral series of these profiles creates a cross-sectional image (B scan) or a three-dimensional reconstruction when a stack of B scans is combined. Scanning approaches with full-field illumination allow the acquisition of stacks of "en face" scans. Typically, penetration depths of 1–2 mm can be reached, at a resolution of 4–10 μm [30].

The capability of OCT to create high-resolution tomography first piqued the interest of the ophthalmological community, where it is now a staple technique in retinal assessment. Naturally, attributes like fast acquisition time, high-resolution images, noninvasiveness, and multifaceted structural assessment make OCT an interesting technique for dermatology. Moreover, OCT devices are often manageable handheld scanners, increasing their usability in the clinic.

Polarization-sensitive OCT (PS-OCT) has been described as a quantification tool for collagen density and alignment by means of tissue birefringence [31]. Jaspers et al. compared burn scars and healthy skin using a volume-based birefringence method, which showed strong correlation to histologically determined collagen content [32]. By applying speckle decorrelation, Liew et al. visualized the microvasculature of burn scars in three dimensions [33]. A similar strategy was used in the clinical follow-up of burn scars undergoing laser ablation [34], allowing the authors to distinguish mature and immature scars [35]. Comparable strategies have been applied to lymph vessels [36]. Combined vascularity, lymph vessels, and birefringence analyses were used by Park et al. to longitudinally follow wound healing in a mouse model, showing angiogenetic changes and realignment of birefringent signals [37].

Simultaneous mechanical testing allows the correlation of local structural changes to variations in stiffness. Es'haghian et al. showed that combining a handheld OCT probe with a mechanical loading device permits concurrent imaging of the in vivo scars and stiffness mapping [38, 39]. Vibrational perturbation of the skin and the analysis of resonance frequencies while imaging the layers of the skin have also received some attention recently for bulk measurements of mechanical properties [40, 41].

OCT has been described as a tool for measuring thickness of individual skin layers. Because the limited penetration depth makes full thickness imaging impossible, its application is limited to the epidermal thickness [42, 43].

Confocal Microscopy

Higher-resolution images to assess structures with submicron resolution in 3D can be obtained using various microscopic techniques. In confocal fluorescence microscopy, the addition of a set of pinholes to a traditional fluorescence microscope allows for the selection and detection of a small focal volume. Selective labeling with a fluorophore allows for the imaging of a particular substance of interest by excitation of the fluorophore by a lamp or laser and detection of the fluorescence emission signals. Images are obtained by scanning the laser or the sample, yielding images with a resolution of 0.4 λ/NA where λ is the wavelenght of the emitted light and NA is the numerical aperture of the objective, which is an improvement of ~30% compared to traditional fluorescence microscopy. Another advantage over widefield microscopy is that the labeling with fluorophores can be sparser, allowing for a fairer comparison of relative quantities of structures.

Confocal microscopy has been used to determine the ratios of collagen of different scar types [44], cell-signaling molecules [45] or innervation [46] of different scar types and as an ex vivo tool in evaluation of microneedling penetration depth [47]. Furthermore, the superior resolution allows for quantitative collagen orientation analysis [29, 48]. Devices like the VivaScope (MAVIG, Munich, Germany) [49] are based on reflectance confocal microscopy (RCM), in which backscattered light from unlabeled structures is analyzed, based on changes in refractive index. The in vivo applications of RCM lie predominantly in the diagnosis of various skin cancers [50], as its penetration depth is limited to the epidermis and upper part of the dermis. However, attempts to analyze collagen production after micro-needling of acne scars have been described in vivo with a combination of dermoscopy and RCM [51]. The limited penetration depth seems a significant hurdle in scar research; however, combining the device with an OCT arm allowed Iftimia et al. to analyze both structural and birefringence properties in burn scars [52].

Nonlinear Optical Microscopy

Introduction

As discussed above, confocal microscopy allows for three-dimensional imaging; however in this technique, samples require specific staining and sometimes also fixation and slicing, which may affect ECM structure and organization. Nonlinear optical (NLO) microscopy involves label-free imaging of unfixed tissue in three dimensions and has strong potential in the visualization of the scar microstructure. Here, we discuss several types of NLO microscopy, namely, higher harmonic generation microscopy (HHG) and multiphoton excited autofluorescence (MEA), and explain their strengths in label-free imaging of scars.

Nonlinear microscopy can be described as the conversion of multiple photons into a single photon, based on the specific nonlinear behavior of certain molecules or structures. This process occurs only when the intensity of the incident light is sufficiently high. To keep the average laser power on the sample sufficiently low, short-pulsed lasers are used (generally femtosecond lasers) [53].

MEA involves the absorption of two or more photons by an intrinsic fluorophore and the recording of the subsequent fluorescence emission, which is then at a wavelength shorter than of the excitation light. Alternatively, external fluorophores can be applied to the sample to label specific structures. In contrast to single-photon fluorescence, excitation wavelengths typically lie in the infrared region, allowing deeper tissue penetration of up to 1.6 mm [54].

Comparably, in the HHG processes, two or three photons are converted into a single photon. No energy transfer takes place however, and the emitted photons have exactly half (second harmonic generation, SHG) or a third (third harmonic generation, THG) of the wavelength of the incident photons and exactly double or triple the energy, respectively. This allows the detection of the specific signal using narrow-banded filters, improving contrast between structures. Simultaneous registration of these signals using one system allows for label-free visualization of the most important structural proteins of the ECM.

Two-Photon Excited Autofluorescence (2PEF)

MEP involves two or three photons being absorbed by a fluorophore and the subsequent emission of a single photon of a shorter wavelength. Two-photon excited autofluorescence (2PEF) has been described extensively in skin research.

2PEF is applicable to fluorophores used in single-photon fluorescence. As this is a fundamentally different process, excitation wavelengths will not equate to exactly double the wavelength of the single-photon excitation. The emission spectrum however will be identical. Fluorophores naturally present in biological tissue have well-described excitation and emission spectra, and extrapolation to the two-photon excitation wavelength is usually warranted. Although penetration depths more than one millimeter have been described in the context of brain tissue [54], the density of the skin and the relevant excitation wavelengths do not permit such deep penetration. Imaging systems are conventionally limited to several hundred micrometers in depth.

Both collagen and elastin, the most important structural proteins of the extracellular matrix (ECM), have convenient 2PEF profiles [55]. On the cellular level, the abundantly present cytoplasmic metabolites NADH and FAD are prolific emitters in their reduced and oxidized states, respectively. An example of 2PEF imaging of dermal fibroblasts can be seen in ◘ Fig. 19.1.

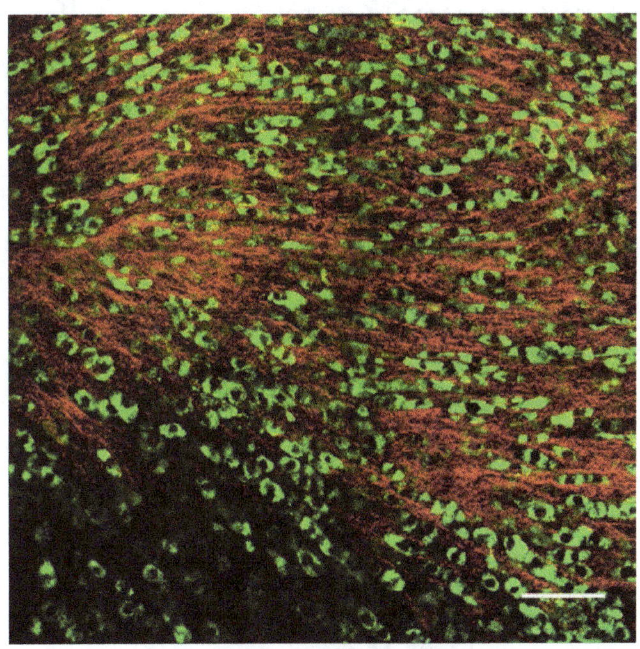

◘ **Fig. 19.1** Combined two-photon excited fluorescence image (2PEF, green) and second harmonic generation image (SHG, red) of cultured human dermal cells and their derived collagen matrix, respectively. Collagen fibers induce a bright SHG signal, whereas intrinsic fluorophores in the cytoplasm of the dermal cells outline the cells. In vitro images were acquired using a previously described setup [87]. Scale bar: 500 µm

Simultaneous recording allows a redox ratio to be calculated. The feasibility of this strategy was shown in an in vivo mouse model by Quinn et al. [56], visualizing metabolic changes during wound healing. Another in vivo study used the same concept to investigate the depth-dependent metabolism of keratinocytes [57]. Melanin content has been used as an in vivo marker for several dermatological disorders [58].

Second Harmonic Generation (SHG) Microscopy

The introduction of SHG microscopy has sparked a slew of research in dermatology. Also known as frequency doubling, it involves the interaction of two photons of the same wavelength with a nonlinear material and the subsequent creation of a single photon with double the frequency and energy. The ability of a material for second harmonic generation, described by the nonlinear susceptibility coefficient $\chi(2)$, depends on the non-centrosymmetric structure. Biologically significant harmonophores include collagen [59], myosin [60], and microtubules [61].

In the case of fibrillar collagen, the repeating dipoles of peptide bonds and the structural alignment on all levels of the molecular and supramolecular structure (parallel peptide bonds are assembled into parallel fibrils; fibrils are aligned into fibers) result in coherent amplification of the emitted second harmonic signal refs. This also means that the structural alignment of collagen fibers influences the SHG signal intensity [62]. As this is not the case for non-fibrillar collagen types, SHG microscopy is specific for type I and II collagens and forms a highly specific tool for 3D imaging of unprocessed skin samples as showed in ◘ Fig. 19.2 Abnormal ratios of collagen I:III have been described in multiple fibrotic processes [63]. Although collagen type III, often deposited alongside type I, is a fibrillar collagen, it produces only weak SHG signals [64]. As the SHG signal is dependent on phase-matching conditions, most of the signal forwardly propagated. The thin scattered fibers of collagen type III and their associated reduction in phase matching appear to be distinguishable from type I by comparing forward- and backward-scattered SHG images [65, 66]. The opacity of collagenous tissues however makes the detection of this signal impractical, rendering this technique possible only in thin specimens.

Multiple strategies to distinguish scar types using SHG images have been described. Most of these focus on software-based analysis of collagen fiber orientation and density [67–69]. Matrix organization and orientation have been described as abnormal in scars [29]. Non-software-based approaches rely on the dependence of the nonlinear susceptibility of collagen on the polarization of the incident light. Polarization-sensitive SHG (PS-SHG) probes the organization of collagen fibers by sequentially rotating the polarization relative to the optical axis and probing the SHG response. By analyzing the SHG intensity at different angles of polarization, orientation vectors can be reconstructed [70, 71]. Note that because of the strong dependence of SHG on polarization, software-based analyses should be performed on images from circularly polarized light sources.

Using unstained tissue allows simultaneous biomechanical testing during imaging. For example, Rosin et al. assessed the scarring capacity of healing split-thickness skin grafts by microstructural SHG imaging of collagen and biaxial stretch testing [72]. The authors correlate the loss of waviness patterns to increased stiffness.

The reduced phototoxicity (as no external fluorophores are used) from these optical processes allows in vitro and even in vivo imaging, for example, skin equivalents [73], lab-grown wound models [74], and antifibrotic treatments [75].

Several research groups have made attempts to include SHG in clinical decision-making. Predominately applied to neoplastic lesions, consecutive follow-up of

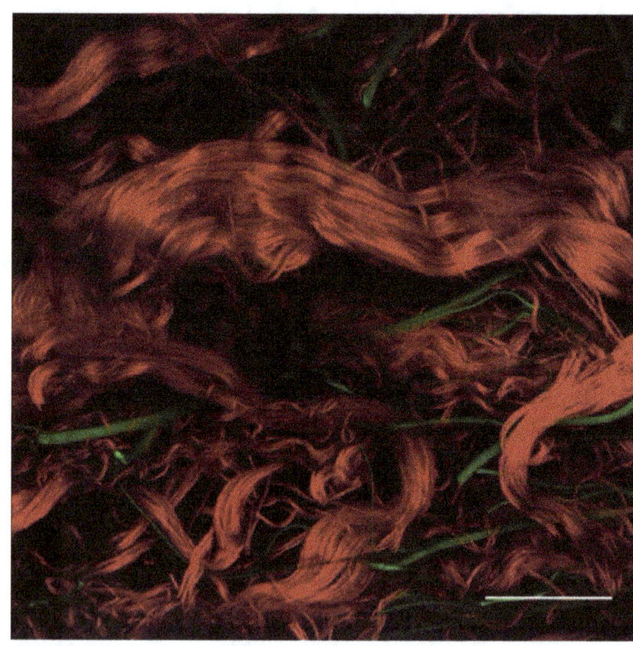

◘ **Fig. 19.2** Combined 2PEF (green) and SHG (red) image of elastin and collagen fibers, respectively. Unprocessed ex vivo human skin, specifically the reticular dermis, was imaged using the setup described in [87]. A stack of 35 images was acquired in the Z-axis. Image processing in ImageJ resulted in the 3D projection seen here [88]. Scale bar: 500 μm

scars and topical therapies has also been described. Commercial translation has already resulted in multiple devices marketed for in vivo dermatological applications. The Dermaspect (JenLab GmbH, Berlin, Germany) device entails a multimodal (2PEF, CARS, SHG) microscope with an adjustable scan head for in vivo skin imaging [76]. Innovations in laser technology allow for increasingly smaller and cheaper devices [77, 78].

Third Harmonic Generation (THG) Microscopy

The propensity of a material for third harmonic generation depends not only on its nonlinear susceptibility coefficient $\chi(3)$ but also on whether partial phase matching can be achieved by a small inhomogeneity at the focus, making THG an interface-sensitive technique [79]. THG is less specific than SHG, increasing the number of possible applications. By setting the focal volume of the incident laser beam to several times the size of a typical tissue structure, a geometry can be created where the phase-matching conditions enable efficient THG. As the THG contrast comes from inhomogeneities and tissue interfaces with a high $\chi(3)$, cell membranes and cell nuclei are clearly displayed with THG microscopy, since they contain lipids which are known to have a high $\chi(3)$ [80]. Not surprisingly, the multilayered structure of the epidermis provides excellent contrast. ◘ Figure 19.3 shows a THG cross section of the epidermis in a drug penetration experiment. To illustrate the potential in dermatology, THG was shown to be a viable imaging technique for label-free tracking of melanoma cells [81]. The THG contrast from melanin and structural features allowed differentiation of skin cancers [82].

In the context of scar tissue, the surface of elastin fibers is an adequate THG emitter [83]; thus, combining SHG and THG potentially allows for three-dimensional imaging of unstained, unfixed, and unsliced tissue.

Although an analysis of scar tissue has not been described yet, THG has strong potential as a label-free imaging technique because of reduced phototoxicity. Indeed, several articles describe the in vivo "optical biopsy" technique in the skin [78, 84].

Coherent Anti-Stokes Raman Spectroscopy (CARS)

The structural information provided by SHG and THG can be supplemented by chemical information using another nonlinear process, Coherent anti-Stokes Raman Spectroscopy (CARS). Here, two lasers with different frequencies are focused on the sample, to probe the vibrational fingerprint of the molecules in the focal point. The CH2 content of lipids provides excellent contrast when imaging phospholipid-rich cell membranes and adipocytes. The OH signal from water molecules makes this technique especially applicable for research into transepidermal water loss [76, 85].

Future Perspectives

The enormous increase in available devices for volumetric analysis is indicative for the increased attention for quantification tools in scar research. Technological advances and the need for point of care solutions have already resulted in smaller and manageable devices suitable for bedside use. This trend can be expected to continue with smartphone-based solutions already being investigated in wound evaluation [86]. Both researcher and clinicians should however be mindful of the fact that most devices are not adequately tested on their clinimetric properties.

This trend is also applicable to experimental techniques. As image acquisition times decrease and devices get smaller, we can expect integration of different imaging techniques, each bringing their own strengths in elucidating the multifaceted issue of pathological scarring.

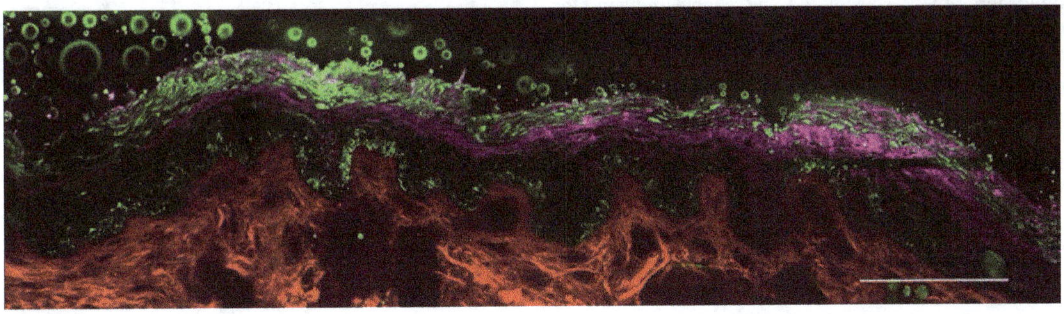

◘ **Fig.** Nonlinear microscopy image of a cross section of ex vivo skin. The THG signal (green) depicts the layers of the epider-mis; collagen fibers in the papillary dermis give rise to the SHG signal in red. In this experiment, fluorescently labeled (magenta) hyaluronic acid (250 kDa) was applied to the skin's surface to quantify epidermal skin penetration. Scale bar: 500 μm

Take Home Messages

- Technological advances will increase the number of devices for scar assessment, while reducing their size.
- The integration of multiple techniques has the potential to improve scar assessment.
- For most devices, the clinimetric properties are insufficiently determined.
- SHG microscopy is a valuable tool for experimental research into scar pathophysiology and potential therapeutics.

References

1. Spronk I, Polinder S, Haagsma J, Nieuwenhuis M, Pijpe A, Van der Vlies C, et al. Patient-reported scar quality of adults after burn injuries: a five-year multicenter follow-up study. Wound Repair Regen. 2019;27(4):406–14.
2. Gardien KLM, Baas DC, de Vet HCW, Middelkoop E. Transepidermal water loss measured with the Tewameter TM300 in burn scars. Burns 2016; 42 (7), 1455–62.
3. Brown BC, Mckenna SP, Siddhi K, Mcgrouther DA, Bayat A. The hidden cost of skin scars: quality of life after skin scarring. J Plast Reconstr Aesthet Surg. 2008;61:1049–58.
4. Lee KC, Dretzke J, Grover L, Logan A, Moiemen N. A systematic review of objective burn scar measurements. Burns Trauma 2016;4:14.
5. Feldstein S, Wilken R, Wang JZ, Taylor SL, Eisen DB. Development and initial validation of the trace-to-tape method: an objective outcome measure for linear postoperative scars. Br J Dermatol. 2019;181(3):633–4.
6. Van Zuijlen PPM, Angeles AP, Suijker MH, Kreis RW, Middelkoop E. Reliability and accuracy of techniques for surface area measurements of wounds and scars. Int J Low Extrem Wounds. 2004;3(1):7–11.
7. Stekelenburg CM, Van Der Wal MBA, Knol DL, De Vet HCW, Van Zuijlen PPM. Three-dimensional digital stereophotogrammetry: a reliable and valid technique for measuring scar surface area. Plast Reconstr Surg. 2013;132(1):204–11.
8. Stekelenburg CM, Jaspers MEH, Niessen FB, Knol DL, Van Der Wal MBA, De Vet HCW, et al. In a clinimetric analysis, 3D stereophotogrammetry was found to be reliable and valid for measuring scar volume in clinical research. J Clin Epidemiol. 2015;68(7):782–7.
9. Verhiel SHWL, Piatkowski de Grzymala AA, Van den Kerckhove E, Colla C, van der Hulst RRWJ. Three-dimensional imaging for volume measurement of hypertrophic and keloid scars, reliability of a previously validated simplified technique in clinical setting. Skin Res Technol. 2016;22(4):513–8.
10. Su S, Sinha S, Gabriel V. Evaluating accuracy and reliability of active stereophotogrammetry using MAVIS III Wound Camera for three-dimensional assessment of hypertrophic scars. Burns. 2017;43(6):1263–70.
11. Rashaan ZM, Stekelenburg CM, van der Wal MBA, Euser AM, Hagendoorn BJM, van Zuijlen PPM, et al. Three-dimensional imaging: a novel, valid, and reliable technique for measuring wound surface area. Skin Res Technol. 2016;22(4):443–50.
12. Hoogewerf CJ, Van Baar ME, Middelkoop E, Van Loey NE. Patient reported facial scar assessment: directions for the professional. Burns. 2013;40(2):347–53.
13. Goei H, Van Der Vlies CH, Tuinebreijer WE, Van Zuijlen P, Middelkoop E, Van Baar M. Predictive validity of short term scar quality on final burn scar outcome using the Patient and Observer Scar Assessment Scale in patients with minor to moderate burn severity. Burns. 2017;43(4):715–23.
14. Fischer TW, Peter WW. Direct and non-direct measurement techniques for analysis of skin surface topography. Ski Pharmacol Appl Ski Physiol. 1999;12:1–11.
15. Bloemen MCT, Van Gerven MS, Van Der Wal MBA, Verhaegen PDHM, Middelkoop E. An objective device for measuring surface roughness of skin and scars. J Am Acad Dermatol. 2010;64(4):706–15.
16. Trojahn C, Schario M, Dobos G, Kottner J. Reliability and validity of two in vivo measurements for skin surface topography in aged adults. Skin Res Technol. 2015;21:54–60.
17. Petit L, Bettoli DZV, Kang BDS, Martel P. Validation of 3D skin imaging for objective repeatable quantification of severity of atrophic acne scarring. Skin Res Technol. 2018;24(4):542–50.
18. Lumenta DB, Kitzinger H, Selig H. Objective quantification of subjective parameters in scars by use of a portable stereophotographic system. Ann Plast Surg. 2011;67(6):641–5.
19. Askaruly S, Ahn Y, Kim H, Vavilin A, Ban S, Kim PU, et al. Quantitative evaluation of skin surface roughness using optical coherence tomography in vivo. IEEE J Sel Top Quantum Electron. 2019;25(1):1–8.
20. Gankande TU, Duke JM, Danielsen PL, Dejong HM, Wood FM, Wallace HJ. Reliability of scar assessments performed with an integrated skin testing device – the DermaLab Combo. Burns. 2014;40(8):1521–9.
21. Lau JCM, Li-tsang CWP, Zheng YP. Application of tissue ultrasound palpation system (TUPS) in objective scar evaluation. Burns. 2005;31:445–52.
22. Nedelec B, Correa JA, Rachelska G, Armour A, LaSalle L. Quantitative measurement of hypertrophic scar: interrater reliability and concurrent validity. J Burn Care Res. 2008;29(3):501–11.
23. Simons M, Kee EG, Kimble R, Tyack Z. Ultrasound is a reproducible and valid tool for measuring scar height in children with burn scars: a cross-sectional study of the psychometric properties and utility of the ultrasound and 3D camera. Burns. 2017;43(5):993–1001.
24. Li JQ, Li-tsang CWP, Huang YP, Chen Y, Zheng YP. Detection of changes of scar thickness under mechanical loading using ultrasonic measurement. Burns. 2013;39:89–97.
25. Nedelec B, Correa JA, Rachelska G, Armour A, LaSalle L. Quantitative measurement of hypertrophic scar: intrarater reliability, sensitivity, and specificity. J Burn Care Res. 2008;29(3):489–500.
26. Agabalyan NA, Su S, Sinha S, Gabriel V. Comparison between high-frequency ultrasonography and histological assessment reveals weak correlation for measurements of scar tissue thickness. Burns. 2017;43(3):531–8.
27. Andrews CJ, Kempf M, Kimble R, Cuttle L. Skin thickness measurements increase with excision and biopsy processing procedures. Wound Repair Regen. 2017;25:338–40.
28. Tyack Z, Simons M, Kimble RM, Muller MJ, Leung K. The reproducibility and clinical utility of the 3D camera for measuring scar height, with a protocol for administration. Skin Res Technol. 2017;23(4):463–70.
29. Verhaegen PDHM, van Zuijlen PP, Pennings NM, van Marle J, Niessen FB, Van Der Horst CMAM, et al. Differences in collagen architecture between keloid, hypertrophic scar, normotrophic scar, and normal skin: an objective histopathological analysis. Wound Repair Regen. 2009;17:649–56.
30. Babalola O, Mamalis A, Lev-Tov H, Jagdeo J. Optical coherence tomography (OCT) of collagen in normal skin and skin fibrosis. Arch Dermatol Res. 2014;306(1):1–9.

31. Gong P, Wood FM, Sampson DD, Mclaughlin RA. Imaging of skin birefringence for human scar assessment using polarization-sensitive optical coherence tomography aided by vascular masking assessment using polarization-sensitive optical. J Biomed Opt. 2014;19(12).
32. Jaspers MEH, Feroldi F, Vlig M, De Boer JF, Van Zuijlen PPM. In vivo polarization-sensitive optical coherence tomography of human burn scars: birefringence quantification and correspondence with histologically determined collagen density. J Biomed Opt. 2017;22(12).
33. Liew YM, Mclaughlin RA, Gong P, Wood FM, Sampson DD. In vivo assessment of human burn scars through automated quantification of vascularity using optical coherence tomography automated quantification of vascularity using. J Biomed Opt. 2013;18(6).
34. Es'haghian S, Gong P, Chin L, Harms K, Murray A, Rea S, et al. Investigation of optical attenuation imaging using optical coherence tomography for monitoring of scars undergoing fractional laser treatment. J Biophotonics. 2017;10:511–22.
35. Gong P, Es S, Harms K, Murray A, Rea S, Kennedy BF, et al. Optical coherence tomography for longitudinal monitoring of vasculature in scars treated with laser fractionation. J Biophotonics. 2016;9(6):626–36.
36. Gong P, Es'haghian S, Harms K-A, Murray A, Rea S, Wood FM, et al. In vivo label-free lymphangiography of cutaneous lymphatic vessels in human burn scars using optical coherence tomography. Biomed Opt Express. 2016;7(12):1219–23.
37. Park KS, Choi WJ, Song S, Xu J, Wang RK. Multifunctional in vivo imaging for monitoring wound healing using swept-source polarization-sensitive optical coherence tomography. Lasers Surg Med. 2017;50(3):213–21.
38. Es'haghian S, Kennedy KM, Gong P, Li Q, Chin L, Wijesinghe P, et al. In vivo volumetric quantitative micro- elastography of human skin. Biomed Opt Express. 2017;8(5):121–8.
39. Es'haghian S, Kennedy KM, Gong P, Sampson DD, Mclaughlin RA, Kennedy BF. Optical palpation in vivo: imaging human skin lesions using mechanical contrast. J Biomed Opt. 2015; 20(1).
40. Shah RG, Devore D, Silver FH. Biomechanical analysis of decellularized dermis and skin: initial in vivo observations using OCT and vibrational analysis. J Biomed Mater Res Part A. 2018;106(5):1421–7.
41. Silver FH, Shah RG. Mechanical spectroscopy and imaging of skin components in vivo: assignment of the observed moduli. Skin Res Technol. 2019;25(1):47–53.
42. Reinholz M, Schwaiger H, Poetschke J, Epple A, Ruzicka T, Von Braunmuhl T, et al. Objective and subjective treatment evaluation of scars using optical coherence tomography, sonography, photography, and standardised questionnaires. Eur J Dermatol. 2016;26(December):599–608.
43. Ud-Din S, Foden P, Stocking K, Mazhari M, Al-Habba S, Baguneid M, et al. Objective assessment of dermal fibrosis in cutaneous scarring: using optical coherence tomography, high frequency ultrasound and immuno-histo-morphometry of human skin. Br J Dermatol. 2019;6
44. Oliveira GV, Hawkins HK, Chinkes D, Burke A, Luiz A, Tavares P, et al. Hypertrophic versus non hypertrophic scars compared by immunohistochemistry and laser confocal microscopy: type I and III collagens. Int Wound J. 2009;6(6):445–52.
45. Sideek MA, Teia A, Kopecki Z, Cowin AJ, Gibson MA. Co-localization of LTBP-2 with FGF-2 in fibrotic human keloid and hypertrophic scar. J Mol Histol. 2016;47(1).
46. Tey HL, Maddison B, Wang H, Ishiju Y, Mcmichaef A, Marks M, et al. Cutaneous innervation and itch in keloids. Acta Derm Venereol. 2012;92(5):529–31.
47. Sasaki GH. Micro-needling depth penetration, presence of pigment particles, and fluorescein-stained platelets: clinical usage for aesthetic concerns. Aesthetic Surg J. 2017;37(1):71–83.
48. Van Zuijlen PPM, Ruurda JJB, Van Veen HA, Van Marle J, Van Trier AJM, Groenevelt F, et al. Collagen morphology in human skin and scar tissue: no adaptations in response to mechanical loading at joints. Burns. 2003;29:423–31.
49. Edwards SJ, Patalay R, Wakefield V, Karner C. Diagnostic accuracy of reflectance confocal microscopy using VivaScope for detecting and monitoring skin lesions: a systematic review. Clin Exp Dermatol. 2017;42(3):266–75.
50. Waddell A, Star P, Guitera P. Advances in the use of reflectance confocal microscopy in melanoma. Melanoma Manag. 2018;10(5).
51. Fabbrocini G, Ardigò M, Mordente I, Ayala F, Cacciapuoti S, Monfrecola G. Confocal microscopy images to monitor skin needling in the treatment of acne scars. J Clin Exp Dermatol Res. 2015;6(6).
52. Iftimia N, Ferguson RD, Mujat M, Patel AH, Zhang EZ, Fox W, et al. Combined reflectance confocal microscopy/optical coherence tomography imaging for skin burn assessment. Biomed Opt Express. 2013;4(5):178–87.
53. Hockberger PE, Skimina TA, Centonze VE, Lavin C, Chu S, Dadras S, et al. Activation of flavin-containing oxidases underlies light-induced production of H 2 O 2 in mammalian cells. Proc Natl Acad Sci U S A. 1999;96(May):6255–60.
54. Kobat D, Horton NG, Xu C. In vivo two-photon microscopy to 1.6-mm mouse cortex. J Biomed Opt. 2011;16(10).
55. Zoumi A, Yeh A, Tromberg BJ. Imaging cells and extracellular matrix in vivo by using second-harmonic generation and two-photon excited fluorescence. PNAS. 2002;99(17):11014–9.
56. Quinn KP, Leal EC, Tellechea A, Kafanas A, Auster ME, Veves A, et al. Diabetic wounds exhibit distinct microstructural and metabolic heterogeneity through label-free multiphoton microscopy. J Invest Dermatol. 2016;136(1):342–4.
57. Jones JD, Ramser HE, Woessner AE, Quinn KP. In vivo multiphoton microscopy detects longitudinal metabolic changes associated with delayed skin wound healing. Commun Biol. 2018;19(1):198.
58. Lentsch G, Balu M, Williams J, Lee S, Harris RM, König K, et al. In vivo multiphoton microscopy of melasma. Pigment Cell Melanoma Res. 2019;32(3):403–11.
59. Campagnola PJ, Millard AC, Terasaki M, Hoppe PE, Malone CJ, Mohler WA. Imaging of endogenous structural proteins in biological tissues. Biophys J. 2002;82(1):493–508.
60. Plotnikov SV, Millard AC, Campagnola PJ, Mohler WA. Characterization of the myosin-based source for second-harmonic generation from muscle sarcomeres. Biophys J. 2006;90(2):693–703.
61. Dombeck DA, Kasischke KA, Vishwasrao HD, Ingelsson M, Hyman BT, Webb WW. Uniform polarity microtubule assemblies imaged in native brain tissue by second-harmonic generation microscopy. PNAS. 2003;100(12):7087–6.
62. Bueno JM, Ávila FJ, Artal P. Second harmonic generation microscopy: a tool for quantitative analysis of tissues. In: Stanciu SG, editor. Microscopy and analysis. IntechOpen, 2016, pp. 99–220.
63. Huang C, Murphy GF, Akaishi S, Ogawa R. Keloids and hypertrophic scars: update and future directions. Plast Reconstr Surg Glob Open. 2013;1(25):1–7.
64. Cox G, Kable E, Jones A, Fraser I, Manconi F, Gorrell MD. 3-Dimensional imaging of collagen using second harmonic generation. J Strucutral Biol. 2006;141(2003):53–62.
65. Kottmann RM, Sharp J, Owens K, Salzman P, Xiao G, Phipps RP, et al. Second harmonic generation microscopy reveals altered collagen microstructure in usual interstitial pneumonia versus healthy lung. Respir Res. 2015;16(61).

66. Tilbury K, Lien C, Chen S, Campagnola PJ. Differentiation of col I and col III isoforms in stromal models of ovarian cancer by analysis of second harmonic generation polarization and emission directionality. Biophys J. 2014;106(2):354–65.
67. Liu Y, Zhu X, Huang Z, Cai J, Chen R, Xiong S, et al. Texture analysis of collagen second- harmonic generation images based on local difference local binary pattern and wavelets differentiates human skin abnormal scars from normal scars. J Biomed Opt. 2015;20(1):16021.
68. Chen G, Liu Y, Zhu X, Huang Z, Cai J, Chen R. Phase and texture characterizations of scar collagen second-harmonic generation images varied with scar duration. Microsc Microanal. 2015;21(4):855–62.
69. Yildirim M, Quinn KP, Kobler JB, Zeitels SM, Georgakoudi I, Ben-Yakar A. Quantitative differentiation of normal and scarred tissues using second-harmonic generation microscopy. Scanning. 2016;38(6):684–93.
70. Mazumder N, Deka G, Wu W, Gogoi A, Zhuo G, Kao F. Polarization resolved second harmonic microscopy. Methods. 2017;128:105–18.
71. Hristu R, Stanciu SG, Tranca DE, Stanciu GA. Improved quantification of collagen anisotropy with polarization-resolved second harmonic generation microscopy. J Biophotonics. 2017;10:1171–9.
72. Rosin NL, Agabalyan N, Olsen K, Martufi G, Gabriel V, Biernaskie J, et al. Collagen structural alterations contribute to stiffening of tissue after split-thickness skin grafting. Wound Repair Regen. 2016;24:263–74.
73. Meleshina AV, Rogovaya OS, Dudenkova VV, Sirotkina MA, Lukina MM, Bystrova AS, et al. Multimodal label-free imaging of living dermal equivalents including dermal papilla cells. Stem Cell Res Ther. 2018;9(84):1–12.
74. Torkian BA, Yeh AT, Engel R, Sun C, Tromberg BJ, Wong BJ. Modeling aberrant wound healing using tissue-engineered skin constructs and multiphoton microscopy. Arch Facial Plast Surg. 2004;6:180–7.
75. Qian HS, Weldon SM, Matera D, Lee C, Yang H, Fryer RM, et al. Quantification and comparison of anti- fibrotic therapies by polarized SRM and SHG- based morphometry in rat UUO model. PLoS One. 2016;11(6):1–13.
76. Weinigel M, Breunig HG, Uchugonova A, Konig K. Multipurpose nonlinear optical imaging system for in vivo and ex vivo multimodal histology in vivo and ex vivo multimodal histology. J Med Imaging. 2015;2(1):16003.
77. Rolopp A, Sákányi A, Aluszka D, Csati D, Vass L, Kolonics A, et al. Handheld nonlinear microscope system comprising a 2 MHz repetition rate, mode- locked Yb-fiber laser for in vivo biomedical imaging. Biomed Opt Express. 2016;7(9):49–53.
78. Chung H-Y, Greinert R, Kartner FX, Chang G. Multimodal imaging platform for optical virtual skin biopsy enabled by a fiber-based two- color ultrafast laser source. Biomed Opt Express. 2019;10(2):514–25.
79. Debarre D, Beaurepaire E. Quantitative characterization of biological liquids for third-harmonic generation microscopy. Biophys J. 2007;92:603–312.
80. Witte S, Negrean A, Lodder JC, De Kock CPJ, Testa Silva G, Mansvelder HD, et al. Label-free live brain imaging and targeted patching with third-harmonic generation microscopy. Proc Natl Acad Sci U S A. 2011;108(15):5970–5.
81. Weigelin B, Bakker G, Friedl P. Principles of interface guidance and microvesicle dynamics Intravital third harmonic generation microscopy of collective melanoma cell invasion. Intra Vital. 2012;1(1):32–43.
82. Tsai M, Cheng Y, Chen J, Liao Y, Sun C. Differential diagnosis of nonmelanoma pigmented skin lesions based on harmonic generation microscopy. J Biomed Opt. 2014;19(3).
83. Yu C, Tai S, Kung C, Wang I, Yu H, Lee W, et al. In vivo and ex vivo imaging of intra-tissue elastic fibers using third-harmonic-generation microscopy. Opt Express. 2007;15(18): 527–32.
84. Chen S, Wu H, Sun C. In vivo harmonic generation biopsy of human skin. JBO Lett. 2009;14(6):25–7.
85. Osseiran S, Dela Cruz J, Jeong S, Wang H, Fthenakis C, Evans CL. Characterizing the stratum corneum structure, barrier function, and chemical content of human skin with coherent Raman scattering imaging. Biomed Opt Express. 2018;9(12).
86. Foltynski P. Ways to increase precision and accuracy of wound area measurement using smart devices: advanced app Planimator. PLoS One. 2018;13(3):1–16.
87. Van Huizen L, Kuzmin N, Barbe E, Van der Velde S, Te Velde E, Groot M. Second and third harmonic generation microscopy visualizes key structural components in fresh unprocessed healthy human breast tissue. J Biophotonics. 2019;12(6):e201800297.
88. Schindelin J, Arganda-carreras I, Frise E, Kaynig V, Longair M, Pietzsch T, et al. Fiji: an open-source platform for biological-image analysis. Nat Methods. 2012;9(7):676–82.

13

Ideal Wound Closure Methods for Minimizing Scarring After Surgery

Rei Ogawa

Contents

Background

The healing of open cutaneous wounds involves the generation of vascularized granulation tissue that closes the gap in the skin. Thereafter, an effective epidermal barrier is created over the granulation tissue. Wounds in which sutures have approximated the edges also undergo granulation, albeit less than in open wounds that must heal by secondary intention. In both cases, the adherence of the wound edges becomes stronger over time: in general, wounded skin acquires 80% of the dermal strength of the surrounding normal skin by 3 months post-wounding [1].

Cutaneous Wound Healing and Mechanobiology

These wound-healing phenomena are the result of a cascade of complex biochemical events that can be categorized into four general overlapping phases: coagulation, inflammation, proliferation, and remodeling. Significantly, all four phases of wound healing are influenced by both intrinsic and extrinsic mechanical forces. For example, the formation of granulation tissue in the proliferating phase is driven by intrinsic and extrinsic mechanical stimulation of the fibroblasts, myofibroblasts, endothelial cells, and epithelial cells that are in and near the wound. Similarly, myofibroblasts contract the wound in the proliferative phase by mechanical forces that are themselves shaped by many extrinsic forces, including the natural tension in the skin. The remodeling phase can also be influenced by extrinsic mechanical forces [2]. During this phase, fibroblasts secrete collagen and fibronectin, which are key components of the extracellular matrix (ECM). These cells then regulate the volume of the ECM by secreting collagenase. This repeated synthesis and enzymatic breakdown of ECM proteins remodels the three-dimensional structure of the ECM. For proper remodeling, the synthesis and degradation processes must be carefully balanced: if there is too much ECM synthesis, scars can become hypertrophic. Conversely, if there is excessive ECM degradation, the scar can become atrophic. Multiple lines of evidence show that this ECM remodeling process can become deranged by extrinsic forces on the ECM [3]. For example, wounds on the major joints tend to develop hypertrophic scars because the joint movements place strong cyclical tension on the wound. This tension provokes chronic inflammation of the dermis, namely, the unceasing influx and activation of inflammatory cells, the persistent generation of blood vessels and nerve fibers, and the constant production of collagen by the activated fibroblasts. This chronic inflammation blocks the conversion of the granulation tissue into dermis-like tissue by the remodeling process and results in an immature hypertrophic scar that is red, elevated, hard, and painful.

These observations suggest that, to prevent pathological scarring after surgery, it is necessary to ensure that the sutures cause the wound edges to adhere to each other without any tension, even when strong extrinsic forces are placed on the wound. This will allow the granulation tissue to convert smoothly into dermis-like tissue, thereby yielding minimal scarring.

Surgical Techniques that Can Minimize Dermal Tension

The risk of pathological scarring can be greatly reduced by using subcutaneous/fascial tensile reduction sutures [4]. This is because dermal sutures do not effectively reduce tension on the dermis: rather, to achieve this, we must access much deeper structures, namely, the superficial and deep fascia, and suture them. This type of suturing will elevate the wound edges smoothly while placing minimal tension on the dermis. In other words, it will cause the wound edges to attach naturally to each. Only then should dermal and superficial sutures be used. It is very important to realize that dermal sutures on their own cannot reduce the tension on the dermis: this concept is the key to preventing the formation of pathological scars after surgery.

Thus, in the case of benign tumor excision or scar revision surgery in high-tension areas such as the chest wall, the cutaneous mass should be completely excised along with a minimum of normal skin margin and all fatty tissues under the mass. Hence, all tissues above the deep fascia of the muscle are removed. The wound edges are then undermined under the deep fascia, and the deep fascia is sutured with 0 polydioxanone sutures such as PDS®II (Ethicon, Inc., Somerville, New Jersey). Thereafter, the fibrous membrane in the fatty tissues, namely, the superficial fascia, is sutured using 2–0 and 3–0 PDS®II. This approach causes the wound edges to adhere naturally to each other. Our previous study

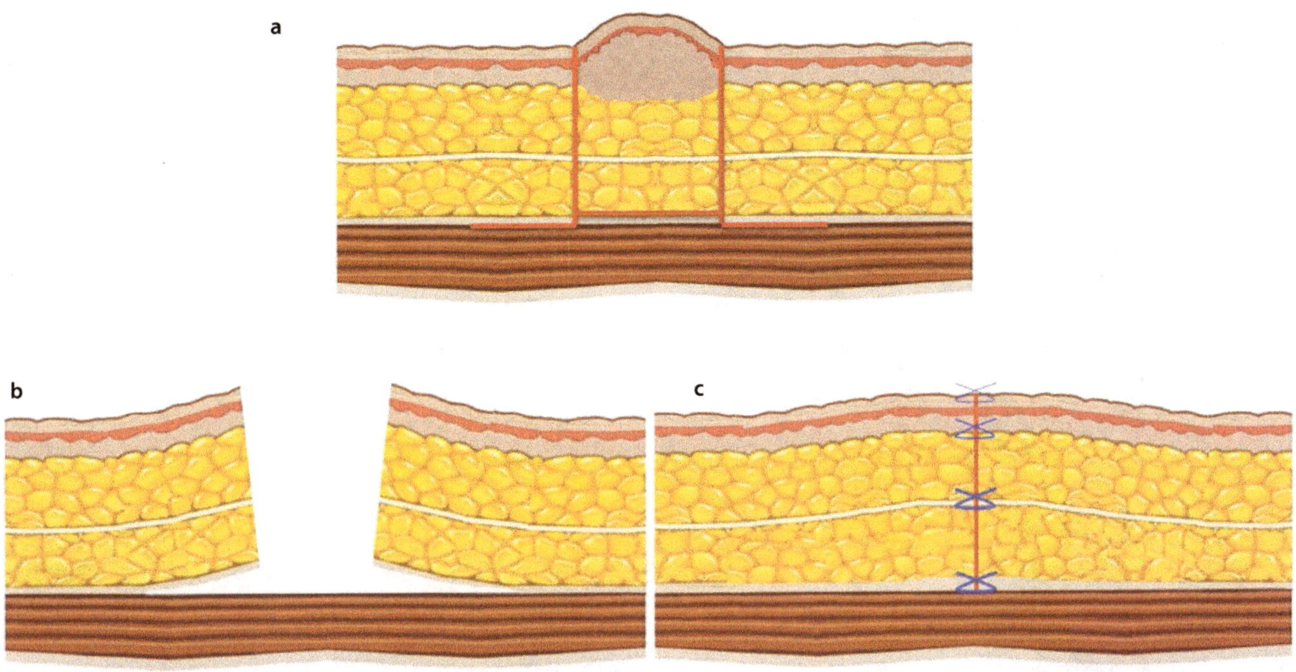

◘ Fig. The ideal closure method for minimizing the tension on the dermis. **a** The fatty tissues are removed along with the scar or tumor. **b** Undermining between the deep fascia and the muscle is performed. **c** The deep and superficial fasciae are then sutured to release the tension on the dermis. The red lines in **a** indicate where the tissue is incised and undermined. Dermal sutures themselves do not effectively reduce tension on the dermis. To achieve this, we must access much deeper structures, namely, the superficial and deep fasciae, and suture them

showed that deep fascia suturing reduced about 90% of the tension on the wound edge, while superficial fascia suturing reduced the remaining 10% [5]. After fascial suturing, dermal sutures using 4–0 PDS®II are started. This is followed by superficial sutures with 6–0 polypropylene or nylon sutures such as Proline® or Ethilon® (Ethicon, Inc., Somerville, New Jersey) (◘ Figs. 21.1, 21.2, and 21.3).

Z-Plasty

Another way to prevent pathological scar formation in high-tension areas is to use zigzag suturing techniques such as the Z-plasty [5]. This is particularly suitable for joint or limb surgery because the fatty tissue layers in these areas are thin: this means that it is difficult to find the superficial fascia and apply the subcutaneous/fascial tensile reduction sutures. Zigzag suturing is also good for long suture wounds because it effectively disrupts the tension on the resulting scar. As a result, zigzag suturing is an effective approach for releasing linear scar contractures. Another major benefit of Z-plasties is that segmented scars mature faster than long linear scars. Thus, if a scar or wound crosses a joint, zigzag incision and suturing will significantly reduce the risk of pathological scar recurrence or development (◘ Fig. 21.4).

In terms of Z-plasty design, the sides of each triangular flap should be 7–10 mm long and the pitch between each z-plasty should be 2–4 cm, depending on the total length of the wound [5]. In our experience, this pitch yields the most satisfactory results (personal observations). Dermal sutures can be started after confirming that the triangular flaps are fully elevated and can be transposed with each other.

It should be noted that, because keloids have much stronger inflammation than hypertrophic scars, it is best to use both tension reduction sutures and Z-plasties during keloid revision surgery [5]. This significantly reduces the risk of recurrence (◘ Fig. 21.5). This risk is also strongly ameliorated by postoperative radiotherapy.

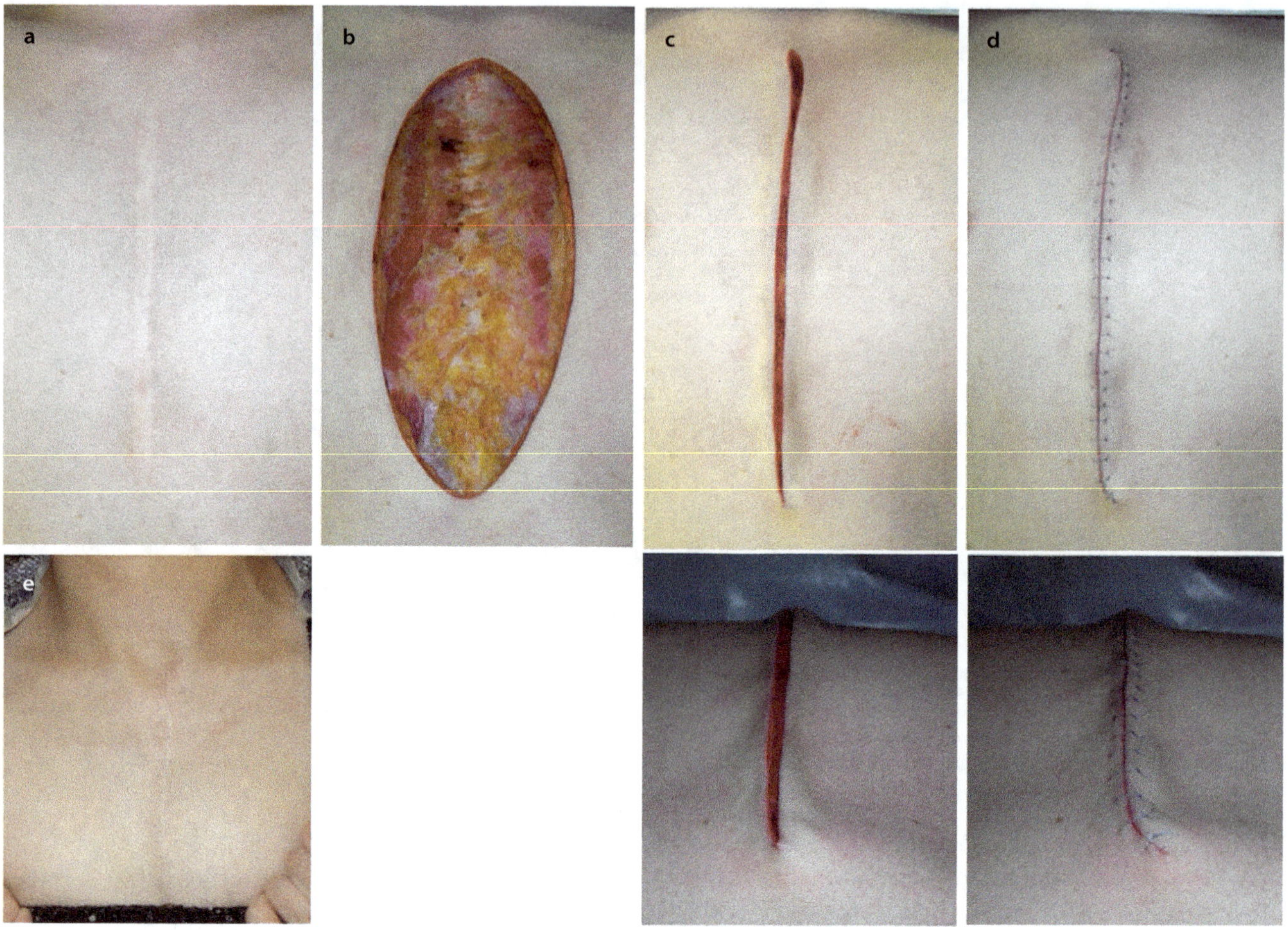

Fig. Chest wall scar revision. **a** Preoperative appearance of the scar. **b** View after the scar and fatty tissues were removed. **c** View after the deep and superficial fasciae of the pectoralis major muscle were sutured. **d** View immediately after the dermal sutures and superficial sutures were placed. **e** View 2 years after surgery. The wound edges were undermined under the deep fascia, after which the deep fascia was strongly sutured. These deep sutures absorb 90% of the tension on the wound

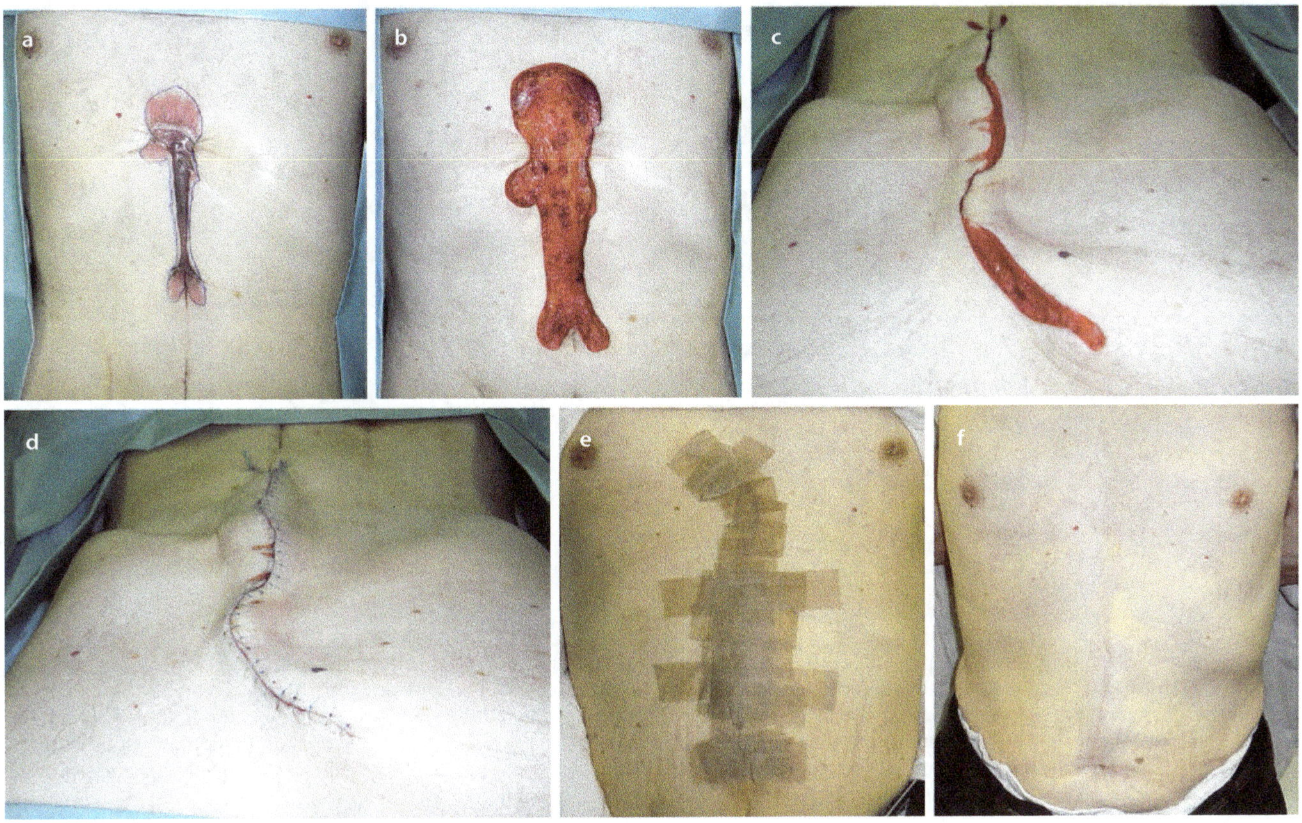

◘ **Fig.** Abdominal wall scar revision. **a** Preoperative appear-ance of the scar and the design of the incisions. **b** View after the scar and fatty tissues were removed. **c** View after the deep and superficial fasciae were sutured. **d** View immediately after dermal sutures and superficial sutures were placed. **e** View of the postoperative taping fixation that was used to stabilize the wound and protect it from extrinsic mechanical forces. **f** View 2 years after surgery. The anterior sheath of the rectus abdominis muscle was strongly sutured. The wound edges were smoothly elevated so that they attached naturally to each other. Dermal sutures could then be placed

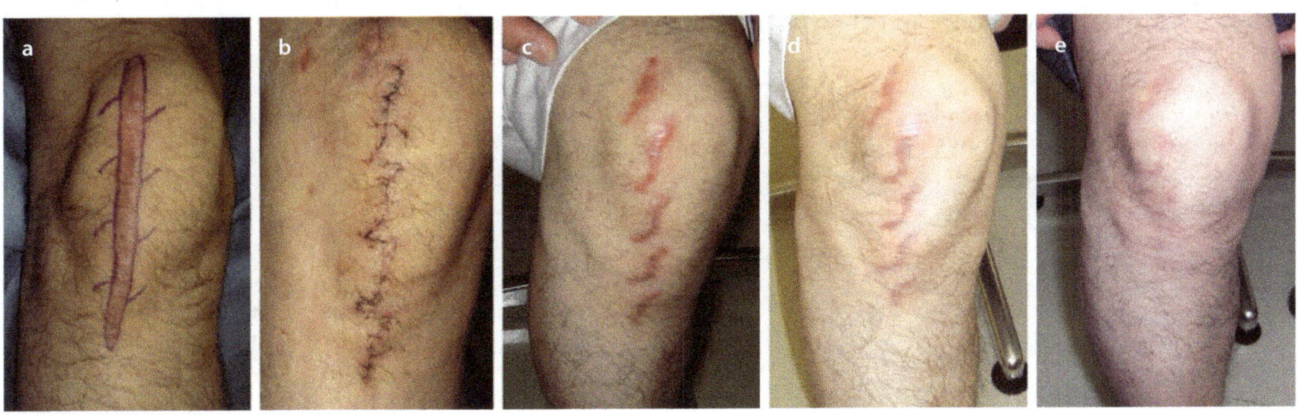

◘ **Fig.** Knee joint scar revision. **a** Preoperative appearance of the scar and the design of the incisions and Z-plasties. **b** View immediately after the operation. **c** View 3 months after surgery. **d** View 6 months after surgery. **e** View 1 year after surgery. In the case of limb surgery, it is difficult to place deep tissue sutures. Therefore, it is necessary to dissipate the tension on the wound by using zigzag line suturing methods such as the Z-plasty: this approach segments the scar and thereby releases its tension. This in turn causes the chronic tension-induced inflammation that is driving pathological scar growth to wane over time

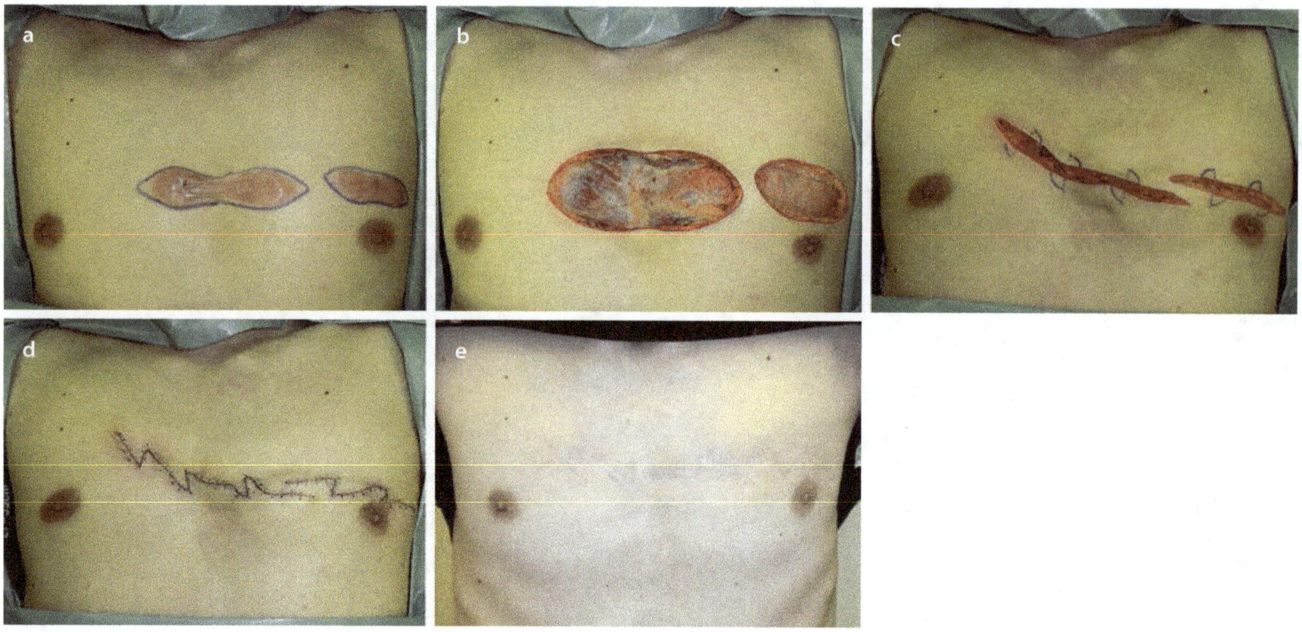

Fig. Anterior chest keloid treatment using tension reduc-tion sutures, Z-plasties, and postoperative radiotherapy. **a** Preopera-tive appearance of the keloid and the design of the incisions. **b** View after the scar and fatty tissues were removed. **c** View immediately after the deep and superficial fascial sutures were placed and the Z-plasties were designed. **d** View immediately after the dermal sutures and superficial sutures were placed. **e** View 2 years after surgery. In cases of keloid revision surgery, great care is needed to decrease the powerful chronic inflammation that is driving the growth of the scar. A combination of tension reduction sutures, Z-plasty, and postoperative radiotherapy can effectively prevent keloid recurrence after revision surgery

Conclusion

All four phases of wound healing are influenced by mechanical forces. These mechanical forces provoke chronic inflammation of the dermis and cause pathological scars. Dermal sutures do not effectively reduce tension on the dermis: rather, to achieve this, we must access much deeper structures, namely, the superficial and deep fascia, and suture them. Another way to prevent pathological scar formation in high-tension areas is to use zigzag suturing techniques such as the Z-plasty.

Take-Home Messages

- The risk of pathological scarring can be greatly reduced by using subcutaneous/fascial tensile reduction sutures.
- Dermal sutures do not effectively reduce tension on the dermis: rather, to achieve this, we must access much deeper structures, namely, the superficial and deep fascia, and suture them.
- A study showed that deep fascia suturing reduced about 90% of the tension on the wound edge, while superficial fascia suturing reduced the remaining 10%.
- Z-plasty is particularly suitable for joint or limb surgery because the fatty tissues layers in these areas are thin: this means that it is difficult to find the superficial fascia and apply the subcutaneous/fascial tensile reduction sutures.

References

1. Levenson SM, Geever EF, Crowley LV, Oates JF III, Berard CW, Rosen H. The healing of rat skin wounds. Ann Surg. 1965;161:293–308.
2. Ogawa R. Mechanobiology of scarring. Wound Repair Regen. 2011;19(Suppl 1):s2–9.
3. Harn HI, Ogawa R, Hsu CK, Hughes MW, Tang MJ, Chuong CM. The tension biology of wound healing. Exp Dermatol. 2017.
4. Ogawa R, Akaishi S, Huang C, Dohi T, Aoki M, Omori Y, Koike S, Kobe K, Akimoto M, Hyakusoku H. Clinical applications of basic research that shows reducing skin tension could prevent and treat abnormal scarring: the importance of fascial/subcutaneous tensile reduction sutures and flap surgery for keloid and hypertrophic scar reconstruction. J Nippon Med Sch. 2011;78(2):68–76.
5. Arima J, Dohi T, Kuribayashi S, Akaishi S, Ogawa R. Z-plasty and postoperative radiation therapy for anterior chest wall keloids: an analysis of 141 patients. Plast Reconstr Surg Glob Open. IN PRESS 2019.

14

Objective Assessment Tools: Physical Parameters in Scar Assessment

M. E. H. Jaspers and P. Moortgat

Contents

Background

Several types of problematic scars can be identified: hypertrophic scars, keloids, contractures, and adherent scars (◘ Fig. 17.1). All these scars require specialized treatment. However, the need for innovation and novel treatment is paramount to further reduce the burden of these scars and to ultimately attain scarless healing. Critical to the development of novel treatment modalities are objective assessment tools that evaluate whether scar treatment is effective and successful. Secondly, assessment tools can be used to monitor the scar's response to interventions. One important aspect to take into account when using tools in clinical practice is to ascertain that the chosen tool is "clinimetrically approved."

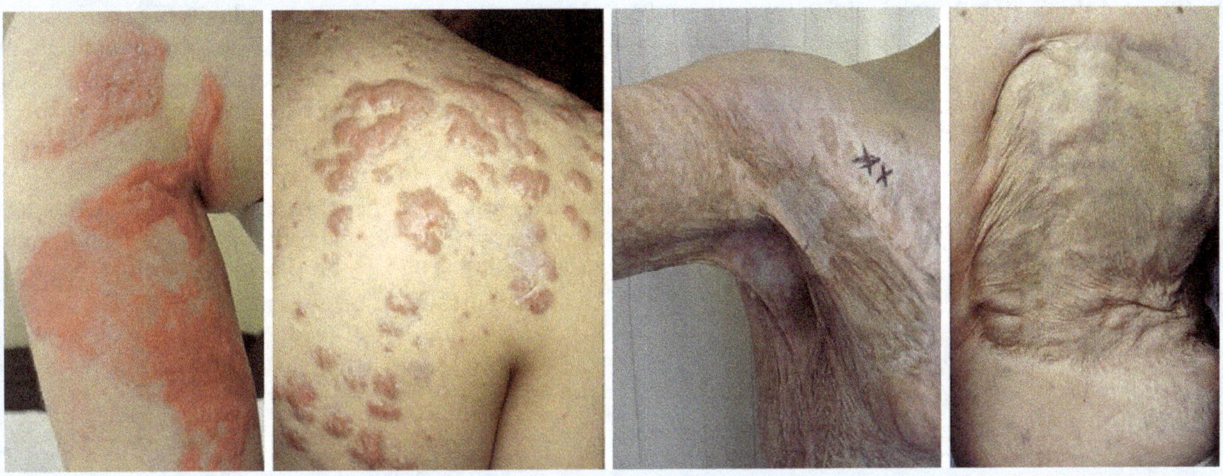

◘ **Fig.** Several types of pathological scars. **a** Hypertrophic scar on the right upper arm, **b** keloids on the right scapula and shoulder, **c** contracture of the right axilla, and **d** widespread adherent scarring on a patient's back and spine. (Reproduced with permission from 'Beyond the skin, new insights in burn care'" by M. E. H. Jaspers, 2017. ISBN: 978-94-6233-852-4. © All rights reserved)

Clinimetrics

The discipline of "clinimetrics" (i.e., measurement in medicine) aims to improve the quality of measurements by assessment of the properties of existing tools or by development of new tools. Before implementation of a new measurement tool in either clinical practice or in research can be considered, two essential properties need to be evaluated: reliability and validity. All measurement tools are required to produce reliable and valid scores.

The general definition of reliability is "the degree to which the measurement is free from measurement error" [1, 2]. In addition, there is an extended definition of reliability: "the extent to which scores for patients who have not changed are the same for repeated measurements under several conditions," which makes clear that repeated measurements are a key point. The variation that may arise between repeated measurements decreases the reliability. This can be attributed either to the measurement tool, the persons performing the measurement, the patients undergoing the measurement, or the circumstances under which the measurements are performed. The measurement error comprises both the systematic and random error of a patient's score that cannot be attributed to true changes in the scar. So, parameters of measurement error are relevant for the measurements of changes in scar status. Moreover, these parameters are of great value for clinicians as they are expressed in the units of measurement, which facilitates interpretation. Finally, to determine whether changes are clinically relevant, the minimally important change (MIC) can be calculated, which is defined as "the smallest change in score which patients, clinicians or relevant others perceive as important" [2, 3]. To monitor the scar of an individual patient, it is of paramount importance that the MIC is smaller than the measurement error of the tool.

Validity is defined as "the degree to which an instrument truly measures what it purports to measure" [1]. Validity can be divided into three types: content validity, construct validity, and criterion validity. Content validity focuses on the correspondence of the content of the measurement tool with the construct that is intended to measure. Content validity is assessed qualitatively during development by pretesting, expert opinion, and literature review. Construct validity is applicable in situations in which there is no gold standard, and therefore this type of validity refers to whether the measurement tool provides the expected scores, based on knowledge about the construct. Criterion validity focuses on the correspondence of the (new) measurement tool with the gold standard (i.e., criterion). In theory, the gold standard is a perfectly valid assessment, but this rarely exists in practice. Also in scar care, it is challenging to identify a suitable criterion. In light of this chapter and of using tools in the future, it is important to take this into account and to be aware of the reliability and validity of the gold standard or comparator instrument itself.

Over the years, the number of available tools has increased rapidly. However, it is important to realize that not every scar parameter can be assessed and that the use of technologies and corresponding terminology is not standardized yet. Hereby, an overview is provided for three important physical scar parameters that can be assessed by (noninvasive) objective tools: color, elasticity, and perfusion.

Color

Erythema and Pigmentation

When looking at hypertrophic scars, one could ask the question: Which feature makes these scars so obvious and therefore problematic? Besides increased thickness or an irregular surface, the amount of erythema and pigmentation appear to have a major impact on the judgment of scar quality by both clinicians and patients. Moreover, the assessment of erythema could be imperative to predict the end of the remodeling phase [4]. Therefore, color measurements are an essential part of scar evaluation, and the associated measurement outcomes are common parameters in scar research.

It is beyond the scope of this chapter to state the underlying causes of the formation of erythema and pigmentation. However, it is important to realize how these aberrant scar features are constituted, to consequentially assess them in the right way. Moreover, it is underlined that the terminology regarding color measurements is not standardized yet. In clinical practice and in research, the measurement outcomes blood flow, scar color, erythema, and redness are used interchangeably or often replaced by the umbrella term "vascularization," which is not appropriate [5].

For the purpose of clarity, it is beneficial to provide a detailed description of every feature when assessed by a certain tool. Erythema is a complex characteristic that may be defined as the level of oxygenated hemoglobin measured at 660 nm, which shows to have a correlation with subjectively assessed redness [5]. Furthermore, scar color is also constituted by the amount of pigmentation, expressed by the outcome measurement melanin.

Reflectance Spectroscopy

Reflectance spectroscopy has been in use for over 60 years to assess skin color. At present, many affordable handheld devices are available that can easily be used in daily clinical settings. The most commonly used principles for measuring scar color are tristimulus reflectance colorimetry and narrow-band reflectance spectrophotometry. Both principles determine color by measuring the intensity of reflected light of specific wavelengths. The main chromophores in human scar tissue, hemoglobin and melanin, are primary determinants of the color. It has to be taken into account that these chromophores can be measured separately, but may influence each other. It is suggested that a scar with high hemoglobin values can mask the amount of melanin and vice versa.

Tristimulus Colorimetry

Tools based on the principle of tristimulus reflectance colorimetry are the Chroma Meter CR-400 (Konica Minolta Sensing Inc., Osaka, Japan) and the Skin-Colorimeter CL 400 (Courage and Khazaka electronic GmbH, Köln, Germany). This principle was developed to objectively represent color in a manner analogous to how color is perceived by the human eye. As well as with narrow-band spectrophotometry, white light is sent to the skin by LEDs in a probe. Light is scattered in all directions whereas the light reflected from the skin or scar is measured through three particular wavelength filters and expressed accordingly. This technique expresses XYZ-values, which can be calculated into RGB (red/green/blue) values or the related three L∗a∗b components: L∗ (brightness), a∗ (amount of red-green), and b∗ (amount of yellow-blue) [6, 7]. These components are based on the color system of the Commission International d'Eclairage (CIE) Lab system.

Concerning the clinimetric properties, the parameter LAB2 by the Colorimeter shows and ICC of 0.95 for the interrater reliability [6]. The Chroma Meter was first investigated on *healthy skin*, showing ICC values >0.92 for all parameters (L∗, a∗, and b∗) during measurements by two observers, thereby reporting the interrater reliability [8]. The latter study also reports standard error of measurement (SEM) values, which are between 0.38 and 0.59 and thereby low. In addition, a preceding type of the Chroma Meter (CR-221) was evaluated on scar tissue and shows ICC values >0.73 for a single measurement by one observer (test–retest) and ICC values >0.91 when the measurements of four observers are averaged [9]. In this study, SEM values are between 1.26 and 4.33, which is rather high.

Narrow-Band Spectrophotometry

Narrow-band tools are based on the fact that hemoglobin and melanin show different spectral curves for the absorption of light. The tools offer read-out of erythema and melanin values as well as CIE L∗a∗b values. The erythema and melanin index values are based on the differences in light absorption of red and green by hemoglobin and melanocytes, respectively. The erythema index is defined as: E = 100 × log (intensity of reflected red light/intensity of reflected green light) and the melanin index can be defined as: M = 100 × log (1/intensity of reflected red light). It has to be taken into account that the index values can be measured separately, but may influence each other.

In the DSM III ColorMeter (Cortex Technology, Hadsund, Denmark) this is achieved by two light-emitting diodes (LEDs) (green 568 nm and red 655 nm) that illuminate a surface and record the intensity of reflected light using a photodetector. The Mexameter MX 18 (Courage and Khazaka electronic GmbH, Köln, Germany) uses 16 light-emitting diodes that emit light at three wavelengths (green: 568 nm; red 660 nm; infrared 880 nm), where after the reflected light is measured by a receiver unit. Erythema is measured by the green and red wavelengths, whereas melanin is determined by the red and infrared wavelengths. Readings are expressed between 0 and 1000, corresponding to white and black respectively.

Both tools are examined in several clinical studies and provide reliable data on scars [10]. The most common reliability parameter examined is the intraclass correlation coefficient (ICC) for ratings performed by several observers (i.e., interrater reliability). Erythema measured by the Mexameter shows an ICC between 0.82 and 0.97 and for the DSM II ColorMeter an ICC of 0.84 is reported [6, 11]. In addition, the DSM II ColorMeter also offers read-out of CIE L∗a∗b values, which will be described in the next paragraph. Investigation of the parameter a∗ by the DSM II ColorMeter shows an ICC of 0.94 [6]. Unfortunately, information on parameters concerning the measurement error of these color tools is lacking. Furthermore, attempts are made to assort the most *valid* parameter of each tool [6]. However, as previously mentioned, it is often difficult to appoint an adequate comparator instrument that exactly measures the same feature (i.e., construct) of a scar as the tool under study. This is underscored by the poor correlations reported between color-measuring tools and scar assessment scales [10, 12]. Overall, the correlation between erythema assessed by a tool and redness assessed by a scar assessment scale is between 0.4 and 0.7 [5, 11, 12].

Ultimately, the DermaLab Combo (Cortex Technology, Hadsund, Denmark) will be mentioned here. This device offers a combination of measurement possibilities. The color probe uses the principle of reflectance spectrometry to measure scar color and all above-mentioned parameters can be reproduced: erythema, melanin, L∗, a∗, and b∗. As previously stated, the parameters erythema and a∗ can be used to indicate scar erythema. A weak to moderate correlation is found between erythema values and redness scored by a subjective tool and in terms of reliability, the ICC varies between 0.66 and 0.84 for measurements by two observers, whereas the test–retest reliability is even lower: 0.29–0.42 [13, 14].

Several studies show that erythema index scores decline over time [15, 16] and all clinical studies report that distinction between scar tissue and healthy skin can be made with color-measuring tools. Therefore, it is stated that objective color measurements appear reliable to determine change over time in a (heterogeneous) study population, which merits their scientific use. However, for the clinical follow up of an individual patient, SEM values need to be very low. Moreover, concerning the validity, it is challenging to define the exact measured construct, which is becoming even more complex given that the tools can reflect various parameters. This has to be taken into account when a color-measuring tool is selected to monitor the scar's response to interventions.

From a practical point of view, it is important to notice that pressure on the scars will change the color toward the white spectrum. Therefore, users are required to lightly put a color-measuring tool on the scar to reduce the influence of pressure. Another limitation, which also accounts for elasticity-measuring tools, is the small size of the probe's measurement area. To comprehensively present the color or elasticity of a scar as a whole, the proposed solution is to work with a predefined algorithm, covering several measurement areas within the borders of one scar. For example, by drawing an imaginary line through the horizontal and vertical axis of the scar, resulting in five measurement points: one on the intersection of both lines and four halfway the intersection and the border of the scar. In this way, also selection bias by the observer is avoided.

Spectrophotometric Analysis (SIA)

To provide information on color outside the visible spectrum, relating to deeper structures of the scar, infrared light can be used. Spectrophotometric intracutaneous analysis (SIA) can be performed via a clinical device, the SIAscope, which utilizes a probe that exerts radiation ranging from 400 to 1000 nm and produces 8 narrowband spectrally filtered images of the skin. These images are processed by software algorithms and allow subsequently visualization and quantification of blood, collagen, and melanin. It already has been used to monitor changes in scar tissue in response to treatment [17].

Elasticity

The second physical parameter that causes poor functional scar quality is a loss of elasticity, which is due to increased collagen synthesis and lack of elastin in the dermal layer. However, as will be emphasized in this paragraph, certain tools quantify the opposite of elasticity, which is tissue *hardness*.

Cutometer

The Cutometer MPA-580 is designed to measure elasticity (i.e., elevation) of the upper skin or scar layer using a predefined negative pressure setting, which mechanically deforms the skin. Negative pressure (i.e., vacuum) is instantly created in the device where after the skin is drawn into the aperture of the probe (◘ Fig. 17.2). Subsequently, after a defined time, the skin is released. Inside the probe, the vertical deformation of the skin is determined by a noncontact optical measuring system. This optical measuring system consists of a light source and a light receptor and two prisms facing each other that project the light from transmitter to receptor. The light intensity varies due to the penetration depth of the skin. The resistance of the skin to the negative pressure (rigidity) and its ability to return to its original position (elasticity) are displayed as curves (penetration depth in mm/time) in real time during the measurement. This measurement principle allows data collection on the elastic and mechanical properties of skin or scar surface and enables objective quantification.

The Cutometer is a feasible device containing a probe, which is available in several aperture sizes (2, 4, 6 and 8 mm Ø) to fit different skin sites and different study requirements (◘ Fig. 17.2). The smaller apertures mainly measure the elastic properties of the epidermis. With a larger aperture (6 and 8 mm), the measurement also comprises the dermal component, which is designated for scar assessment. As with the color-measuring tools, it is important to ensure light contact is made between the scar and the probe to avoid alterations in outcome measure. Measurements can be monitored as live curves on the screen of a connected laptop. The software of the Cutometer MPA 580 allows calculation of many parameters of interest from the different portions of the measurement curve. The two most relevant parameters are labelled as R and U (◘ Figs. 17.3 and 17.4).

R-Parameters:

- R0: Behavior of the skin/scar to force (rigidity), maximum amplitude of the curve in mm
- R1/R4: Ability of the skin/scar to return to its original state, minimum amplitude after relaxation
- R2: Viscoelasticity: Resistance to mechanical force versus ability of returning in %
- R3/R9: Tiring effect (fatigue) visible with repeated suction/relaxation
- R5: Net elasticity: Elastic portion of the suction part versus the elastic portion of the relaxation part in %

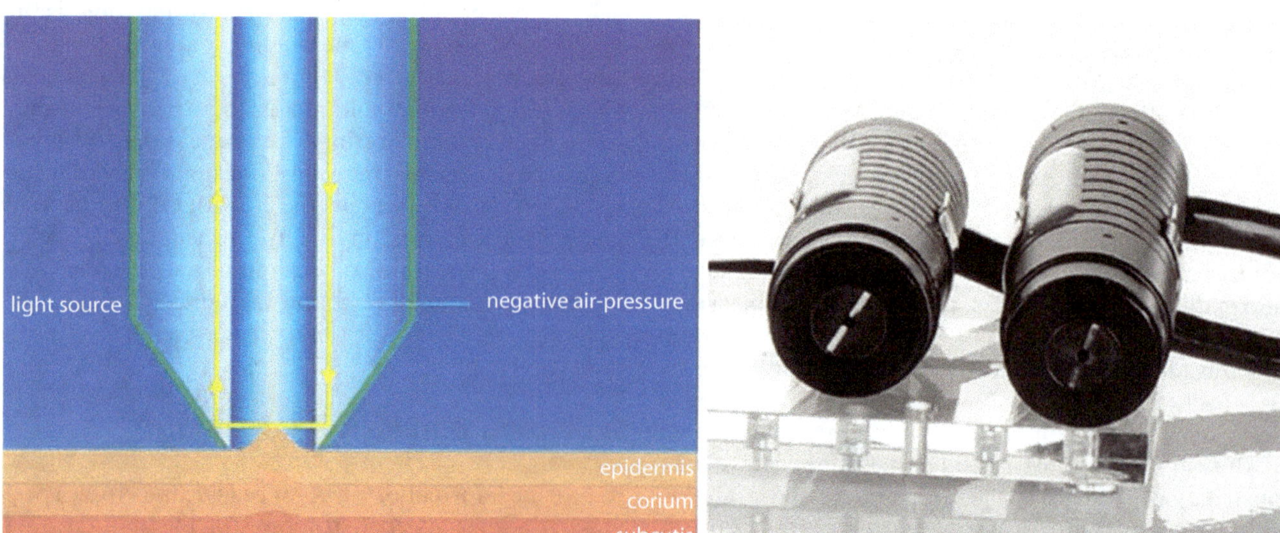

◘ **Fig.** Left: measuring principle of the Cutometer. Right: different aperture sizes of the probes. Reused with permission from Courage + Khazaka electronic GmbH. © All rights reserved

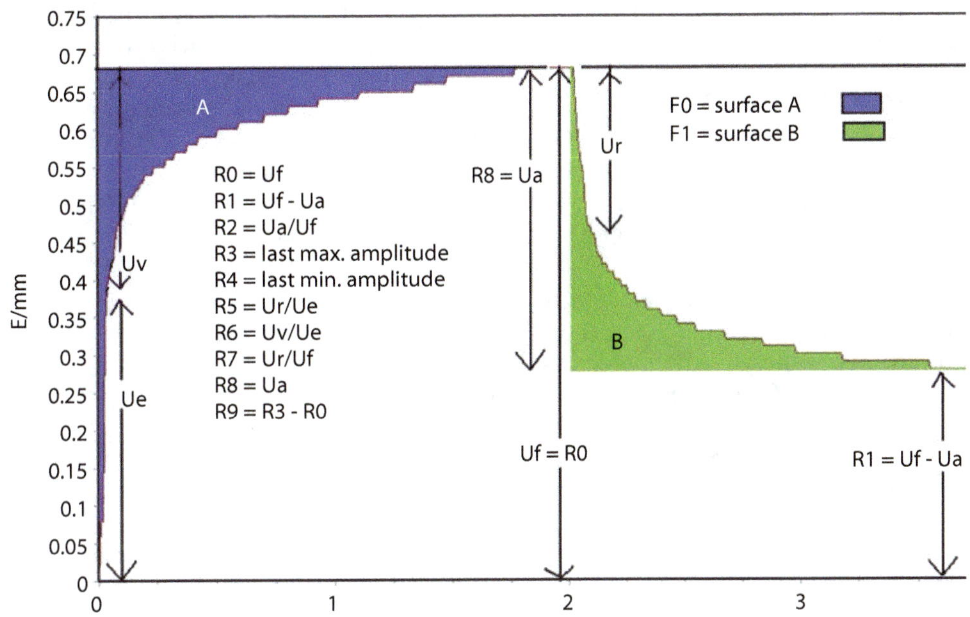

Fig. The R-parameters of the Cutometer. Reused with permission from Courage + Khazaka electronic GmbH. © All rights reserved

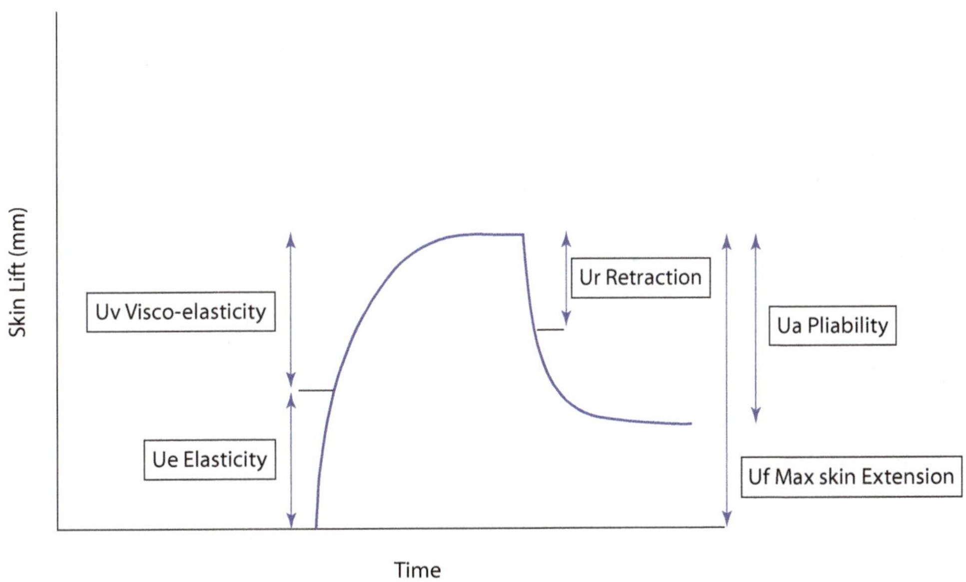

Fig. The U-parameters of the Cutometer

- R6: Portion of the viscoelasticity of the curve in %
- R7: Portion of the elasticity compared to the complete curve in %
- R8: Complete relaxation after the pressure is removed in mm

U-Parameters:

- Uf (maximal skin extension): Deformation at the end of the vacuum period
- Ue (elasticity): Extent of skin stretching within the first 0.1 s of the vacuum period
- Ua (pliability): Difference between the maximum deformation and the deformation after 1 s of normal pressure
- Ur (retraction): Relaxation of the skin within the first 0.1 s after the ending of the vacuum, that is, the ability of the skin to return to its initial position after deformation and is related to the function of elastic fibers
- Uv (viscoelasticity): Difference between the deformation after the 0.1 s and the maximal deformation

The different parameters and their terms (i.e., elasticity, skin extension, pliability, retraction, and viscoelasticity) suggest that each parameter measures a different aspect of skin or scar deformation. However, the parameters are highly correlated when tested on scars, hence, a single parameter is sufficient to use in the evaluation of scar elasticity (see below) [18].

Clinimetric Properties

The reliability of a single measurement performed by a single observer is good for extensibility (Uf) and elasticity (Ue) and ranges $r = 0.74–0.76$. For viscoelasticity, pliability, and retraction the reliability is low to moderate: $r = 0.35–0.69$. The Coefficient of Variation (CV = S.E.meas/mean × 100) for measurements on scars, based on the measurements of four observers, shows the lowest variation for extensibility (22.5%), whereas the highest variation is calculated for viscoelasticity measurements (36.0%) [18]. The concurrent validity was estimated by calculating the correlation between subjective evaluation of pliability and each of the Cutometer parameters. The correlations were moderate ($r > 0.46$) and statistically significant for each parameter except for viscoelasticity for which the correlation was low.

In general, it is stated that the reliability of the 2 mm probe is worse than the reliability of larger probes, because the small probe only reflects low values (small skin deformation). This is easily explained by the fact that the ICC or correlation is highly influenced by a wide range in measured values and by a heterogeneous population. So, when higher values or a range of values within a population are measured, this positively affects reliability as expressed by relative parameters. Of all parameters, either maximal skin extension (R0/Uf) or elasticity (Ue) appears to be influenced the least by variations in force applied to the probe and therefore it is the most reliable parameter to detect change in scar elasticity over time or after treatment.

DermaLab

The DermaLab elasticity probe (Cortex Technology, Hadsund, Denmark), which is the successor of the Dermaflex, consists of a light plastic probe that is much smaller than that of the Cutometer. This probe is attached to the skin using double-sided adhesive rings to form a closed chamber. Within this chamber, two narrow beams of light run at different heights parallel to the skin surface and serve as elevation detectors. A controlled vacuum is created in the closed chamber in over 30–60 s. In contrast to the Cutometer, the DermaLab probe measures the amount of suction required (in megapascal, MPa) to achieve an elevation of the skin of 1.5 mm. In pronounced adherent scars, this may cause a problem, as the scar is sometimes too stiff to be elevated sufficiently to reach the level of the detectors. The DermaLab shows an excellent ICC for test–retest reliability on scars (0.76–0.91); however, on healthy skin the ICC is much lower (ICC 0.45) [14].

Both the DermaLab and the Cutometer show advances of being a "hub," to which other measurement probes can be attached. The DermaLab Combo, for example, provides several probes, considering nine skin parameters (e.g., elasticity, color, transepidermal water loss, temperature), including ultrasound measurement of dermal scar thickness.

Tonometers

Tonometry works by exerting pressure on the skin and therefore quantifies predominantly firmness or hardness of tissue. Two types of tonometers can be distinguished: one type is based on air that flows through the system, which is blocked at a certain pressure (e.g., the Tissue Tonometer), and the second type provides an indentation load in the vertical direction (e.g., the Durometer). The Tissue Tonometer (Flinders Biomedical Engineering, Adelaide, Australia) is a weight-loaded device that exerts pressure directly on the area to be measured. The weight drives a blunt probe into the tissue with a tissue deformation as a result. This tissue deformation can be measured in millimeters, with a sensitivity of 0.01 mm. The readings are directly proportional to the firmness of the tissue being measured.

The Tissue Tonometer shows good intra-observer reliability, but a moderate correlation ($r = 0.44–0.46$) with the pliability score of a subjective scoring system (the VSS scale) is found. Additionally, the measurement requires a contralateral reference point, making it a relative measure [Lye 2006]. Another study, using a modified Tissue Tonometer, shows excellent interobserver reliability (ICC = 0.95) for healthy skin, accompanied by a low SEM of 0.025 mm [19]. A significant difference between scars and normal tissue was also demonstrated in the latter study. The Durometer (Rex Gauge Company, Inc., Glenview, Ill.) also shows good ICCs for the interobserver reliability (0.82–0.91) in one study, however, this is on sclerodermal skin [20].

Important to mention is that tonometers are influenced by the hardness of underlying tissue, which may limit the compression of the skin. This has to be taken into account when measuring locations where bone structures are situated directly under the area of interest. Possibly, measurements in these areas are not reflecting the condition of the skin/scar but instead of the underlying structure. Another shortcoming of tonometers include the need to place the device accurately, which must be within 5° of upright position to measure correctly.

Perfusion

Hypertrophic scars result from a wide array of derailed wound healing processes. It is suggested that new blood vessel formation, mainly apparent as angiogenic sprouting of preexisting blood vessels, is an essential process in the development of hypertrophic scars. Therefore, several treatment regimens (e.g., laser, pressure garments, and cryotherapy) work by destructing the microvasculature and/or reducing the blood flow. This may result in hypoxia that would lead to fibroblast degeneration and collagen degradation, both enhancing shrinkage of the hypertrophic scar tissue. As a result, it is of interest to measure scar blood flow (i.e., perfusion).

Laser Doppler Imaging

Laser Doppler imaging, a noninvasive flow measurement technique, can be used to quantify and visualize blood flow in scars [15, 21]. Laser Doppler imaging can be divided in the older technique, laser Doppler flowmetry (LDF), in which the fiber optic probe is in contact with the tissue, and the newer laser Doppler imaging (LDI) devices. The working mechanism is based on the Doppler principle. In LDF, a single-point measure of the cutaneous blood flow in a scar is obtained. LDF systems are therefore more limited compared to the other systems and unsuitable to use in larger heterogeneous scars. However, there are currently modern and high performance LDF systems such as the moorVMS-LDF (Moor Instruments Ltd., Axminster, United Kingdom) or the PeriFlux 5000 (Perimed AB, Järfälla, Sweden) that are ideal for laboratory or scientific use. In LDI, laser light directed at moving erythrocytes in sampled tissue exhibits a frequency change, which is photo detected and processed to generate a line-by-line color-coded map that is proportional to the amount of perfusion in the tissue. After completion of a LDI measurement, data can be analyzed offline using software to calculate the blood flow automatically, where after it is expressed in perfusion units (PU).

To assess blood flow in a scar, the moorLDI Imaging System (Moor Instruments Ltd., Axminster, United Kingdom) can be used. Previous studies show that hypertrophic scars sustain an elevated blood flow compared to normal skin [15, 22]. Another clinical study also presents a statistically significant increase in blood flow values of scars compared to healthy skin [5]. In more detail, the latter study shows increased LDI blood flow values in 29/32 included patients. Interestingly, this study also compares the association between the outcomes of LDI and colorimetry using the DSM II ColorMeter. The results indicate that blood flow and erythema values are not correlated. During measurements of 32 hypertrophic scars, a widespread in erythema values is observed, whereas the accompanying blood flow values are mostly beneath 300 PU and thereby low. These data are in agreement with a previous study, presenting that erythema (measured using the skin-colorimeter expressing L∗a∗b index values) is associated with blood flow, but this correlation is not consistent at different test moments [4]. As a result, it is concluded that LDI and colorimetry are non-interchangeable measurement tools.

LDI can be a valuable adjunct in the research setting, where it might be useful to monitor scar development and/or response to treatment that is directed at lowering blood flow. However, although new laser Doppler instruments became available over the last years, it is important to keep in mind that the tool has some limitations in terms of feasibility (e.g., high cost, long assessment time, and moderate ease of use). Therefore, LDI seems less suitable for the follow-up of scars in daily practice.

Laser Speckle Imaging

Laser speckle imaging (LSI) or laser speckle perfusion imaging (LSPI) are alternative perfusion monitoring techniques that generate high-resolution images of tissue in a shorter assessment time than LDI. In addition, these devices provide the possibility to zoom in with increased resolution of a smaller area of interest. The moorFLPI-2 blood flow imager (Moor Instruments Ltd., Axminster, United Kingdom) and the PeriCam PSI (Perimed AB, Järfälla, Sweden) both use the laser speckle contrast technique to deliver real-time high-resolution blood flow images. The latter system contains an invisible near infrared laser (785 nm), spreading the beam over the area of interest by a diffuser, creating a speckle pattern. Subsequently, blood perfusion is calculated by analyzing the variations (i.e., interference) in the speckle pattern. High values reflect high blood flow and should thereby indicate immature or hypertrophic scars.

A clinical study comparing the ability of LSPI with LDI in determining and monitoring hypertrophic scar perfusion shows a positive correlation ($r^2 = 0.86$) [23]. Moreover, in terms of feasibility, the LSPI device demonstrates a faster scan time and higher resolution, which may be an advantage for usage in clinical practice. Also, reactions to mechanical or pharmacological interventions can be studied nearly real time, allowing a dynamic way of studying scars. Perfusion rates within keloids are also assessed by LSI, showing significantly higher perfusion in keloids and adjacent skin compared with nonadjacent healthy skin [24]. However, a thorough clinimetric evaluation of LSI in scars is currently not available.

Conclusion

Color, elasticity, and perfusion are scar characteristics with a high clinical relevance. Two features, erythema and pigmentation, determine the color of the scar. Erythema is a complex characteristic that may be defined as the level of oxygenated hemoglobin measured at 660 nm. Pigmentation is often referred to as the level of melanin, which can be excessively present (hyperpigmentation) or underrepresented (hypopigmentation). Reflectance spectroscopy is the most widely used measurement technique to assess scar color. Perfusion of vascularization and scar color are often bracketed together but both represent totally different features. The mixture of terms can also be found in literature where vascularization is described as scar color, blood flow, the presence of microvessels, as well as the amount of redness [9, 12, 15, 25]. Conform definitions in several dictionaries and physiology textbooks, we would like to propose that vascularization is defined as the formation of blood vessels and capillaries in living tissue, which reflects a process. The presence of microvessels is a physical result of this process, and blood flow fulfils the functional role of perfusion. Scar redness is likely to be a derivative of all features that is assessed subjectively. For the purpose of clarity, it would be beneficial to provide a detailed description of every feature when assessed in research as well as in clinical practice, as we feel that the various scar features cannot be generalized into the umbrella term "vascularization." The term elasticity is most probably related to the lack of elastin in the dermal layer of scar tissue, but can also be considered as an umbrella term including extensibility, pliability, or suppleness of the scar. The most reliable assessment technique here measures vertical elasticity or extensibility by means of suction.

All tools are able to differentiate between scar tissue and healthy skin; however, this can also easily be determined by subjective evaluation. Objective tools should be able to monitor an individual patient in clinical practice, thereby distinguishing small scar changes. Thus, the measurement error of the tool must be smaller than the desired scar change to be measured. Taking into account reliability, patient friendliness, and feasibility in terms of cost and portability, a recommended panel of devices for the assessment of color, elasticity, and perfusion of scars consists of the DSM III ColorMeter for scar color, the Cutometer for scar elasticity and laser speckle imaging to assess scar perfusion.

Take-Home Messages

- A range of handheld tools is available to objectively assess physical scar parameters.
- When using a tool in clinical practice or for scientific use, take the clinimetric properties into account.
- To monitor scars in an individual patient, it is of paramount importance that the minimally important change (MIC) is smaller than the measurement error of the tool.
- It is showed that erythema and blood flow are not directly related to each other and therefore seem two different scar parameters (i.e., constructs).
- It is essential to provide a precise description of which scar parameter is aimed to assess.
- To assess scar color, the most widely used tool is the DSM III ColorMeter, offering read-out of erythema and melanin index values as well as CIE L*a*b values.
- Elasticity can be best measured using the Cutometer, reflecting absolute and relative parameters of which Uf and Ue are recommended.
- To assess scar perfusion, laser Doppler imaging and laser Speckle imaging are available.

References

1. Mokkink LB, Terwee CB, Patrick DL, Alonso J, Stratford PW, Knol DL, et al. The COSMIN study reached international consensus on taxonomy, terminology, and definitions of measurement properties for health-related patient-reported outcomes. J Clin Epidemiol. 2010;63(7):737–45.
2. De Vet HCW, Terwee CB, Mokkink LB, Knol DL. Measurement in medicine. A practical guide. 1st ed. Cambridge: Cambridge Univ Press; 2011.
3. Crosby RD, Kolotkin RL, Williams GR. Defining clinically meaningful change in health-related quality of life. J Clin Epidemiol. 2003;56(5):395–407.
4. Mermans JF, Peeters WJ, Dikmans R, Serroyen J, van der Hulst RR, Van den Kerckhove E. A comparative study of colour and perfusion between two different post surgical scars. Do the laser Doppler imager and the colorimeter measure the same features of a scar? Skin Res Technol. 2013;19(2):107–14.
5. Jaspers MEH, Stekelenburg CM, Simons JM, Brouwer KM, Vlig M, van den Kerckhove E, et al. Assessing blood flow, microvasculature, erythema and redness in hypertrophic scars: a cross sectional study showing different features that require precise definitions. Burns. 2017;43(5):1044–50.
6. van der Wal M, Bloemen M, Verhaegen P, Tuinebreijer W, de Vet H, van Zuijlen P, et al. Objective color measurements: clinimetric performance of three devices on normal skin and scar tissue. J Burn Care Res. 2013;34(3):e187–94.
7. Chardon A, Cretois I, Hourseau C. Skin colour typology and suntanning pathways. Int J Cosmet Sci. 1991;13(4):191–208.
8. Van den Kerckhove E, Staes F, Flour M, Stappaerts K, Boeckx W. Reproducibility of repeated measurements on healthy skin with Minolta Chromameter CR-300. Skin Res Technol. 2001;7(1):56–9.

9. Draaijers LJ, Tempelman FR, Botman YA, Kreis RW, Middelkoop E, van Zuijlen PP. Colour evaluation in scars: tristimulus colorimeter, narrow-band simple reflectance meter or subjective evaluation? Burns. 2004;30(2):103–7.
10. Deng H, Li-Tsang CWP. Measurement of vascularity in the scar: a systematic review. Burns. 2018;45(6):1253–65.
11. Nedelec B, Correa JA, Rachelska G, Armour A, LaSalle L. Quantitative measurement of hypertrophic scar: interrater reliability and concurrent validity. J Burn Care Res. 2008;29(3):501–11.
12. Verhaegen PD, van der Wal MB, Middelkoop E, van Zuijlen PP. Objective scar assessment tools: a clinimetric appraisal. Plast Reconstr Surg. 2011;127(4):1561–70.
13. Gankande TU, Duke JM, Wood FM, Wallace HJ. Interpretation of the DermaLab Combo(R) pigmentation and vascularity measurements in burn scar assessment: an exploratory analysis. Burns. 2015;41(6):1176–85.
14. Gankande TU, Duke JM, Danielsen PL, DeJong HM, Wood FM, Wallace HJ. Reliability of scar assessments performed with an integrated skin testing device – the DermaLab Combo((R)). Burns. 2014;40(8):1521–9.
15. Oliveira GV, Chinkes D, Mitchell C, Oliveras G, Hawkins HK, Herndon DN. Objective assessment of burn scar vascularity, erythema, pliability, thickness, and planimetry. Dermatol Surg. 2005;31(1):48–58.
16. van der Wal MB, Vloemans JF, Tuinebreijer WE, van de Ven P, van Unen E, van Zuijlen PP, et al. Outcome after burns: an observational study on burn scar maturation and predictors for severe scarring. Wound Repair Regen. 2012;20(5):676–87.
17. Moncrieff M, Cotton S, Claridge E, Hall P. Spectrophotometric intracutaneous analysis: a new technique for imaging pigmented skin lesions. Br J Dermatol. 2002;146(3):448–57.
18. Draaijers LJ, Botman YA, Tempelman FR, Kreis RW, Middelkoop E, van Zuijlen PP. Skin elasticity meter or subjective evaluation in scars: a reliability assessment. Burns. 2004;30(2):109–14.
19. Corica GF, Wigger NC, Edgar DW, Wood FM, Carroll S. Objective measurement of scarring by multiple assessors: is the tissue tonometer a reliable option? J Burn Care Res. 2006;27(4):520–3.
20. Merkel PA, Silliman NP, Denton CP, Furst DE, Khanna D, Emery P, et al. Validity, reliability, and feasibility of durometer measurements of scleroderma skin disease in a multicenter treatment trial. Arthritis Rheum. 2008;59(5):699–705.
21. Bray R, Forrester K, Leonard C, McArthur R, Tulip J, Lindsay R. Laser Doppler imaging of burn scars: a comparison of wavelength and scanning methods. Burns. 2003;29(3):199–206.
22. Ehrlich HP, Kelley SF. Hypertrophic scar: an interruption in the remodeling of repair--a laser Doppler blood flow study. Plast Reconstr Surg. 1992;90(6):993–8.
23. Stewart CJ, Frank R, Forrester KR, Tulip J, Lindsay R, Bray RC. A comparison of two laser-based methods for determination of burn scar perfusion: laser Doppler versus laser speckle imaging. Burns. 2005;31(6):744–52.
24. Liu Q, Wang X, Jia Y, Long X, Yu N, Wang Y, et al. Increased blood flow in keloids and adjacent skin revealed by laser speckle contrast imaging. Lasers Surg Med. 2016;48(4):360–4.
25. Brusselaers N, Pirayesh A, Hoeksema H, Verbelen J, Blot S, Monstrey S. Burn scar assessment: a systematic review of objective scar assessment tools. Burns. 2010;36(8):1157–64.

15

Scar Contractures

Marguerite Guillot Masanovic and Luc Téot

Contents

Introduction

The prevalence of contractures is high, especially after burns and may vary, depending on the age, the depth of the initial burns, and the time between burns and the occurrence of the contractures. Young patients and children are more likely candidates to develop contractures. When skin grafting after burn is performed in due time, the prevalence is lower. Contractures are more likely to occur in more severe burns, flame burns, children, females, on the cervical spine and in the upper extremity. The absence of physiotherapy and an abnormal long period awaiting spontaneous healing without skin grafting will progressively induce severe contractures. This is still frequently observed on the upper limbs in burn patients in developing countries. Early excision and skin grafting is the best option to reduce the incidence of contractures. Other causes of contractures are less frequently observed, but may be seen after trauma or infection, linked to noncompliance, a too long immobilization, a joint destruction, an epiphysiodesis in children. This chapter proposes to give an overview of the functional limitations of the skin contractures and the need for an adapted early rehabilitation program starting during the healing stage and carried on during the next 2 years post burns and other causes of skin limitation.

General Features

Incidence of contractures has been recently analyzed [1, 2] on patients presenting acute burns across or adjacent to the neck, shoulder, elbow, wrist, hip, knee, and ankle. Passive range of motion was measured at 3–6–9–12 months after burn. Limited range of motion of non-operated burned joints was restored back to normal within 6–9 months. From the operated burned joints, 58.6% demonstrated a limited range of motion at 3–6 weeks declining to 20.9% at 12 months. The upper part of the body was affected more often by scar contracture than the lower part. Reconstructive surgery was performed in 13.3% of the operated burned joints. This study confirms that a quick skin grafting is a good option to prevent severe contractures, but not enough to prevent all of them.

Contractures may clinically present with different characteristics, like bands of skin partially limiting the range of joint movements to a complete impossibility to move, all joints being glued in deep stiffness. Contractures are more or less severe, depending if the deep structures (tendons, aponeurosis, subcutaneous muscles, or fascia) are involved in the process, and the type of contracture, static or dynamic.

Skin capacity is particularly limited in burns of the dorsal aspect of the hand, if an adapted rehabilitation program including staged splinting of the hand before, during, and after skin grafting, as well as slow movements during the inflammation stage and more active after some months is not properly done. The usual limitation is observed at the level of the metartarsophalangeal joints (in flexion) and the grip is impacted.

Contractures may variably limit the amplitude of movements, some of them being only observed during full movements, others imposing a severe stiffness and a blockade of any movement. Neck contractures may simply affect the extreme degrees of lateral movements or realize a vertical contracture (chin to thorax) imposing strong difficulties to maintain the horizontal sight, a situation extremely difficult to live with.

Web contractures may limit multidirectional movements on the neck or the shoulder, others will limit opening of orifices (mouth, nostrils, perineal areas) with concentric contractures, a cause of difficulties to feeding.

Contractures may vary along time. An early inflammation is frequently observed in children or young adults after burns, lasting some months especially on mobile areas like the thorax and the upper limb. This situation may be transiently observed during the first 2 years and may disappear afterward. This period should be covered by adapted physiotherapy programs, aiming at an augmented range of movements and a less red skin.

Contractures of the Neck

Neck skin is extremely mobile over the underlying structures. This mobility will be quickly limited in burns, due to a skin retraction linked to wound healing and particularly to the mechanical action of myofibroblasts, but also to the pain during movements inducing a voluntary restriction of movement during the healing stage. These combined factors induce a centripetal retraction and may lead to different situations, ranging from a single line of skin tension in the lateral movements (◘ Fig. 13.1) to severe vertical and horizontal loss of movements. The subcutaneous muscles, embedded in the scarring process,

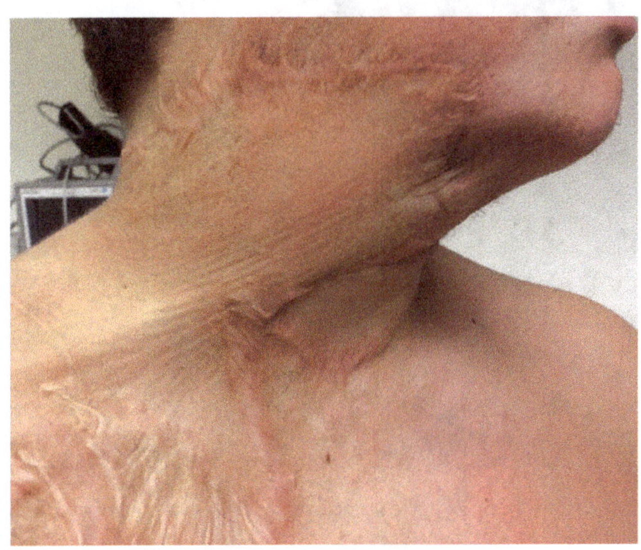

◘ **Fig. 13.1** Neck contracture persistent in spite of several surgical procedures

contribute to skin limitation. In severe situations the horizontal sight may be impacted, bending permanently the neck and imposing a difficult surgery.

Axillar Contractures

Three different areas may be impacted by retractile scars, the anterior and posterior pillars, and the central axilla. Skin contractures may affect any one or the three of these areas, with different possible extensions on the anterior or posterior thorax. The shoulder is mobile anteriorly, posteriorly, and laterally, needing a full skin mobility in all aspects of the region. A large range of functional deficits may be encountered in burns, with a good reactivity to early physiotherapy and specifically to range axilla orthotic, as demonstrated [3] (◘ Figs. 13.2, 13.3, and 13.4).

Hand Contractures

Burns usually affect the dorsal aspect of the hand, with a centripetal retraction impairing the complete combined flexion of all digits together. The deficit in terms of grip may be crucial; other situations may limit one or two digits in flexion. When the situation has become chronic, tendon shortening and bone deformities may be observed, imposing complex surgical procedures including bone shortening, joint arthrodesis, and tendon lengthening to restore function.

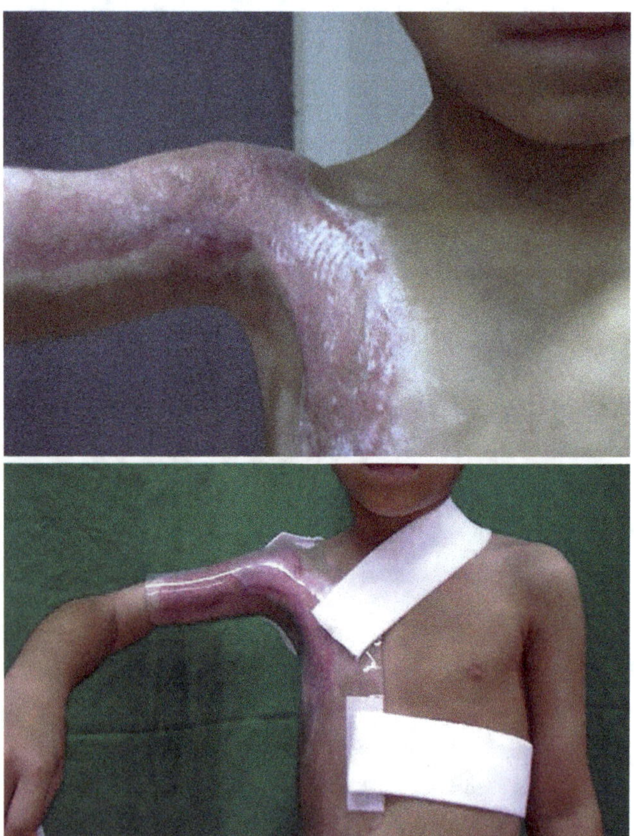

◘ **Figs.** Postburn axillar contracture treated by an orthotic orlen realized at fashion

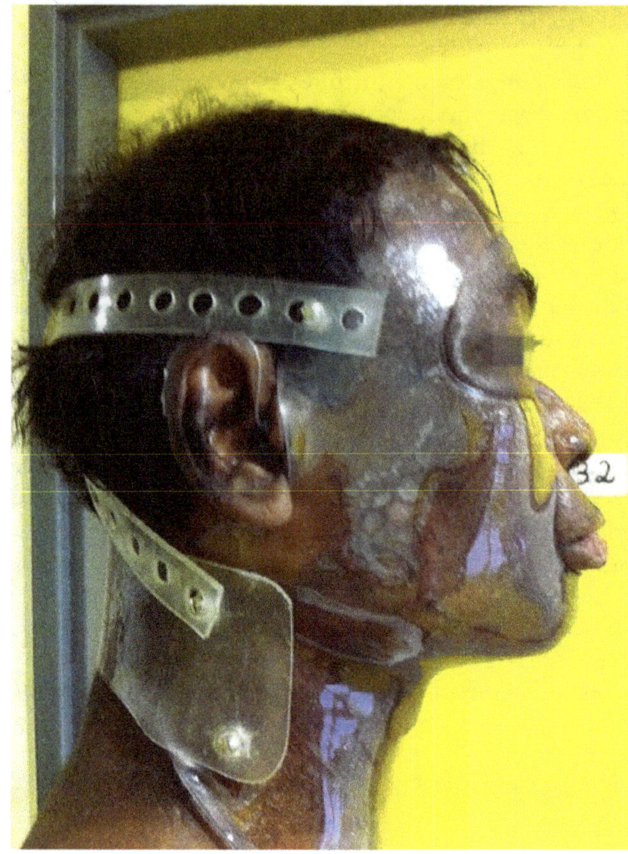

◘ **Fig.** Severe postburn neck contracture on a young female treated by an orthesis worn initially 24/7 during 2 months and then at night

The dorsal aspects of the interdigital webs are frequently involved, with consequences on the separate movements of each digit, a quadrige effect often observed in poorly managed deep burns.

The palmar aspect of the hand is less frequently touched but more frequent in children, but the very deep scarring tissues may sometimes reach more than 2 cm depth, inducing tendons blockade. Usually these severe scars embed totally the underlying structures, nerves, vessels, tendons, and muscles (◘ Fig. 13.5).

Persistent contractures observed in young adults having been submitted to burns that occurred during childhood, with retracted wrists and elbows or completely locked axillas, which sometimes require bone resection or amputation, are less observed now with the development and diffusion of NGO programs acting in underdeveloped countries.

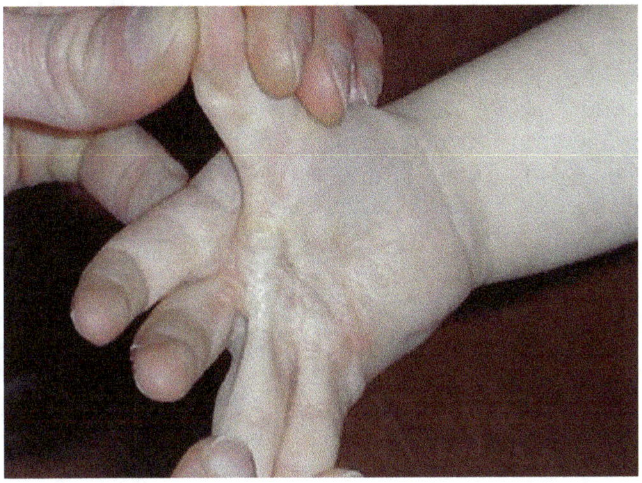

Fig. Palmar contracture embedding the whole palmar area, creating a maximal web between the I and the IV. Surgery is needed

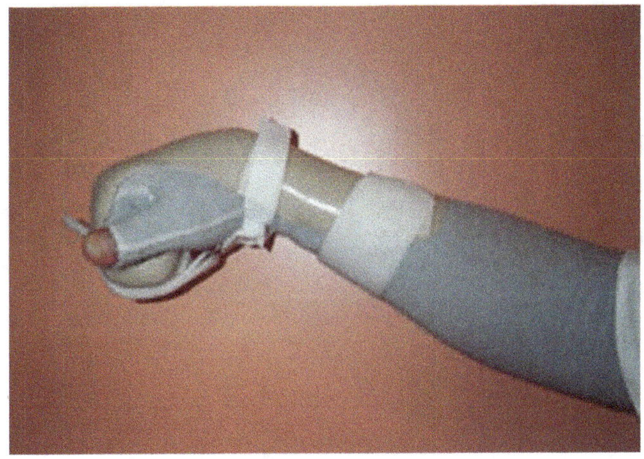

Fig. Hand splint in complete digital flexion used for mechanical tension over the dorsal aspect

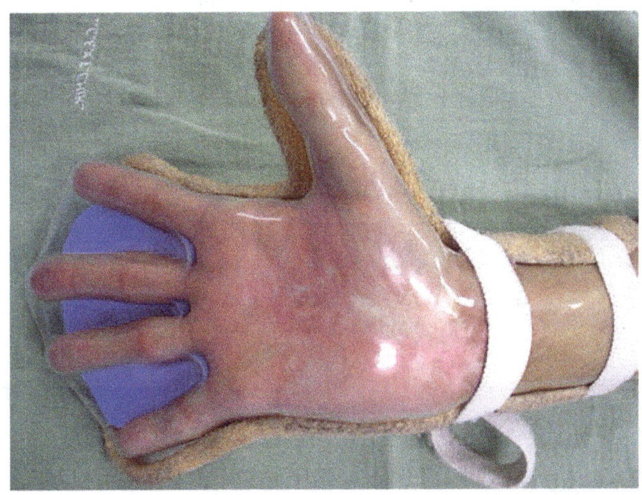

Fig. Hand splint in complete digital extension used for mechanical tension on the palmar aspect. In case of contracture touching both the aspects of the hand, alternative positioning in flexion during night and in extension during the day may be proposed

Other Anatomical Sites of Scar Contractures

Lower limbs may develop contractures at the level of hips (in flexion), knee, and foot (dorsal positioning of toes). These contractures are better managed by an adapted rehabilitation, completed by surgical procedures if needed.

Rehabilitation Programs

During the wound-healing stage, splinting of the burned hands, the neck, the axillar, and the lower limbs are needed to prevent contractures. Most of the burns centers benefit of a specific rehabilitation team included in the organization of the center. Passive movements during the dressing change and positioning of joints into adapted customized splints in position of maximum extension capacity will efficiently limit the development of contractures (Fig. 13.6). Exercise is allowed as soon as the inflammatory period is under control, immobilization being the most anti-inflammatory agent.

After skin closure, active and passive movements will be encouraged but it is essential not to exert an excessive mechanical tension on contractures, relayed and completed by the design of compressive garments, and mechanical compression of the involved areas. Specific rehabilitation centers for severely burned patients exist in some countries, proposing multiprograms to soften the scar, manipulate joints, and efficiently prevent the occurrence of the contractures using positioning, especially on the axillar region, the neck, and the hands (Figs. 13.7 and 13.8).

Pruritus and the risk of stretching are prevented using hydration and drugs. Capsaicin and cooling are frequently used to limit pain and inflammation. These programs are long, painful, and psychologically demanding. A limited compliance of the patients may explain some of the poor results sometimes observed, but most of the patients get benefit of these treatments.

Once the inflammation stage is completed, more active compressive techniques like endermology, motorized skin manipulations (LPG), stretching posture, high power jets, or other types of physiotherapy are proposed, with good results at 2 years. More than 90% of the patients come back to a normal function if the program is done properly.

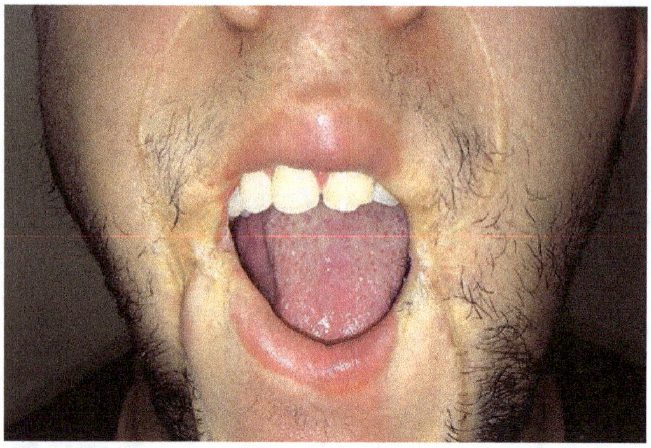

Fig. Bilateral contracture of the mouth web, combined with a red lip loss of substance. Surgery using W–Y-5 plasties, plus advancement of the mucosa will be proposed

Despite clear international recommendations [4] the studies on the modalities of application and the type of splints cover only a limited number of cases, therefore the evidence for these strategies is limited [5].

Surgical Strategies

Contracture release creates a large skin defect, and the aim of surgery is to restore as far as possible a full skin disponibility after surgery and to prevent recurrence.

Z Plasties

Z plasty is the most frequently used surgical technique [6]. Based on the principle of skin disponibility and softness of adjacent areas, the triangles designed by the Z-shape incisions break the linear scar contracture with a new scar without any mechanical tension. The cosmetic result is usually acceptable. Linear contractures are better managed using Z plasties, multiple Z plasties. Web contracture may be treated using W–Y 5 plasties combing 2 Z plasties and an advancement flap, or omega plasties using the contracted skin but needing two small full skin grafts on the edges.

Skin Grafts

Skin grafts are by definition free skin transfers from one site to another without any vascular connection. Depending on their thickness, skin grafts form two different techniques, split-thickness skin grafts (STG) limited to epidermis and a thin layer of dermis, harvested using a dermatome and full-thickness skin grafts (FTG), which include the epidermis and the entire dermis; harvested with a scalpel and needing a defatting before application. The donor sites of STG heal by rapid re-epithelialization (like a superficial abrasion) while the donor site of FTG must be closed primarily for healing, so their use is limited to smaller defects. The main disadvantage of STG is the lack of dermal component, meaning a risk of recurrence higher than when using a flap.

Dermal Substitutes

Since three decades the introduction of acellular dermal substitute has changed the profile of skin grafting. The dermal component brought by the use of collagen (and elastin) inside the dermal substitute limits the secondary retraction of the thin skin graft applied to cover it, even if some shrinking is sometimes observed [7]. Different devices are proposed, with or without elastin, the collagen coming from different animals like cows, sharks, or pigs with different combination with elastin, and with or without a protective film in silicone, depending if the product is immediately covered by skin graft or secondarily after 3 weeks, the device being slowly incorporated in the new dermis before skin coverage. Hori et al. recently compared the contraction capacity, pores size, and shape of the different proposed devices [7] which may induce a secondary contraction.

Flaps

Large contractures have to be excised and replacement using different types of flaps.

Random skin flaps are frequently used [8], coming from the adjacent area when scar-free, but pedicled fasciocutaneous flaps bring a rich vascular network. Branches from this plexus reach the skin as direct or indirect perforators. They can be used locally or regionally, and rotated into the defect [9].

Perforator flaps, more recently developed, are based on a fine dissection of the perforator vessels going through the fascia to vascularize the overlying skin island. This increases the range of motion of these pedicled flaps and it reduces significantly the donor site morbidity.

Free flaps enlarge even further the armamentarium for tissue transfer. In principle, all axial flaps can be transferred as a free vascularized flap: the artery and the vein (eventually also the nerve) are transected at the donor site and re-anastomosed microsurgically with a recipient vessel at another part of the body. Till recently, free fasciocutaneous flaps and perforator flaps were most frequently used for coverage of contracture defects. Both can however result in significant donor site morbidity by harvesting structurally important fascia.

Conclusion

In summary, contractures after burns are difficult to prevent, some areas like axilla, neck, and upper limbs being predominantly affected. Early skin grafting may prevent contractures, but an adapted rehabilitation program should be established and redefined during the regular check-up done by the burns team. When constituted, a precise analysis of the lacking skin surface should be done by the surgical team, issuing to a covering program depending on the area involved and the expertise of the team. Function may efficiently be restored using different techniques, skin grafting and dermal substitutes being more adapted in term of volumes, flap providing a suppler skin.

Take-Home Message

Contractures may form a severe functional deficit. Early prevention is mandatory, with a combination of exercise and positioning to prevent skin retraction. In specific situations like the burned hand immobilization can be done in both positions: flexion during the night and extension during the day. Treatment is difficult, and a balance should be sought between surgery, which always means a restart in the rehabilitation process, and the rehabilitation limits which should be established in close conjunction together with the team in charge. Recurrence is a risk if the postoperative management is not properly realized.

References

1. Kwan PO, Tredget EE. Etiological principles of scar and contracture. Hand Clin. 2017;33(2):277–92. https://doi.org/10.1016/j.hcl.2016.12.004. Epub 2017 Mar 1.
2. Schouten HJ, Nieuwenhuis MK, van Baar ME, van der Schans CP, Niemeijer AS, van Zuijlen PPM. The prevalence and development of burn scar contractures: a prospective multicenter cohort study. Burns. 2019;45(4):783–90. https://doi.org/10.1016/j.burns.2019.03.007, pii: S0305-4179(19)30144-5.
3. Thomas R, Wicks S, Toose C, Pacey V. Outcomes of early use of an end of range axilla orthotic in children following burn injury. J Burns Care Res. 2019;40(5):678–88. https://doi.org/10.1093/jbcr/irz058.
4. Monstrey S, Middelkoop E, Vranckx JJ, Bassetto F, Ziegler UE, Meaume S, Téot L. Updated scar management practical guidelines: non-invasive and invasive measures. J Plast Reconstr Aesthet Surg. 2014;67:1017–25.
5. Richard R, Wards RS. Splinting and controversies. J Burn Care Rehabil. 2005;26(5):392–6.
6. Kim YH, Hwang KT, Kim KH, Sung IH, Kim SW. Application of acellular human dermis and skin grafts for lower extremity reconstruction. J Wound Care. 2019;28(Suppl 4):S12–7. https://doi.org/10.12968/jowc.2019.28.Sup4.S12.
7. Hori K, Osada A, Isago T, Sakurai H. Comparison of contraction among three dermal substitutes: morphological differences in scaffolds. Burns. 2017;43(4):846–51. https://doi.org/10.1016/j.burns.2016.10.017. Epub 2016 Nov 17.
8. Hifny MA. The square flap technique for burn contractures: clinical experience and analysis of length gain. Ann Burns Fire Disasters. 2018;31(4):306–12.
9. Teot L, Bosse JP. The use of scapular skin island flaps in the treatment of axillary postburn scar contractures. Br J Plast Surg. 1994;47(2):108–11.

16

Scar Assessment Scales

Michelle E. Carrière, Annekatrien L. van de Kar, and Paul P. M. van Zuijlen

Contents

Background

Over the last decades, standardized measurements of medical treatment outcome have become increasingly important. First of all, application of evidence-based medicine requires that the research field evaluates the effectiveness of new and existing treatments. Therefore, no clinical trial can exist without the appropriate outcome measurement instruments to determine the study outcomes in a reliable and valid way. These outcome measurement instruments are not only vital in the research setting but also indispensable in daily clinical practice to monitor scars in individual patients. Furthermore, standardized scar measurements are performed and recorded in clinical registries with the aim to improve the quality of care and patient health outcomes.

Scar outcome measurement instruments can be either measurement devices or scar assessment scales. Measurement devices are often seen as objective instruments that provide solid quantitative analyses of scar characteristics. However, measurement devices have to be purchased for sometimes high prices and can only be used at one place at a time. Another disadvantage may be that most devices are only able to evaluate one scar characteristic. In addition, cutting-edge measurement technologies often involve time-consuming measurements and analyses that require training of the observer, which might be appropriate in research settings but is less suitable in clinical practice. Contrary to measurement devices, scar assessment scales are qualitative evaluations of multiple scar characteristics provided by an individual, either the patient or the clinician/researcher. Scar assessment scales are sometimes criticized by their subjective nature. However, advantages of scar assessment scales are their ability to provide fast evaluation of multiple scar characteristics, their (usually) free and easy accessibility, and their ability to capture the patient's view on their scars. The latter is especially important as nowadays patients are receiving more information about treatment options and are getting more involved in making treatment decisions and in reporting treatment outcomes. In this chapter, an overview of the content and development of most frequently used scar assessment scales is provided.

Domains

Scars can influence patients in several health domains, ranging from appearance to quality of life. These different domains require different levels of measurements. Measurements acquired with clinician-reported scales are limited to observable aspects of the scar, such as appearance, physical characteristics, and functional impairment of the scar. On the other hand, patient-reported scar scales allow for the evaluation of additional health domains that cannot be observed by clinicians, such as scar symptoms and quality of life.

Scar Assessment Scales

◘ Table 14.1 provides an overview of consecutive developed scar assessment scales, the constructs measured, and whether it is reported by the patient or clinician. ◘ Table 14.2 shows which scar aspects are assessed in the most frequently used scales. The first concepts of scar assessment scales were reported in the late 1980s, but the first widely used, validated scar scale was developed in 1990 by Sullivan et al., which became widely known as the Vancouver Scar Scale (VSS) [1]. The VSS consists of four items: vascularity, pigmentation, thickness, and pliability. Since this first introduction to scar assessment scales, the development of many other scales followed. Various authors modified the original version of the VSS by adding extra items to the scale or altering the answering categories of the existing items [2–4]. This resulted in an abundance of modified VSS versions—of which the modified VSS by Baryza et al. is the most widely used [2]. The Seattle, Hamilton, and Manchester scar scales were consecutively developed from 1997 to 1998 [5–7]. The Seattle and Hamilton scales were both developed for photographic evaluation of scar [5, 6]. The Manchester scar scale introduced two new items: an "overall assessment," rated on a VAS scale (0–10), and if the scar appeared matte or shiny [7]. Until 2000, the focus remained on the clinician/observer, as all developed scales were clinician-reported, focusing on visual and physical scar characteristics. This changed when Nedelec et al. added a symptomatic assessment (i.e., items of pain and itch) to the original VSS [3]. However, it was not until 2004 that in addition to symptoms such as pain and itch, the patient's opinion on visual and physical scar characteristics was incorporated into a scar assessment scale called the *Patient and Observer Scar Assessment Scale* (POSAS) [8]. The POSAS captures both the clinician's (observer's) and the patient's perspective on multiple-characteristics scar quality. A few years after the introduction of the POSAS, Bock et al. made it possible to evaluate the quality of life of patients with keloid and hypertrophic scars by the development of the *Bock Quality of Life Scale* [9]. This was the first patient-reported scar scale measuring at the level of quality of life. Around the same time, the *Stony Brooks Scar Evaluation Scale* was introduced, which is a clinician-reported scar scale specifically designed for the assessment of surgical scars [10]. Therefore, it included an item to evaluate the presence of suture marks. The *Patient Scar Assessment Questionnaire*, *Patient-Reported Impact of Scars Measure* (PSAQ), and *Brisbane Burn*

Table Overview of consecutive developed scar assessment scales

Scar scale	Year	Clinician-reported	Patient-reported	Type of scars	Construct
Vancouver Scar Scale	1990	X		Burn	Physical characteristics and appearance
Modified Vancouver Scar Scale by Baryza et al.	1995	X		Burn	Physical characteristics and appearance
Seattle Scar Scale	1997	X		Burn	Physical characteristics and appearance
Hamilton Scar Scale	1998	X		Mix	Physical characteristics and appearance
Manchester Scar Scale	1998	X		Mix	Physical characteristics and appearance
Modified Vancouver Scar Scale by Nedelec et al.	2000	(X)		Burn	Physical characteristics and appearance, scar sensation
Patient and Observer Scar Assessment Scale	2004	X	X	Mix	Physical characteristics and appearance, scar sensation
Bock Quality of Life	2006		X	Hypertrophic/keloid	Quality of life
Stony Brooks Scar Evaluation Scale	2007	X		Surgical	Scar characteristics and appearance
Patient Scar Assessment Questionnaire	2009		X	Surgical	Scar characteristics and appearance, scar sensation Consciousness (body image and confidence)
Patient-Reported Impact of Scars Measure	2010		X	Surgical	Scar sensation Quality of life
Brisbane Burn Scar Impact Profile	2016		X	Burns	Scar characteristics and appearance Scar sensation Quality of life
Scar Cosmesis Assessment and Rating scale	2016	(X)		Surgical	Scar characteristics and appearance Scar sensation
Scar Q	2018		X	Mix	Scar characteristics and appearance Symptoms Psychological problems

(*X*) = Clinician-reported scale in which the presence of pain and itch is included

Scar Impact Profile (BSSIP) are more recently developed patient-reported scales which measure aspects of quality of life, in addition visual and physical scar characteristics, symptoms, and/or satisfaction [11–13]. Most recently, the *Scar Q* was developed for the evaluation of physical characteristics, scar appearance, symptoms, and physiological problems [14].

Measurement Properties/Clinimetrics

To evaluate the quality of available scar assessment scales, several measurement properties must be considered, i.e. ,validity, reliability, and responsiveness [15]. The most important property is content validity. Content validity is the degree to which the content of a measure is an adequate reflection of the construct to be measured [15]. Good content validity means that all items included in the scale are relevant and no relevant items are missing for the construct of interest (within a specific population and context of use). Furthermore, it means that patients should understand the content as intended. Lack of content validity can influence all other measurement properties [16]. To ensure good content validity, it is important that well-designed scale development studies are performed that use qualitative methods to gain patient/professional input on the content of the scale. In addition, the draft scale must be pilot tested to ensure its content is relevant, comprehensive, and comprehensible for patients. In Table 14.3, it is noted if

Table Overview of the content of most frequently used scar assessment scales

	VSS	Modified VSS by Baryza et al.	Manchester Scar Scale	POSAS (2.0)	Bock Quality of Life	SBSES	PSAQ	PRISM	BBSIP	Scar Q
Number of subscales	1	1	1	2	1	1	5	2	10	2
Number of items[a]	4	4	6	14	15	5	39	37	66	24
Visual and physical scar characteristics										
Vascularity	X	X		X			X			
Pigmentation	X	X		X			X			
Color			X	X		X	X		X	X
Thickness	X	X	X	X		X	X		X	X
Pliability/hardness	X	X	X	X					X	X
Roughness							X		X	
Surface irregularities				X			X		X	X
Distortion			X	X						
Shiny surface			X				X			
Hatch marks						X				
Width						X	X			X
Length							X			X
Overall appearance			X	X		X	X			X
Symptoms										
Pain				X			X	X	X	X
Itch				X	X		X	X	X	X
Stinging								X		
Burning								X		
Discomfort							X		X	

	VSS	Modified VSS by Baryza et al.	Manchester Scar Scale	POSAS (2.0)	Bock Quality of Life	SBSES	PSAQ	PRISM	BBSIP	Scar Q
Numbness							X			X
(Hyper) Sensitivity								X	X	X
Tingling							X	X		X
Tightness							X		X	X
Impaired movement					X				X	X
Dryness									X	X
Sensitive to temperature (changes)					X			X	X	
Swelling										X
Inflammation								X		
Open wounds									X	
Tiredness									X	
Psychosocial										
Self-consciousness							X	X		
Self-confidence					X			X	X	
Embarrassment					X			X		X
Unhappy feelings								X	X	X
Angry feelings								X	X	
Sexual concerns					X			X		
Feeling unattractive					X			X		
Not accepting scars					X					
Hiding scars					X		X			

(continued)

Table (continued)

	VSS	Modified VSS by Baryza et al.	Manchester Scar Scale	POSAS (2.0)	Bock Quality of Life	SBSES	PSAQ	PRISM	BBSIP	Scar Q
Avoid talking about scars					X					
Reactions of others					X		X	X	X	
Impact on social interactions and activities					X			X	X	
Impact of scar treatments									X	
Suicidal thoughts					X					
Satisfaction										
Overall satisfaction										
Appearance							X			
Symptoms							X			

[a]Not all items included in the scales are scored in this table. *VSS* Vancouver Scar Scale, *POSAS* Patient and Observer Scar Assessment Scale, *SBSES* Stony Brooks Scar Evaluation Scale, *PSAQ* Patient Scar Assessment Questionnaire, *PRISM* Patient-Reported Impact of Scars Measure, *BBSIP* Brisbane Burn Scar Impact Profile

Table Methods used for the development of most frequently used scar assessment scales

	VSS	Modified VSS by Baryza et al.	Manchester Scar Scale	POSAS (2.0)	Bock Quality of Life	SBSES	PSAQ	PRISM	BBSIP	Scar Q
Scale development										
Literature search		X		X	X		X	X	X	X
Expert opinion	X	X	X	X	X	X	X	X	X	X
Patient interviews							X	X	X	X
Pilot testing					X		X	X	X	X

VSS Vancouver Scar Scale, *POSAS* Patient and Observer Scar Assessment Scale, *SBSES* Stony Brooks Scar Evaluation Scale, *PSAQ* Patient Scar Assessment Questionnaire, *PRISM* Patient-Reported Impact of Scars Measure, *BBSIP* Brisbane Burn Scar Impact Profile

these requirements were met for the included scar assessment scales. Besides content validity, reliability is an important clinimetric property. Reliability refers to the extent to which scores for patients who have not changed are the same for repeated measurements [15]. Reliability and measurement error are related but distinct measurement properties. Reliability refers to the ability of a measure to distinguish between patients, and measurement error refers to the systematic and random error attributed to the measurement instrument [17]. The responsiveness is the ability of a scale to detect changes over time in the construct to be measured (e.g., scar quality) [15]. All measurement properties should be evaluated in the specific population in which it will be used. The context of use, referring to the application of use (i.e., discriminative, evaluative, or diagnostic application) and to the setting (e.g., hospital or at home), should also be taken into account. Furthermore, the instrument must be practical and user-friendly in order to be easily applicable in clinical practice: an aspect which is defined as feasibility [18]. It is crucial to consider the measurement properties, the context of use, and the feasibility when choosing a measurement instrument. Measurements obtained by poor-quality or non-validated instruments are not trustworthy, and thus, studies that utilize these instruments yield unreliable results and invalid conclusions.

Conclusion

Scar assessment scales are useful tools to measure various domains of scars. This chapter provides an overview of the most frequently used scar scales, including their content and development. It is of paramount importance to evaluate the clinimetric properties of an instrument prior to using it for scar assessments for clinical or research purposes in order to prevent measurements obtained by poor-quality instruments.

Take-Home Messages

- Scar assessment scales are important to evaluate the effectiveness of scar treatments and to monitor patients over time.
- Traditional scar scales are clinician/researcher-reported, focusing on the appearance and physical characteristics of the scar, while more recently, developed scales are patient-reported scales which measure aspects of quality of life.
- (Content) Validity, reliability, and responsiveness are important measurement properties which must be evaluated prior to using a scale for scar assessments.

References

1. Sullivan T, Smith J, Kermode J, McIver E, Courtemanche DJ. Rating the burn scar. J Burn Care Rehabil. 1990;11(3):256–60.
2. Baryza MJ, Baryza GA. The Vancouver Scar Scale: an administration tool and its interrater reliability. J Burn Care Rehabil. 1995;16(5):535–8.
3. Nedelec B, Shankowsky HA, Tredget EE. Rating the resolving hypertrophic scar: comparison of the Vancouver Scar Scale and scar volume. J Burn Care Rehabil. 2000;21(3):205–12.
4. Forbes-Duchart L, Marshall S, Strock A, Cooper JE. Determination of inter-rater reliability in pediatric burn scar

assessment using a modified version of the Vancouver Scar Scale. J Burn Care Research. 2007;28(3):460–7.
5. Yeong EK, Mann R, Engrav LH, Goldberg M, Cain V, Costa B, et al. Improved burn scar assessment with use of a new scar-rating scale. J Burn Care Rehabil. 1997;18(4):353–5.. discussion 2
6. Crowe JM, Simpson K, Johnson W, Allen J. Reliability of photographic analysis in determining change in scar appearance. J Burn Care Rehabil. 1998;19(2):183–6.
7. Beausang E, Floyd H, Dunn KW, Orton CI, Ferguson MW. A new quantitative scale for clinical scar assessment. Plast Reconstr Surg. 1998;102(6):1954–61.
8. Draaijers LJ, Tempelman FR, Botman YA, Tuinebreijer WE, Middelkoop E, Kreis RW, et al. The patient and observer scar assessment scale: a reliable and feasible tool for scar evaluation. Plast Reconstr Surg. 2004;113(7):1960–5; discussion 6–7.
9. Bock O, Schmid-Ott G, Malewski P, Mrowietz U. Quality of life of patients with keloid and hypertrophic scarring. Arch Dermatol Res. 2006; 97:433–38. https://doi.org/10.1007/s00403-006-0651-7.
10. Singer AJ, Arora B, Dagum A, Valentine S, Hollander JE. Development and validation of a novel scar evaluation scale. Plast Reconstr Surg. 2007;120(7):1892–7.
11. Tyack Z, Ziviani J, Kimble R, Plaza A, Jones A, Cuttle L, et al. Measuring the impact of burn scarring on health-related quality of life: development and preliminary content validation of the Brisbane Burn Scar Impact Profile (BBSIP) for children and adults. Burns. 2015;41(7):1405–19.
12. Durani P, McGrouther DA, Ferguson MW. The Patient Scar Assessment Questionnaire: a reliable and valid patient-reported outcomes measure for linear scars. Plast Reconstr Surg. 2009;123(5):1481–9.
13. Brown BC, McKenna SP, Solomon M, Wilburn J, McGrouther DA, Bayat A. The patient-reported impact of scars measure: development and validation. Plast Reconstr Surg. 2010;125(5):1439–49.
14. Klassen AF, Ziolkowski N, Mundy LR, Miller HC, McIlvride A, DiLaura A, et al. Development of a new patient-reported outcome instrument to evaluate treatments for scars: the SCAR-Q. Plast Reconstr Surg Glob Open. 2018;6(4):e1672.
15. Mokkink LB, Terwee CB, Patrick DL, Alonso J, Stratford PW, Knol DL, et al. The COSMIN study reached international consensus on taxonomy, terminology, and definitions of measurement properties for health-related patient-reported outcomes. J Clin Epidemiol. 2010;63(7):737–45.
16. Terwee CB, Prinsen CAC, Chiarotto A, Westerman MJ, Patrick DL, Alonso J, et al. COSMIN methodology for evaluating the content validity of patient-reported outcome measures: a Delphi study. Qual Life Res. 2018;27(5):1159–70.
17. de Vet HC, Terwee CB, Knol DL, Bouter LM. When to use agreement versus reliability measures. J Clin Epidemiol. 2006;59(10):1033–9.
18. De Vet HCW, Terwee CB, Mokkink LB, Knol DL. Measurement in medicine. 1st ed. Cambridge: Cambridge University Press; 2011.

17

Japan Scar Workshop (JSW) Scar Scale (JSS) for Assessing Keloids and Hypertrophic Scars

Rei Ogawa

Contents

Background

The Vancouver scar scale [1], the Manchester scar scale [2], and the Patient and Observer Scar Assessment Scale (POSAS) [3] are all very well-known scar evaluation methods. These tools are based on a number of scar variables, including color, height, and pliability. However, since all were mainly developed to evaluate burn scars, they are difficult to use in clinical practice for keloids and hypertrophic scars. This is because these pathological scars require both differential diagnosis and a way to evaluate their response to therapy. Since the Japan Scar Workshop (JSW) was established in 2006, it has sought to develop a scar assessment scale that meets these clinical needs. The first version of this scar assessment tool was named the JSW scar scale (JSS), and it was reported in 2011 [4]. In 2015, the revised second version was reported (◘ Table 15.1 and ◘ Figs. 15.1, 15.2, 15.3, 15.4, 15.5, 15.6, and 15.7) [5]. This chapter introduces the JSS and discusses its clinical importance and usefulness in scar research.

JSW Scar Scale (JSS) 2015

The JSS consists of two tables. One is a scar classification table that is used to determine whether the scar is a normal mature scar, a hypertrophic scar, or a keloid. This grading system helps the user to select the most appropriate treatment method for the scar. The other table in the JSS is an evaluation table that is used to judge the response to treatment and for follow-up. Both tables contain sample images of each subjective keloid/hypertrophic scar item that allow the user to evaluate each item without hesitation (◘ Figs. 15.1, 15.2, 15.3, 15.4, 15.5, 15.6, and 15.7). Japanese guidelines for the prevention and treatment of keloids and hypertrophic scars [6] include JSS 2015.

Classification Table

The classification table consists of two parts: risk factors and the present symptoms. The risk factors consists of six items, each of which has 2–3 categories: (1) human race (African, Other, Caucasian), (2) whether there is a familial tendency (Clearly exists, Does not clearly exist), (3) the number of scars (Multiple, Solitary), (4) the body region the scar is on (Anterior chest/scapular-shoulder/suprapubic, Other), (5) the age at onset (0–30, 31–60, ≥60 years), and (6) the cause(s) (Unknown/minute, Specific type of wounding such as surgery). The present symptoms also consist of six items, each of which has 2–3 categories: (7) scar size (>20 cm^2, <20 cm^2), (8) whether there is vertical growth (Clearly exists, Does not clearly exist), (9) whether there is horizontal growth (Clearly exists, Does not clearly exist), (10) the shape of the scar (Characteristic shape, Others), (11) whether there is erythema around the scar (Clearly exists, Does not clearly exist), and (12) whether there are subjective symptoms (Always exist, Intermittent, None). Thus, the classification table consists of 12 items in total. The categories in each item are weighted: for example, in Human race, African, Caucasian, and Other races are weighted 2, 0, and 1 points, respectively. The minimum and maximum number of points in the classification table are 0 and 25, respectively. If the classification score is 0–5, the scar is deemed to have mature scar characteristics. If the score is 6–15 or 16–25, the scar is deemed to be a hypertrophic scar and a keloid, respectively.

This grading system is thus used to differentially diagnose keloid and hypertrophic scars. It is necessary to have this system because there are many cases in which the scar bears the growth and histological features of both hypertrophic scars and keloids; as a result, it can be difficult to differentially diagnose these scars in real clinical practice. This reality is not mirrored by the current dogma about pathological scars. Thus, many classical textbooks consider keloids and hypertrophic scars to be completely different types of scar. Clinicians define hypertrophic scars as scars that do not grow beyond the boundaries of the original wound, whereas keloids are defined as scars that spread into the surrounding normal skin. Pathologists have their own definitions; they make a histological distinction between keloids and hypertrophic scars on the basis of thick eosinophilic (hyalinizing) collagen bundles called "keloidal collagen": these are present in the former scar type but rarer in the latter. However, we have observed many cases that do not fit these dichotomic definitions. For example, scars with hypertrophic growth characteristics can bear considerable keloidal collagen. Indeed, it is possible that hypertrophic scars and keloids are manifestations of the same fibroproliferative skin disorder and just differ in the intensity and duration of inflammation. These inflammatory features may be shaped by genetic, systemic, and local risk factors [7].

Evaluation Table

The evaluation table consists of six items: (1) Induration, (2) Elevation, (3) Redness of the scar, (4) Erythema around the scar, (5) Spontaneous and pressing pain, and (6) Itch. Each item has four intensity categories, namely, None, Weak, Mild, and Strong. These categories are weighted 0, 1, 2, and 3, respectively. There are sample

◘ Table JSW Scar Scale (JSS) 2015 (Classification and Evaluation of Keloids and Hypertrophic Scars)

Classification (for grading and selection of appropriate treatment methods)		
Risk factors		
1. Human race	Africans	2
	Others	1
	Caucasians	0
2. Familial tendency	Clearly exists	1
	Not clearly	0
3. Number	Multiple	2
	Solitary	0
4. Region	Anterior chest, scapular-shoulder, suprapubic	2
	Others	0
5. Age at onset	0–30 y/o	2
	31–60 y/o	1
	60 y/o	0
6. Causes	Unknown or minute	3
	Specific wound type such as surgery	0
Present symptoms		
7. Size (cm^2)	Over 20 cm^2	1
	Under 20 cm^2	0
8. Vertical growth (elevation) (◘ Fig. 15.1)	Clearly exists	2
	Not clearly	0
9. Horizontal growth (◘ Fig. 15.2)	Clearly exists	3
	Not clearly	0
10. Shape (◘ Fig. 15.3)	Characteristic shape	3
	Others	0
11. Erythema around scars (◘ Fig. 15.4)	Clearly present	2
	Not present	0
12. Subjective symptoms	Always exist	2
	Intermittent	1
	None	0
Total 0–25		
Remarks		
0–5	Character like matured scars (intractability, low risk)	
6–1	Character like hypertrophic scars (intractability, middle risk)	
16–25	Character like keloids (intractability, high risk)	

Evaluation (for judging treatment results and for following-up)			
1. Induration			
0: None	1: Weak	2: Mild	3: Strong
2. Elevation (◘ Fig. 15.5)			
0: None	1: Weak	2: Mild	3: Strong
3. Redness of scars (◘ Fig. 15.6)			
0: None	1: Weak	2: Mild	3: Strong
4. Erythema around scars (◘ Fig. 15.7)			
0: None	1: Weak	2: Mild	3: Strong
5. Spontaneous and pressing pain			
0: None	1: Weak	2: Mild	3: Strong
6. Itch			
0: None	1: Weak	2: Mild	3: Strong
Total 0–18			
Remarks			
Weak: symptoms exist in less than 1/3 of the area, or are intermittently			
Strong: symptoms exist in the entire region, or are continuous			
Mild: between weak and strong			

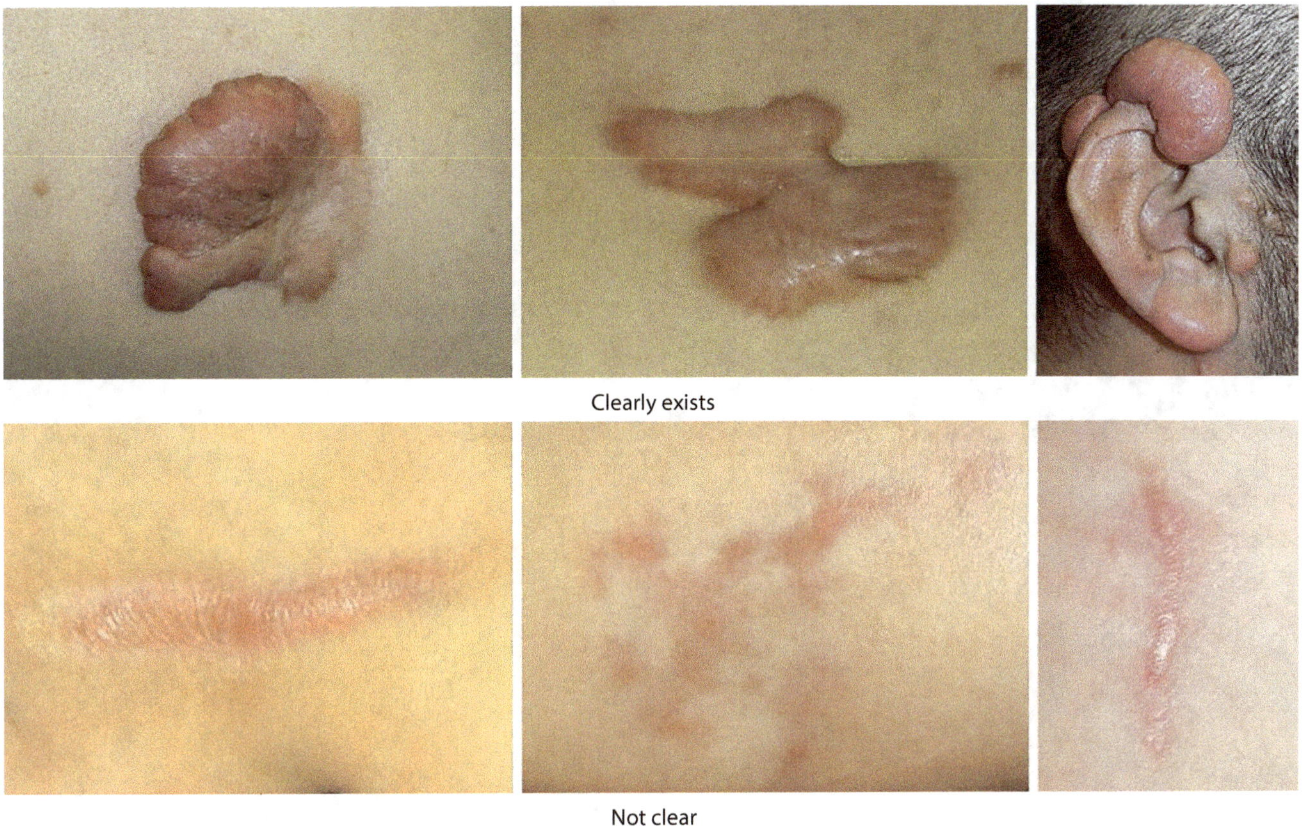

Fig. Vertical growth (elevation)

images of each category in each item that helps the user judge the items. The minimum and maximum total points in the evaluation table are thus 0 and 18, respectively. When the symptoms improve, the total score decreases.

Clinical Suitability and Usefulness of the JSS

We evaluated the clinical suitability of the classification table of JSS2015 with 50 consecutive scar patients in our clinic. The scores of the patients were evenly distributed between 0 and 25 points (Fig. 15.8). This distribution closely reflects our subjective experiences in our scar clinic and those of other Japanese plastic surgeons. As a result, the JSS became a standard classification and evaluation tool for keloid and hypertrophic scars in Japan. The JSS has since been used to evaluate scar severity in several clinical research projects [8–10]. It was also used in a study in Taiwan [9]. However, in our experience, different regions of the world vary in terms of the severity of keloids and hypertrophic scars: in particular, keloids appear to be singularly severe in Africa and East-South Asia, while being rare in western countries. Therefore, in the future, the JSS2015 should be modified to cover other regions of the world.

Conclusion

The Japan Scar Workshop (JSW) developed the JSW scar scale (JSS) to evaluate keloids and hypertrophic scars. The JSS consists of two tables; one is a scar classification table that is used to determine whether the scar is a normal mature scar, a hypertrophic scar, or a keloid, and the other table is an evaluation table that is used to judge the response to treatment and for follow-up. The JSS became a standard classification and evaluation tool for keloid and hypertrophic scars in Japan. In the future, the JSS5 should be modified to cover other regions of the world.

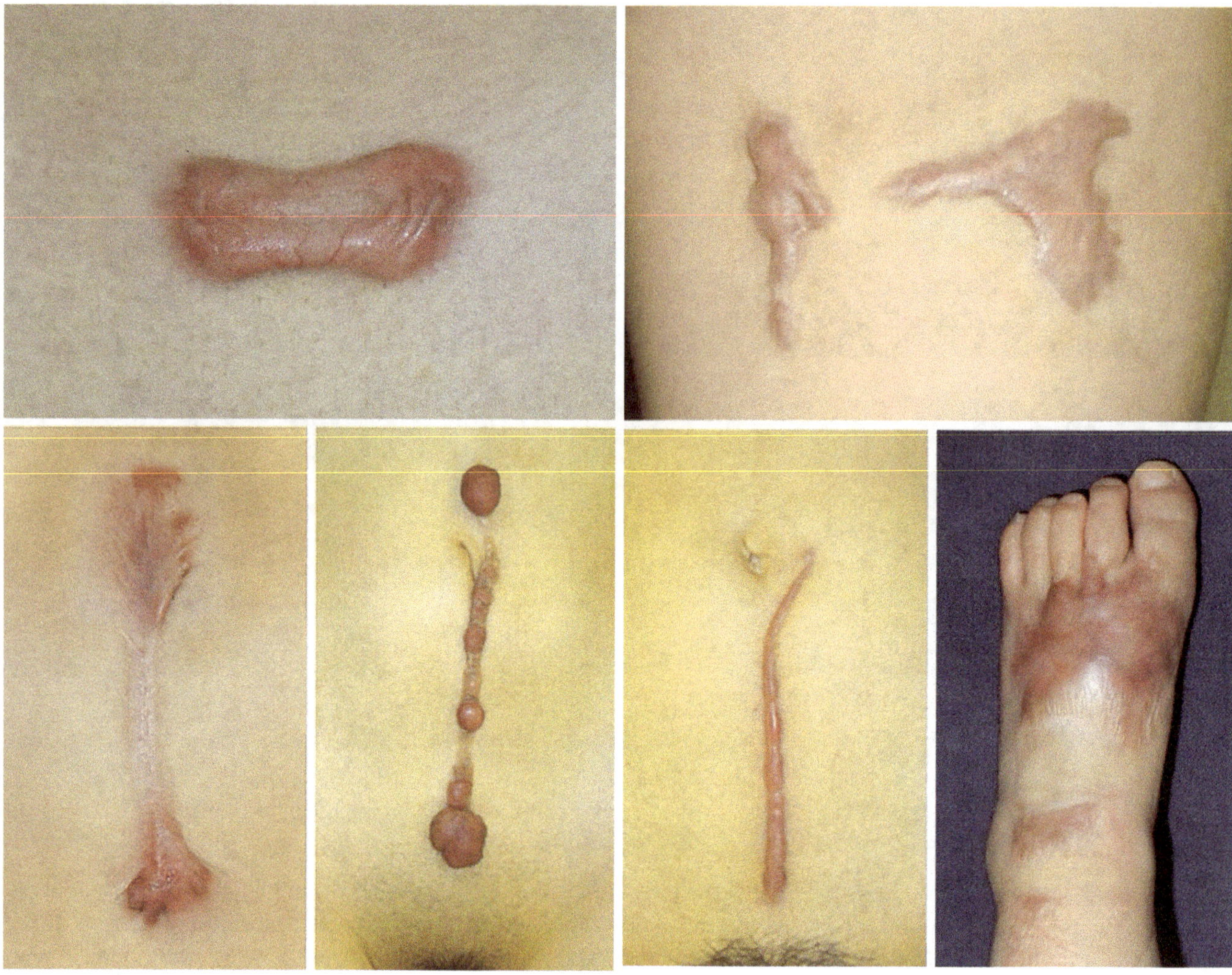

Clearly exists Not clear

Fig. Horizontal growth

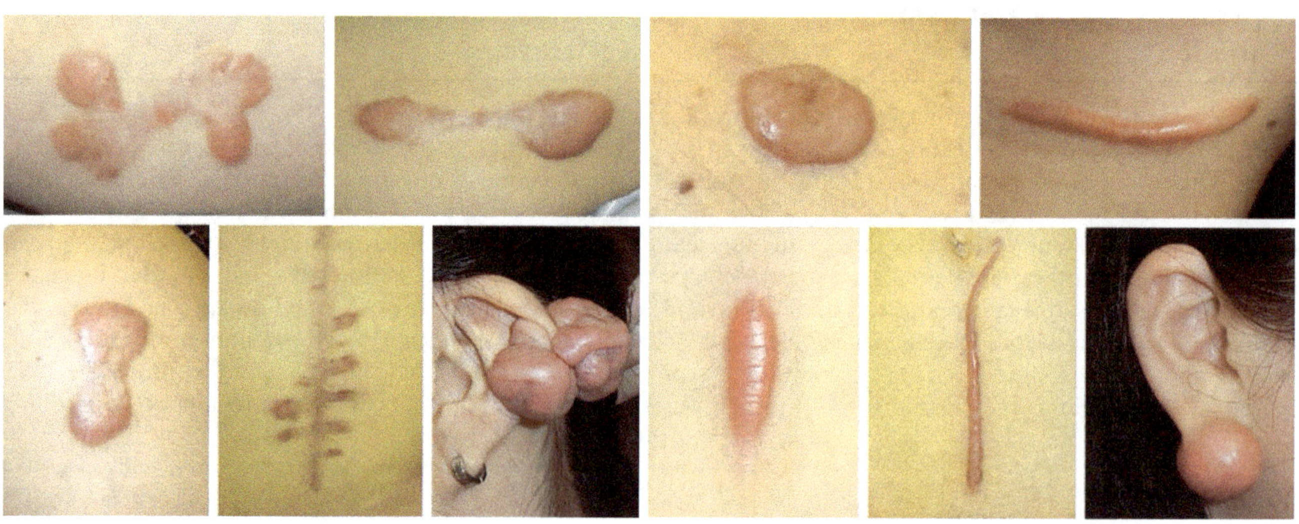

Characteristic shape Others

Fig. Shape

Fig. Erythema around scars

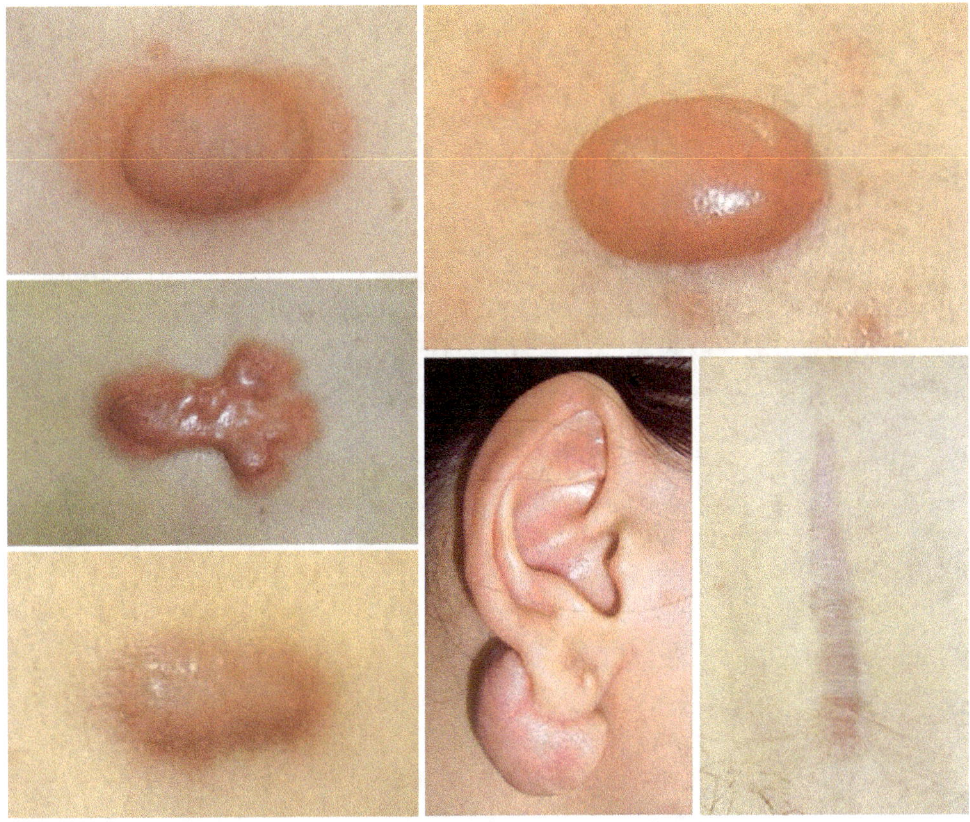

Clearly present

Not present

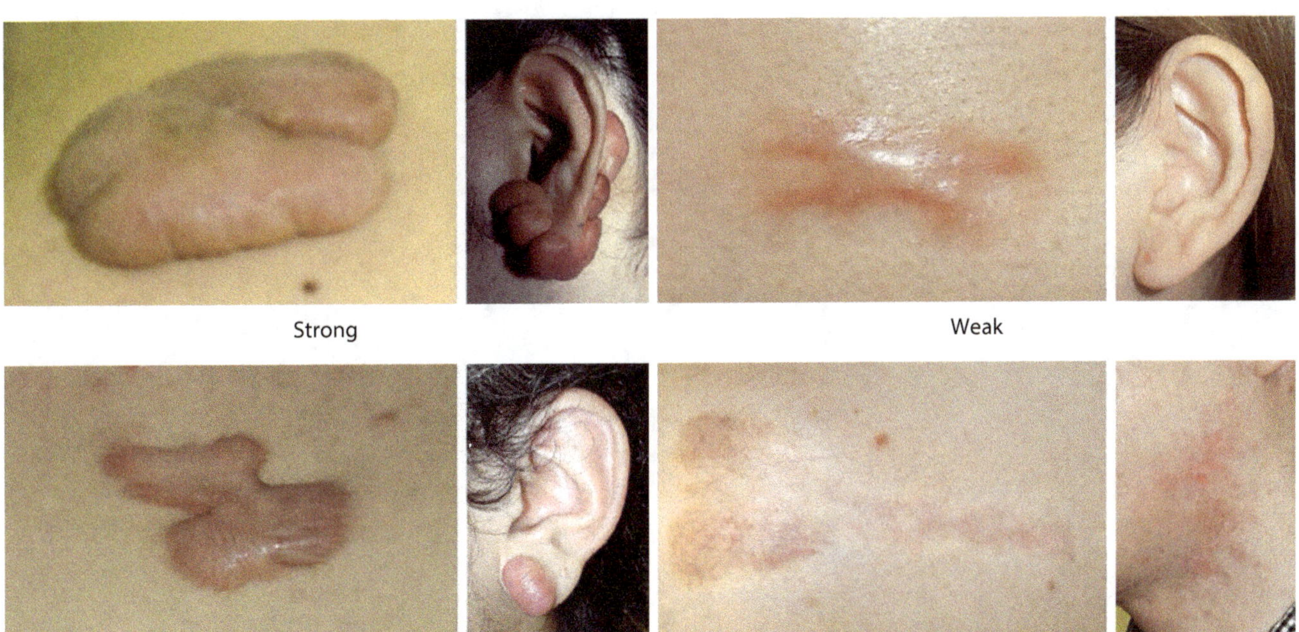

Strong

Weak

Mild

None

Fig. Elevation

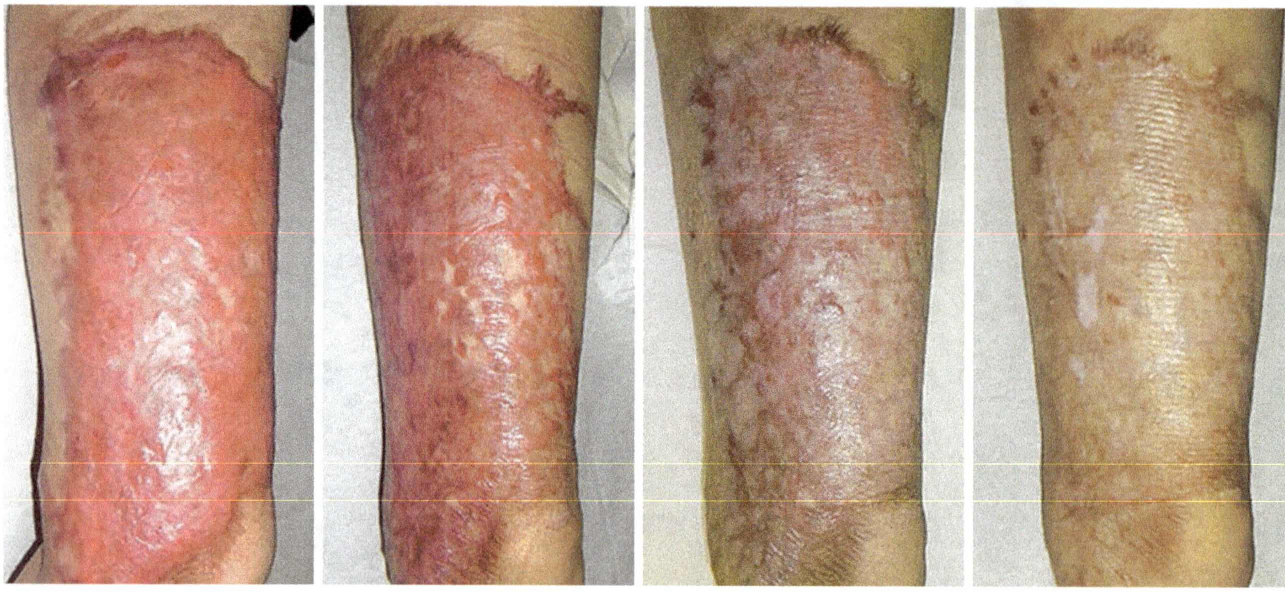

Strong Mild Weak None

Fig. Redness of scars

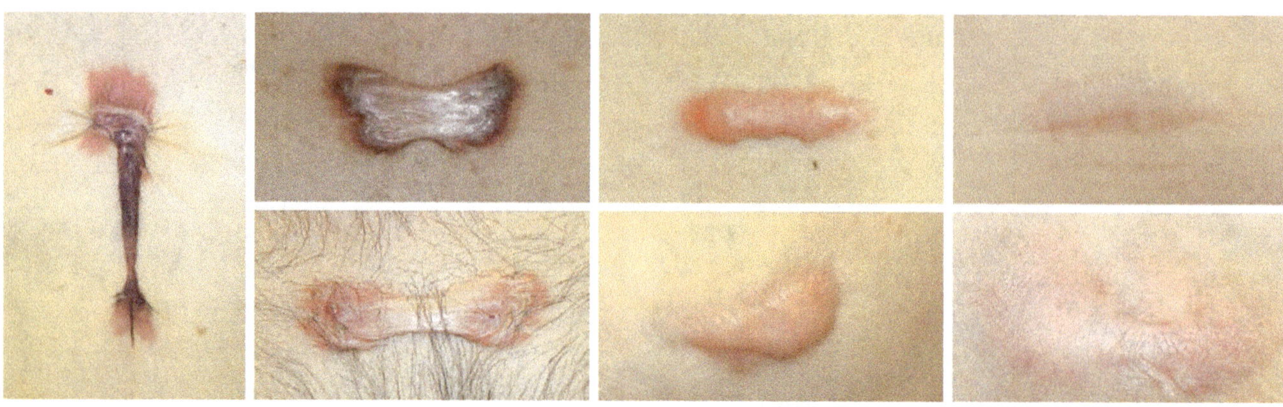

Strong Mild Weak None

Fig. Erythema around scars

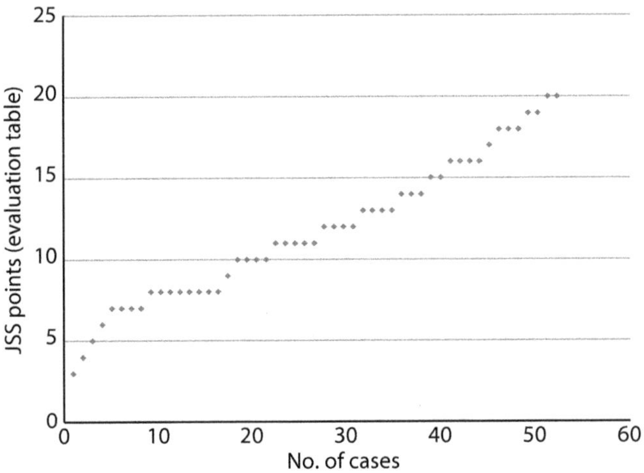

Fig. *Clinical suitability* of the classification table of JSS2015 in consecutive scar patients. We evaluated the clinical suitability of the classification table of JSS2015 by applying it to 50 consecutive scar patients in our clinic. The scores of the patients were evenly distributed between 0 and 25 points. This reflects our general clinical experience

Take-Home Messages

- The Vancouver scar scale, the Manchester scar scale, and the Patient and Observer Scar Assessment Scale (POSAS) were mainly developed to evaluate burn scars.
- The Japan Scar Workshop (JSW) developed the JSW scar scale (JSS) to evaluate keloids and hypertrophic scars.
- The JSS consists of two tables; one is a scar classification table that is used to determine whether the scar is a normal mature scar, a hypertrophic scar, or a keloid, and the other table is an evaluation table that is used to judge the response to treatment and for follow-up.
- The JSS contains sample images of each subjective keloid/hypertrophic scar item that allow the user to evaluate each item without hesitation.

References

1. Baryza MJ, Baryza GA. The Vancouver Scar Scale: an administration tool and its interrater reliability. J Burn Care Rehabil. 1995;16:535–8.
2. Beausang E, Floyd H, Dunn KW, Orton CI, Ferguson MW. A new quantitative scale for clinical scar assessment. Plast Reconstr Surg. 1998;102(6):1954–61.
3. van de Kar AL, Corion LU, Smeulders MJ, et al. Reliable and feasible evaluation of linear scars by the Patient and Observer Scar Assessment Scale. Plast Reconstr Surg. 2005;116:514–22.
4. Ogawa R, Akaishi S, Akita S, Tosa Y, Yamawaki S, Okabe K, Nagao M, Yamamoto J. JSW Scar Scale Working Group. Japan Scar Workshop (JSW) Scar Scale. Available online at: http://www.scar-keloid.com/en/index.html.
5. Ogawa R, Akaishi S, Akita S, Okabe K, Shimizu T, Sunaga A, Tosa Y, Nagao M, Yamawaki S. JSW Scar Scale Working Group. Japan Scar Workshop (JSW) Scar Scale 2015. Available online at: http://www.scar-keloid.com/en/index.html.
6. Ogawa R, Akita S, Akaishi S, et al. Diagnosis and Treatment of Keloids and Hypertrophic Scars-Japan Scar Workshop Consensus Document 2018. Burns Trauma. 2019;7:39.
7. Ogawa R, Akaishi S. Endothelial dysfunction may play a key role in keloid and hypertrophic scar pathogenesis – keloids and hypertrophic scars may be vascular disorders. Med Hypotheses. 2016;96:51–60.
8. Ogawa R, Watanabe A, Than Naing B, Sasaki M, Fujita A, Akaishi S, Hyakusoku H, Shimada T. Associations between keloid severity and single-nucleotide polymorphisms: importance of rs8032158 as a biomarker of keloid severity. J Invest Dermatol. 2014;134(7):2041–3.
9. Koike S, Akaishi S, Nagashima Y, Dohi T, Hyakusoku H, Ogawa R. Nd:YAG laser treatment for keloids and hypertrophic scars: an analysis of 102 cases. Plast Reconstr Surg Glob Open. 2015;2(12):e272.
10. Hsueh WT, Hung KS, Chen YC, Huang YT, Hsu CK, Ogawa R, Hsueh YY. Adjuvant radiotherapy after keloid excision: preliminary experience in Taiwan. Ann Plast Surg. 2019;82(1S Suppl 1):S39–44.

18

Minimal-Invasive Technologies for Treatment of HTS and Keloids: Corticosteroids

Juhee Lee and Jihee Kim

Contents

Background

Hypertrophic scars and keloids represent the consequences are the results of abnormal wound healing. Keloids are characterized by overproduction and deposition of collagen and extracellular matrix (ECM). Keloids often manifest as growing and infiltrative lesions toward the neighboring intact skin beyond the original boundaries. Abnormal fibroblast activity is a histopathological hallmark for keloid pathogenesis leading to prominent accumulation of dermal constituents. Due to sustained proliferation without regression, the patients often experience pruritus and pain which leads to functional impairment affecting quality of life. Recent findings have identified that elevated levels of growth factor and cytokines contribute to aberrant fibroblast activity. Among various singling molecules, transforming growth factor beta (TGF-β) family is a crucial mediator in scar formation.

Management of hypertrophic scars and keloids are yet ill categorized. Unlike keloids, hypertrophic scars may resolve partially without treatment, although treatment is required depending on patient desire for further improvement. The use of steroid for the treatment of excessive scarring was first proposed in the 1950s. The early case reports showed that corticosteroids administered during wound healing halted the growth of granulation tissue. In vitro fibroblasts subject to desoxycorticosterone failed to reach maturation, and there were notable morphologic changes [1]. In the following years, small numbers of patients with keloids were treated with systemic intake and regional injection of ACTH who showed inhibition of recurrence. In 1963, triamcinolone was first used for intralesional injection after surgical excision of keloids [1]. Since then, many groups have reported the successful application of intralesionally injected triamcinolone in scar treatment (◘ Figs. 29.1, 29.2, 29.3, and 29.4).

In the past decades, intralesional injection has been proposed as a standard therapy for hypertrophic scars. The international guidelines on management on keloid scarring have recommended the use of corticosteroids as

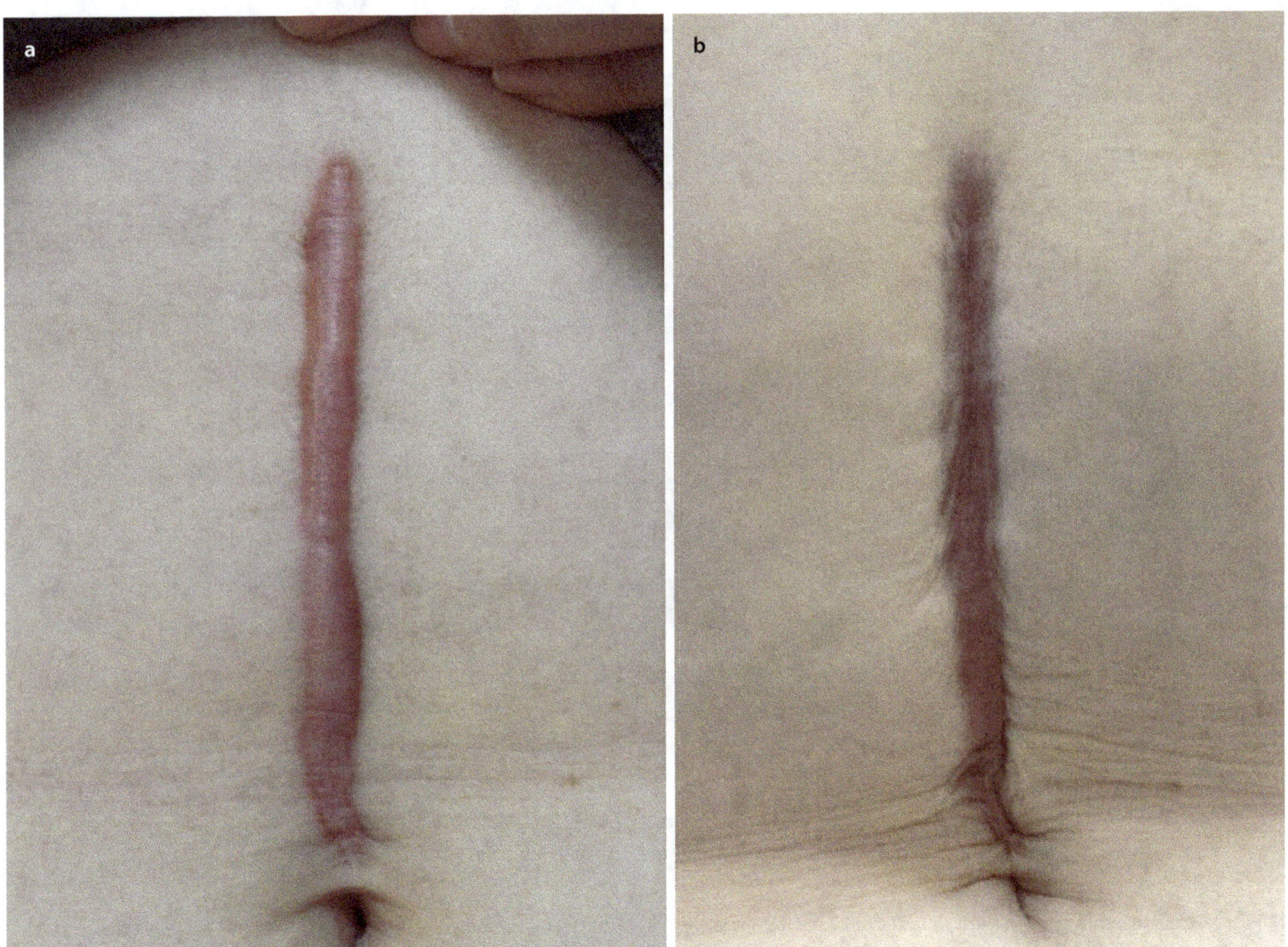

◘ **Fig. a** A 50-year-old man with keloid after total gastrectomy. **b** The patient underwent seven sessions of intralesional injection of triamcinolone (10 mg/ml) in 4 weeks interval

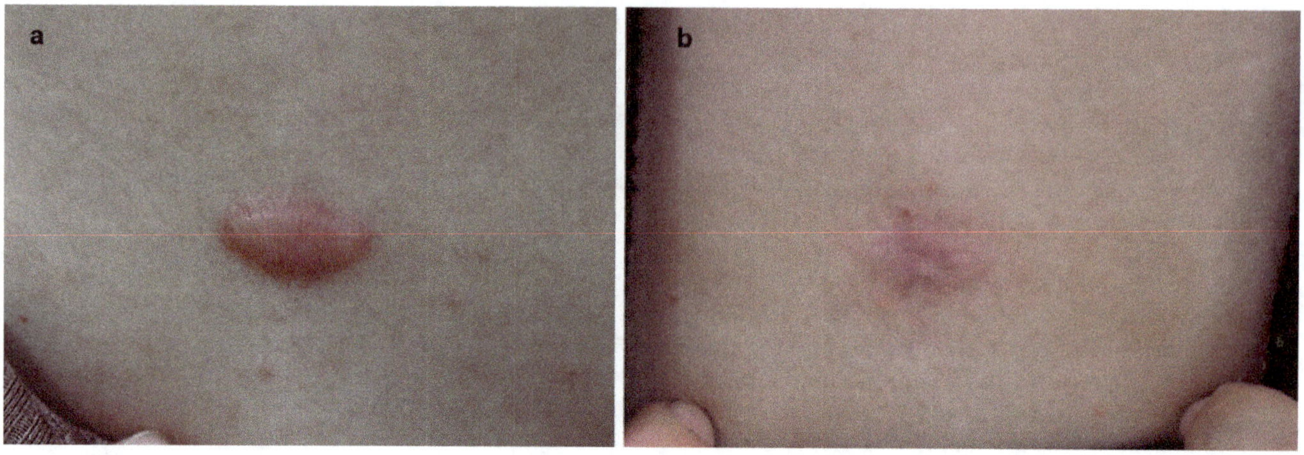

Fig. a A 22-year-old woman with keloid on the chest. **b** The patient underwent four sessions of fractional CO_2 laser (eCO_2 Lutronic, Goyang, Korea. 60 mJ, 15% density) combined with intralesional injection of triamcinolone acetonide suspension of 10 mg/ml

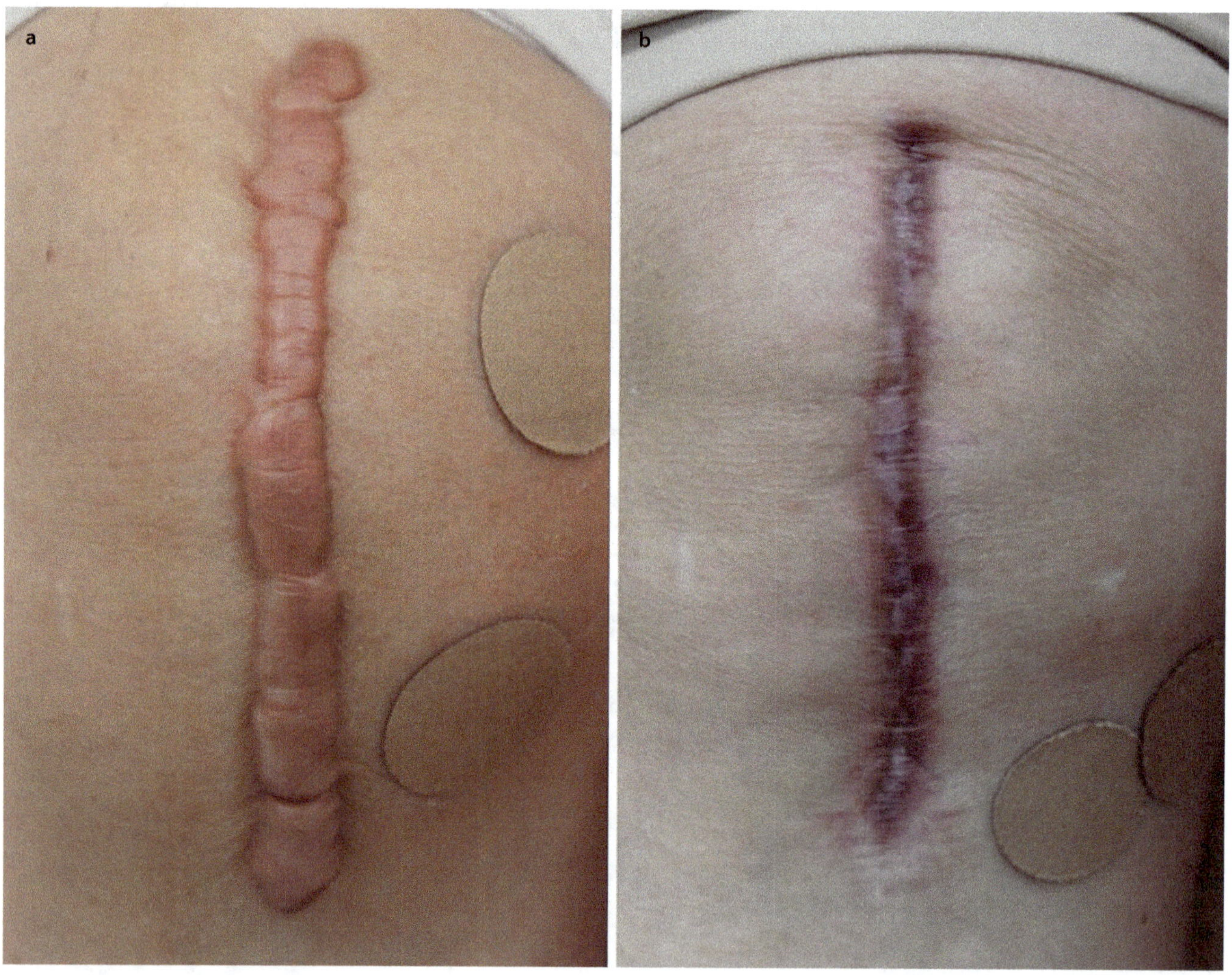

Fig. a A 62-year-old women with keloid after knee replacement surgery. **b** The patient underwent seven sessions of combination cryotherapy and intralesional injection of triamcinolone (10~20 mg/ml) in 4 weeks interval

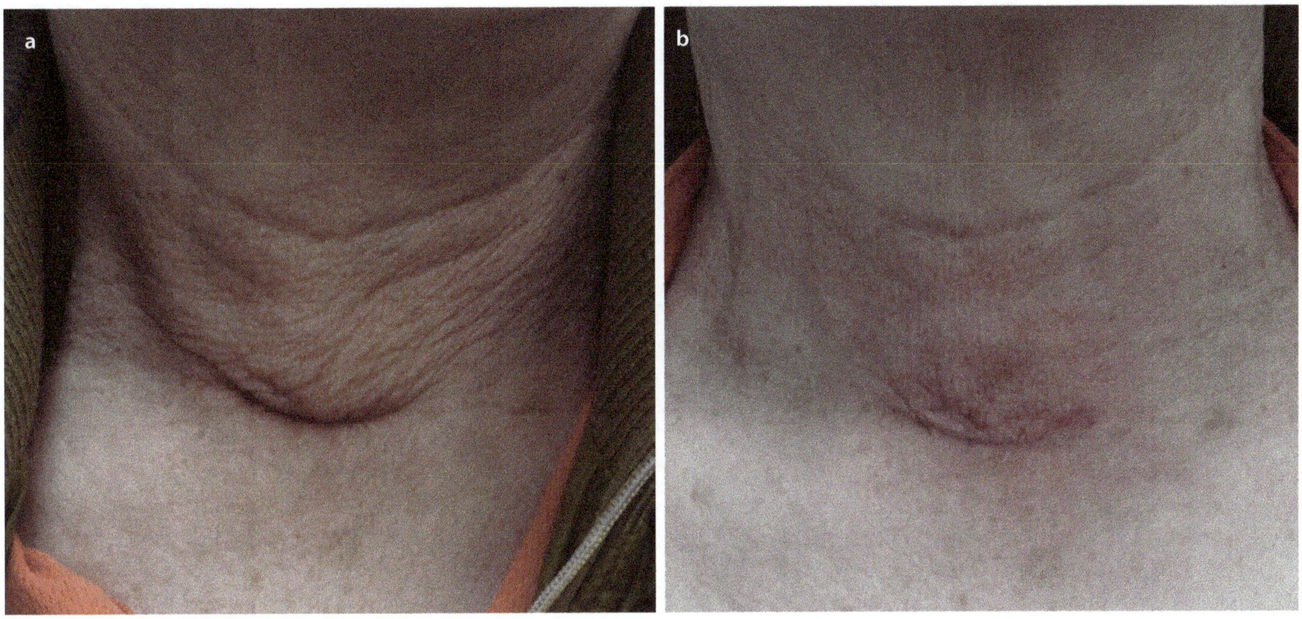

◼ **Fig.** **a** A 60-year-old woman visited 12 weeks after total thyroidectomy. **b** Postoperative lymphedema significantly resolved after single session of intralesional injection of triamcinolone acetonide (10 mg/ml)

a mainstay treatment [2]. Most commonly used corticosteroids for scar treatments are medium- to long-acting agents such as dexamethasone, methylprednisolone, and triamcinolone acetonide. Overall, corticosteroids inhibit all aspects of scar development including inflammation, fibroblast activation, and extracellular matrix accumulations. Thus, the use of corticosteroids efficiently reduces volume of scar tissue and relieves symptoms such as pain and pruritus.

The Corticosteroids

Corticosteroids are the most commonly prescribed anti-inflammatory agent in the medical field. Specific and nonspecific effects of steroids include immunosuppressive, antiproliferative, and vasoconstrictive effects. Besides systemic administration, proper use of topical and intralesional injection requires awareness of its potencies and various formulations.

Pharmacology and Mechanism of Action

All corticosteroids have basic skeletal structure comprising carbon atoms with three hexane rings and one pentane ring. Modifications in the basic cortisol structures result in systemic agents with different potencies, duration of action, metabolism, and mineralocorticoid effects. For example, triamcinolone was synthesized by fluoridation of the hydrocortisone molecule at the 9th position to enhance anti-inflammatory properties.

The free fraction of the corticosteroid enters the cell and exerts its effects by binding to a cytoplasmic glucocorticoid receptor. The glucocorticoid receptor is located within the multi-protein complex consists of heat shock protein and immunophilins. Binding of corticosteroid to its receptor leads to translocation into the nucleus and release from the multiprotein complex. Within the nucleus, the receptor forms a dimer and directly binds to glucocorticoid response elements in the promoter regions of the target genes. Eventually, the intranuclear binding affects the rate of transcription which induces or represses specific target mRNA and protein synthesis. Corticosteroid receptor also interacts with other crucial transcription factors regulating cell metabolism such as cAMP response element binding (CREB) protein. Cellular inflammatory response is modulated via nuclear factor-κB (NF-κB). NF-κB is an important transcription factor that induces the expression of genes regulating inflammatory mediators. Corticosteroids and its receptor inhibit the activity of NF-κB causing reduction of inflammatory process in cell. Additionally, the glucocorticoid receptor has an inhibitory effect on activator protein 1 (AP-1), which controls the expression of various growth factors and cytokine genes. Other key cytokines or proinflammatory molecule inhibited by glucocorticoids includes tumor necrosis factor-α (TNF-α); granulocyte-macrophage colony-stimulating factor (GMCSF); interleukins (IL). IL-1, IL-2, IL-6, IL-8; leukotrienes; and prostaglandins.

Corticosteroid in Scar Treatment

Unlike normal fibroblasts, keloid fibroblasts possess tumor-like properties, showing excessive proliferation and invasion of surrounding tissues. Enhanced migration and invasion of normal fibroblasts are critical factors for the development of keloids. TGF-β signaling has long been considered a pivotal fibrogenic factor in abnormal wound healing. Subsequently, anti-fibrotic strategies based on the blockade or elimination of TGF-β signaling emerged as an important pharmacological target for treating keloids [3]. The clinical response to corticosteroids in scar treatments is mainly achieved by reducing the prolonged inflammatory response during wound healing, inhibiting collagen and reducing excessive ECM synthesis by reducing fibroblast activity. Additionally, intralesional injection of corticosteroids enhances fibroblast and collagen degeneration.

In lesions treated with corticosteroids, thick collagen bundles are dissociated and ECM constituents are markedly reduced. In vivo studies have shown that corticosteroid, especially triamcinolone, can retard synthesis of pro-collagen and TGF-β1 and TGF-β2 expression [4]. Administration of dexamethasone induced reduction in vascular endothelial growth factor and angiogenesis in keloid-derived fibroblasts [5]. Further study on the effect of corticosteroids on keloid pathophysiology is required in the aspect of modulation of chemotaxis immunomodulation controlling fibroblast activity and collagen metabolism.

Topical Steroids

Topical steroids are the most frequently prescribed of all dermatologic drugs, yet its usage has been limited in scar treatment. There are different formulations available in a wide range of potencies and a variety of vehicles. Topical corticosteroids are categorized into four major potency groups and seven classes. The classes are developed based on vasoconstrictor assays and clinical studies which range from class 1 ultra-high potency to class 7 very low potency. Certain formulation is more potent such as ointment formulation, which can enhance percutaneous absorption through increased hydration of the stratum corneum. In selecting a topical glucocorticoid preparation for scar treatment, optimal potency should be selected based on scar extent, location, and thickness. Target site for topical steroids is the viable epidermis or dermis, and the clinical response to a formulation is directly proportional to the concentration of the drug achieved at the target site. When topical application is considered, it is important to monitor potential adverse skin reaction due to continuous application. When skin atrophy or purpura is noted, temporary discontinuation of a topical agent should be considered. For hypertrophic scar or keloid treatment, topical corticosteroids alone have failed to reduce pre-existing scar tissue or prevent scar development and not advocated as a preferred modality.

Intralesional Injection

Keloids and hypertrophic scars are often treated by intralesional injection of therapeutic drugs because the pathogenic target is accumulated collagen and ECM constituents within the dermis. Intralesional administration of corticosteroids allows bypassing the thick stratum corneum barrier and directly treating pathologic dermal lesions with higher concentration of corticosteroids at the site. Triamcinolone acetonide and triamcinolone diacetate are the most widely used corticosteroids for intralesional administration. After its administration, micronized crystals of corticosteroids persist in the skin and released over a period of weeks, thus being the most desirable delivery system for the treatment of chronic inflammatory skin diseases. Triamcinolone agents are available as micronized suspensions of corticosteroid crystals, favored than dexamethasone or betamethasone.

Administration

Typically 27- or 30-gauge needles are the most preferred because it causes less discomfort when penetrating the skin and allow greater precision in injecting the desired quantity. Needles with thicker caliber can be applied for the long-standing lesions with dense tissue. The common therapeutic dosage would be between 10 and 40 mg per mL. Available triamcinolone suspension should be diluted to achieve the final concentration just sufficient to treat the target lesion. Because the injections are administered monthly, the authors favor lower dosage 10 or 20 mg to prevent undesirable effects.

To reduce the discomfort on pain, 1% or 2% lidocaine can be used to dilute triamcinolone in desired concentrations. Lidocaine alone may not induce reduction in pain due to its acidity and sodium bicarbonate can be added. Injection with lidocaine and bupivacaine mixture subcutaneously beneath and around the target lesion few minutes prior to the treatment can be beneficial to minimize pain on administration and after the treatment. Other measures to reduce patient discomfort are to apply ice pack or spray cooling system prior to the injection. Topical lidocaine available in tape or cream formulation can be of benefit.

Before administration, it is important to gently shake to suspend the micronized suspensions evenly. Upon injection, the needle should be introduced to target the

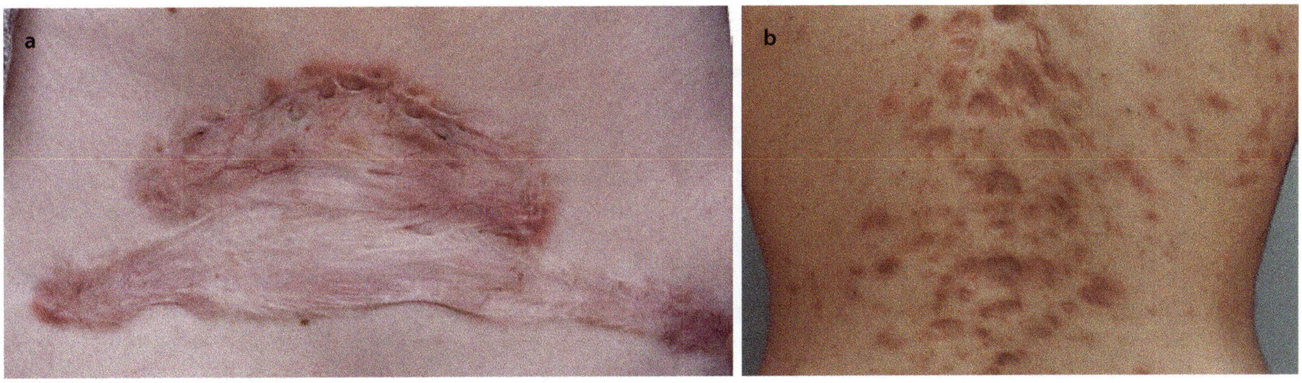

Fig. Localized side effect after corticosteroid intralesional injection. **a** Telangiectasia on the chest. **b** Permanent skin atrophy on the back

dermis where the target tissue is deposited. Resistance is felt when correctly injected to the dermis and when the drug is administered in the upper dermis, slight blanching can be noted. Direct injection to the subcutaneous tissue should be avoided which easily induces lipoatrophy. Long-standing keloid tissue with firm texture should be pretreated with liquid nitrogen to induce edema and subsequent softening of the tissue. Alternatively, injection can be performed to the periphery of the scar tissue directing the needle toward the scar tissue. Most treatment algorithms require multiple serial injections of intralesional steroid. In clinical practice, keloids are treated by a monthly injection until the resolution of clinical symptoms. The clinical response may differ between hypertrophic scars and keloids. While hypertrophic scars tend to be more responsive than keloids and generally flatten with time, keloids may require repeated interventions [6].

Currently, intralesional triamcinolone is the major first-line therapy for treatment of both hypertrophic scars and keloids. Its efficacy is well confirmed by numerous clinical trials and meta-analysis [7]. Intralesional triamcinolone injection effectively induced marked reduction in the size of the keloid. It was particularly efficient when administered after surgical removal of keloid lesions. Intralesional triamcinolone immediately after wound closure and at early postoperative visits, 20 mg/ml and 10 mg/ml respectively, resulted in 76.5% recurrence-free resolutions during a follow-up period of 18 months [8]. Combination treatment regimen with intralesional injection, 20~40 mg/ml, and potent topical steroid application yield favorable results with 85.7% recurrence-free on average of 32-month follow-up period [9]. Given the results of the clinical studies encompass different lesions occurring on different anatomical locations and durations, further clinical trials should be directed to overcome limitations of current repots including differences in timing of intervention, anatomical locations, inclusion and exclusion criteria, and inconsistent outcome measures.

Side Effects and Complications

Steroid-induced side effects include skin atrophy, telangiectasia, hypopigmentation, ulceration, and, rarely, systemic complications. Fortunately, the most commonly encountered side effects of intralesional corticosteroid injection are localized. The incidence of localized side effects is often reported in one-third of patients. Skin atrophy usually occurs over several weeks to months after the injection and may resolve spontaneously without treatment. However, atrophic lesion caused by repeated injection with high dosage persists longer and may induce permanent change. Telangiectasia may occur frequently on the site of injection. In most cases, the lesions do not regress spontaneously and further treatment is required. Laser or light devices such as pulsed dye laser or intensive pulsed light can be successfully applied for its treatment. Foreign body reaction to intralesional triamcinolone is rare but reported. Granulomatous reactions result from the failure of injected crystalized corticosteroid particle to disperse or incomplete absorption. Clinically, prolonged absorption of injected material presents as xanthoma-like lesions and resolves spontaneously over few months (Fig. 29.5).

Systemic complications are rare but occasionally observed. In children, cases of Cushing's syndrome following repeated injection of high dosage intralesional steroid is reported. In adults, the evidence for systemic complication is limited with few reported cases of Cushing's syndrome when patients are subjected to large doses due to extensive keloids. Monthly injection of large dosage of corticosteroids is often brought to account to cause menstrual irregularities. Although there is insufficient clinical evidence, it is unlikely that intralesional corticosteroid alone can cause adrenal complications.

Complications related to intralesional injections can be prevented by using the lowest concentration and the smallest quantity of the drug needed. Increasing the concentration can be adjusted as needed after the repeated course of treatments. For patients with multiple or large lesions, alternating the treatment site or dilution to lower dosage is recommended. Additionally, scars across the joint area and periorbital area can be more susceptible to localized absorption of corticosteroids and higher concentration should be avoided. Although diabetes is not a contraindication to intralesional corticosteroid injection, patients should be approached with caution and appropriate monitoring should be considered.

Further Applications

Enhancing the Effect of Intralesional Corticosteroid

For long-standing hypertrophic scar lesions or large and firm keloids, the combination with cryotherapy can be highly effective. Cryotherapy with liquid nitrogen induces dissociation of accumulated ECM tissue along with possible vascular suppression and apoptosis of fibroblasts. Open spray technique is most commonly used in combination with intralesional injections. When used in combination, injections should be made after defrosting of the lesion. There are several reports showing marked improvement of hypertrophic scars and keloids after either superficial or intralesional cryotherapy. To prevent hypopigmentation from melanocyte destruction or other associated side effects of cryotherapy, shorter exposure (10~30 seconds) is recommended with fewer (two to three) freeze thaw cycles.

In addition to intralesional injection of triamcinolone, localized injection of antimetabolite agents are reported to be beneficial for scar treatments. 5-Fluorouracil (5-FU) is an antimetabolite inhibiting DNA synthesis which increases fibroblast apoptosis and inhibit proliferation. The use of combination triamcinolone and 5-FU has been demonstrated to be as efficacious as triamcinolone alone. Although there are possible side effects from 5-FU including injection site irritation or delayed wound healing, it lacks atrophy or erythema associated with corticosteroid injections. The pain upon administration was a major drawback in 5-FU treatment, while its combination with triamcinolone relieved excruciating pain. Combination of intralesional 5-FU injection with topical corticosteroids yields successful result in scar treatment [3]. Given the requirement for repeated treatment sessions and pain associated with intralesional injection of corticosteroids, other modalities such as lasers and efficient delivery systems are suggested.

Conclusion

The management of keloids and hypertrophic scars continues to challenge clinicians, and there is no universally accepted treatment algorithm. Although there are myriad of treatment options, selection of treatment modality largely depends on the patient desire. The use of corticosteroids has remained mainstay of the treatment for more than half century. While potent topical corticosteroids can be of limited use to address pruritus, intralesional injection of triamcinolone is the mainstay in treatment. Intralesional triamcinolone injection is thought to reduce scar formation by suppressing inflammation, inhibiting fibroblast proliferation, and inducing collagen remodeling. Corticosteroid is cost-effective because it does not require additional equipment, and thus readily applied in patients' regular clinical visits. Further studies are warranted to identify the optimal combination with other modalities for scar treatment.

Take-Home Messages

- Intralesional injection of corticosteroid is effective first-line treatment for the treatment for keloids and hypertrophic scars.
- Corticosteroid inhibits fibroblast growth proliferation and collagen synthesis by effecting on TGF-β signaling and promoting collagen degeneration.
- Intralesional injection of triamcinolone acetonide (10–40 mg/ml) is desired and lower concentration is more favorable for the initial treatments.
- The use of smaller gauge needle and syringe allows better control of the injection and minimize patient discomfort.
- For long-standing and firm scar lesions, combination with cryotherapy is required to achieve optimal penetration.

References

1. Ketchum LD, Smith J, Robinson DW, Masters FW. The treatment of hypertrophic scar, keloid and scar contracture by triamcinolone acetonide. Plast Reconstr Surg. 1966;38(3):209–18.
2. Gold MH, Berman B, Clementoni MT, Gauglitz GG, Nahai F, Murcia C. Updated international clinical recommendations on scar management: part 1-evaluating the evidence. Dermatol Surg. 2014;40(8):817–24. https://doi.org/10.1111/dsu.0000000000000049.
3. Tziotzios C, Profyris C, Sterling J. Cutaneous scarring: pathophysiology, molecular mechanisms, and scar reduction therapeutics Part II. Strategies to reduce scar formation after dermatologic procedures. J Am Acad Dermatol. 2012;66(1):13–24. https://doi.org/10.1016/j.jaad.2011.08.035.

4. Rutkowski D, Syed F, Matthews LC, Ray DW, McGrouther DA, Watson REB, et al. An abnormality in glucocorticoid receptor expression differentiates steroid responders from nonresponders in keloid disease. Br J Dermatol. 2015;173(3):690–700. https://doi.org/10.1111/bjd.13752.
5. Wu WS, Wang FS, Yang KD, Huang CC, Kuo YR. Dexamethasone induction of keloid regression through effective suppression of VEGF expression and keloid fibroblast proliferation. J Invest Dermatol. 2006;126(6):1264–71. https://doi.org/10.1038/sj.jid.5700274.
6. Kim S, Choi TH, Liu W, Ogawa R, Suh JS, Mustoe TA. Update on scar management: guidelines for treating Asian patients. Plast Reconstr Surg. 2013;132(6):1580–9. https://doi.org/10.1097/PRS.0b013e3182a8070c.
7. Wong TS, Li JZ, Chen S, Chan JY, Gao W. The efficacy of triamcinolone acetonide in keloid treatment: a systematic review and meta-analysis. Front Med (Lausanne). 2016;3:71. https://doi.org/10.3389/fmed.2016.00071.
8. Hayashi T, Furukawa H, Oyama A, Funayama E, Saito A, Murao N, et al. A new uniform protocol of combined corticosteroid injections and ointment application reduces recurrence rates after surgical keloid/hypertrophic scar excision. Dermatol Surg. 2012;38(6):893–7. https://doi.org/10.1111/j.1524-4725.2012.02345.x.
9. Ledon JA, Savas J, Franca K, Chacon A, Nouri K. Intralesional treatment for keloids and hypertrophic scars: a review. Dermatol Surg. 2013;39(12):1745–57. https://doi.org/10.1111/dsu.12346.

19

Genetics of Keloid Scarring

Alia Sadiq, Nonhlanhla P. Khumalo, and Ardeshir Bayat

Contents

Background

Overview Keloid disease (KD) is an aesthetically and physically distressing skin disorder [74]. KD is considered a benign tumor of the dermis that develops as a result of a dysregulated healing response to cutaneous wounding [88]. Phenotypically, it is an exophytic proliferative fibrous growth of ill-defined etiopathogenesis [15, 17]. Keloid scarring is an enigma and a challenge to clinicians especially dermatologists and surgeons [87], due to its poor response to clinical management [88].

Keloids are reported to have a high incidence in darker skin races and certain ethnicities of Afro-Caribbean origin [4]. The incidence of keloid cases is 16% in black Africans [15] and keloid predominance in females as compared to the males might be due to more piercing trends in females [82].

This benign skin disease can either occur sporadically, or can exhibit a familial pattern. Keloid disease is considered a genetic disease due to a strong genetic susceptibility to keloid formation as it occurs predominantly in people of African and Asian descent, runs in families, and has been found in twins. However, a well-defined comprehensive mode of inheritance still remains unknown due to insufficient studies to uncover the genetic basis of keloid formation. Nevertheless, inheritance patterns for X-Linked or autosomal dominant trait have been found in families with keloids [71]. Although no specific genes have been identified, that is directly linked to the development of keloids, a few genetic loci have been reported to have a potential role in disease susceptibility. A study conducted in a Japanese population revealed four potential SNPs (single-nucleotide polymorphisms) in three chromosomal regions [76]. Anatomical sites affected with KD also vary in different keloid-prone families [9]. Keloid scarring may comprise of multiple genes, and affected individuals could possess variable genetic susceptibility for a set of genes or gene mutations associated with keloid phenotype [4]. Association studies for keloids such as gene polymorphisms and mutations have been conducted for some genes including SMAD3, SMAD7, and SMAD6, TGF-β1–3, and TGF-βRI-III to investigate the respective genetic basis of disease pathology. Some genetic networks such as cellular apoptosis, MAPKs, TGF-β, IL-6 and PAI-1 have also been studied in keloid pathology [8, 10–13, 15, 99] and also found associated with immunogenic processes as well as other biological pathways (PAI-1, Bcl-2, p53, and collagen deposition) [88]. Complexity and differences in the inheritance modes and familial keloid scarring reflect the variability and heterogeneity in genetic susceptibility, family history, twin genetic makeup, inheritance patterns, linkage, genetic associations, variation in gene expression and respective gene pathways, HLA (human leukocyte antigen) polymorphism, epigenetics, and ethnic populations [88]. Currently, none of hypothesized mechanisms can directly explain the disease pathology. Moreover, the lack of effective treatment options underlines the lack of understanding about disease process and complex and multivariable pathogenesis [74].

Objectives The objectives of this review are to investigate the evidence related to the genetic basis and its association with keloid disease. A comprehensive literature search was performed using PubMed, Google Scholar, CNKI and Embase databases, by applying combinations of relevant MeSH (Medical Subject Headings) words as title. The key search terms included "Keloid, HLA immunogenetics, Linkage, and Large scale population SNP analysis." The appropriate keywords included "Keloid, RNA Sequence analysis, Microarray, Micro RNA, Methylation, Mutation, Epigenetics, and FISH." All retrieved records were compiled in the study for comprehensive review and evaluated based on significance, methodology, evidence, and reproducibility (■Fig. 8.1).

HLA Immunogenetics

Human leukocyte antigen (HLA) is the only complex genetic polymorphic system present on the 6th chromosome (short arm) and is involved in presentation and processing of peptide antigens via HLA class I and II [23]. The association or involvement of HLA in keloid etiology remains elusive as the pathology of dermal fibrosis and poor wound-healing remain ill understood [74].

A study conducted in Caucasians and Chinese Hans populations demonstrated the involvement of immunogenetics (HLA alleles) in keloid etiology. Generally, environmental exposure during the wound-healing process alters the antigen presentation and expression levels of HLA molecules that trigger respective immune response including prolonged inflammation and subsequent release of profibrotic cytokine/chemokines contributing to the excessive extracellular matrix (ECM) deposition, leading to the development of the keloid phenotype. The presence of (altered) immune cells in keloids, provides the insight into the disease pathology. Variable/altered gene and protein expression in keloids supports the contribution of a dysregulated immune system for disease progression or development [4]. The association of immunogenic molecules with the keloid phenotype, has been shown by a study, in which peripheral blood mononuclear cells of keloid patient exhibited increased expression levels of HLA-DR, -DQ, -DP and CD1a molecules in keloid patients [57].

The association of keloids with HLA-I alleles, has been studied in Chinese Han population (192 patients and 252 healthy individuals) to find out the HLA status

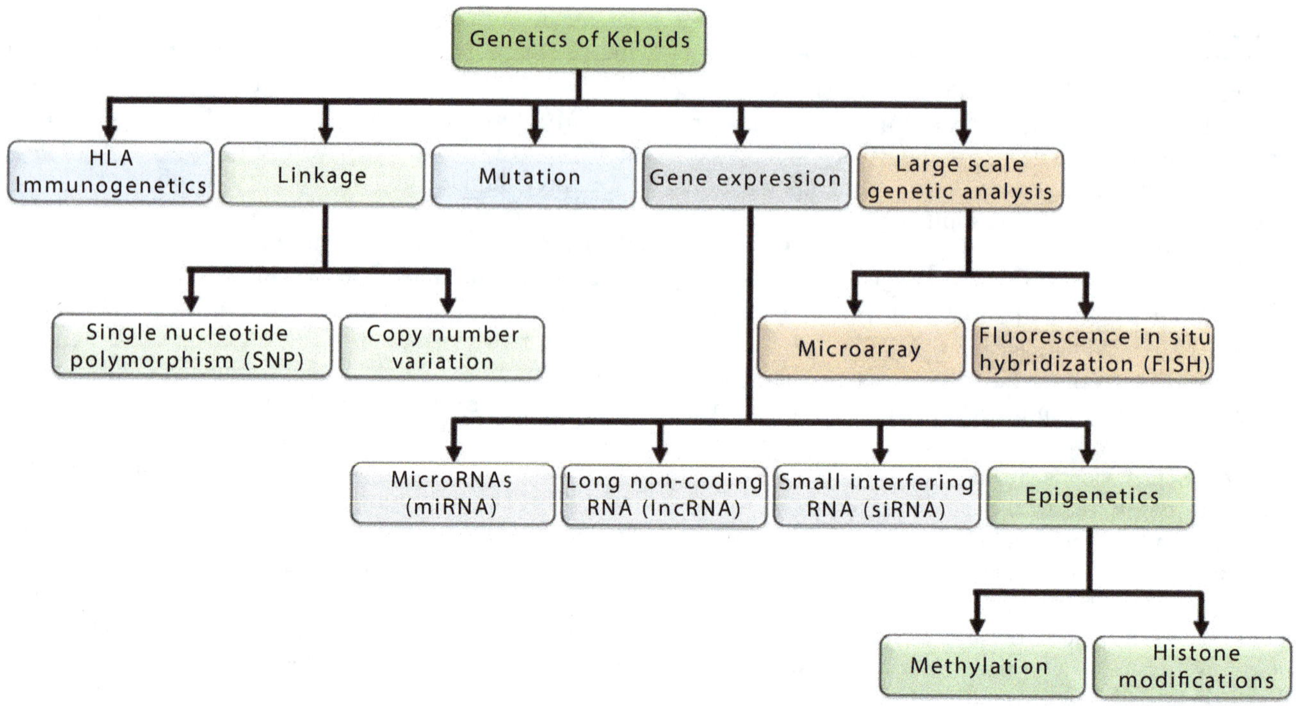

Fig. Association of various genetic elements with keloid development

as a potential contributor to the keloids formation. The frequencies of HLA-A*03, A*25, Cw*0802, and B*07 were significantly high in keloid group but, the frequency of HLA-A*01 was highly decreased in comparison with healthy individuals. This study described high risk haplotypes (A*03-B*07, A*25-B*07, A*03-Cw*0802, A*25-Cw*0802, and B*07-Cw*0802) as contributing components in keloid formation. Interestingly, keloid site specificities, number, severity and details of family inheritance were also associated with specific alleles of HLA class. It shows that maybe these alleles are linked (linkage) with genes, which are responsible for keloid susceptibility [65]. Of note, HLA-I alleles (A*01, A*03, A*25, B*07 and Cw*08:02, HLA-DQA1 and DQB1) previously associated with KD in participants of Chinese ethnicity were shown to have no significant differences in allele frequencies in keloid cases from Jamaican Afro-Caribbean ethnic group [4].

Keloid patients were also found to have an association with blood type A and human leukocyte antigens HLA-B14, HLA-B21, HLA-BW35, HLA–DR5, HLA-DRB1, HLA–DQA1, HLA-DQB1, and HLA-DQW3 [78, 88, 110]. The association of HLA-I histocompatibility antigens, patient's family history with earlobe keloids pathology, has been studied in females of Black ethnic group. This study revealed some factors that appear in high frequency and acts as a risk factor when associated with: (i) HLA-A 9, (ii) HLA-A 23, (iii) HLA-Aw 34, (iv) HLA-Cw 2 antigens, history of (v) hypertension and (vi) post-ear piercing infection [29].

Association between HLA-DRB1 phenotype and keloid etiology has been studied in Caucasians populations of Northern European origin (keloid cases n = 67, control n = 537). It was revealed that frequency of HLA-DRB1*15 was high (38.8%) in Caucasians keloid cases, which appeared as a risk factor of developing KD following injury [17]. Frequencies of serologically detectable HLA antigens, i.e., HLA-B14 and HLA-Bw16, were subsequently found to be more (25%) common as compared to the control, which further suggests that, the individuals having HLA-B14 or HLABwl6 phenotype may be at risk for keloid formation [51].

It seems that most likely there is an association between alleles of HLA class and/or shield against dermal fibrosis, because allele loci (DQ and DR) from class II is a promising genetic marker owing significance contribution in poor wound healing and fibrosis [74]. All of these investigations deliver a strong statement about significant involvement of immunogenic component in keloid pathogenesis [19, 23].

Linkage

The prevalence of KD in identical twins, in families, in certain ethnicities, and at multiple sites strongly supports a genetic predisposition in the development of keloid phenotype [9, 71]. Certainly, the risk of KD occurrence is higher in genetically susceptible individuals (Bayat et al. [8, 12, 16]). In addition to that, recurrence rate (50%) is also higher in the African population with family history having positive keloid cases [9]. The linkage loci of KD were initially found to be on chromosomes 2q23 and 7p11 by Marneros et al. [72], but no putative gene target was further identified.

Single-nucleotide polymorphisms (commonly found to be useful genetic markers in various association studies) may also confer a risk for keloid disease development, such as PTEN (The phosphatase and tensin homolog) gene polymorphisms at rs2299939, rs17431184, rs555895, and rs701848) were found significantly related with high risk of keloid development in Chinese Han population. In addition, it was found that CC genotype from rs2299939 appeared as a risk factor in keloid patients as compared to ACTC haplotype prevalence in population, which seems protective factor against keloid formation [55, 56].

The GWAS (genome-wide association study) identified three keloid susceptibility loci (rs873549 at 1q41, rs8032158 at 15p21.3 and rs940187 and rs1511412 at 3q22.3) in a Japanese population. Furthermore, an association study of these susceptibility loci was also investigated in keloid patients from Chinese Han population. The SNPs 1q41 (rs873549, and rs1442440,) and 15q21.3 (rs2271289 present in NEDD4) revealed significant association with keloid in the Chinese Han population. In addition, AG haplotype was identified as risk factor whereas, GA and AA haplotypes appeared as protective factors from rs1442440 and rs873549 SNPs. It is also suggested that 15q21.3 and 1q41 loci shows genetic association and predisposition for keloid formation in Japanese and Chinese Han populations [116].

Predisposing genes also showed linkage association with keloid susceptibility genes. A study conducted in a selected Han Chinese keloid pedigree, mapped to the region about 1 Mbp on chromosomes 10q23.31, between Fas gene marker D10S1765 and D10S1735, provides the first genetic evidence of a predisposing Fas gene linkage association with keloid susceptibility genes [22].

Another genome-wide association research study (keloid cases =824, Healthy cases= 3205) found strong association of keloid cases with four more SNP loci present at three chromosomal locations (3q22.3–23, 1q41, and 15q21.3) in a Japanese population. It was found that SNP rs873549 at chromosome 1 showed the most significant association with keloid cases [76].

The linkage between the susceptibility locus (18q21.1, SMAD, and PIAS2) to keloid and two loci, 18q21.1and 15q22.31-q23, was also investigated through pedigree linkage analysis in a five-generation Han Chinese keloid family. Seven critical regions of microsatellite markers on chromosomes 18q21.1 and 15q22.31-q23 and were included in analysis. Out of the seven markers, only two (D18S460, D18S467) showed linkage to the disease locus [108]. SMAD genes 3, 6, and 7 are known to be involved in fibrotic disorders, and their association with keloid disease susceptibility was also studied in Jamaican keloid patients. Thirty-five SNPs across these genes were genotyped using time-of-flight mass spectrometry (MALDI-TOF MS) and iPLEX assay. Linkage disequilibrium (LD) was established between several of the SNPs investigated. These findings indicated that the SMAD SNPs were not significantly associated with high risk of keloid formation in the Jamaican population. This study also highlighted the importance of identification of genetic bio-markers as a candidate such as SMAD, which can be helpful diagnostic, prognostic tool and can provide hope for development of new therapeutics for keloid scar management [15].

Keloid predisposition loci at chromosome 7p11 was studied in a Chinese population pedigree [21] consisting of 5 affected generations and a total of 32 members. Four microsatellites on chromosome 7p11 were selected as the genetic markers. This study provided the first genetic indication that keloid predisposition loci did not locate on chromosome 7p11 in Chinese population, furthermore, it suggested that familial keloid predisposition loci are heterogeneous.

Recently in another research study, analysis was conducted through whole genome sequence data, and identified "Leu401Pro variant" in ASAH1 (N-acylsphingosine amidohydrolase) gene, that revealed co-segregation pattern with keloid phenotype in a large population of Yoruba family. This genetic variant is known to play a role in tumor formation, inflammation and cell proliferation, which suggested that it may be involve in keloid development through various other mechanisms. This study also found some rare coding variants but their susceptibility for non-syndromic development of keloid is not known [85].

Large-Scale Population Single-Nucleotide Polymorphism (SNP)

Researchers have started to investigate deeper into the human genome by using high-throughput microarray genotyping technologies with an objective to develop high-density SNPs map arrays in families with keloid history. Previously genome-wide case-control association study described three susceptibility loci (i) 1q41, (ii) 3q22.3-23, and (iii) 15q21.3 in association with keloid disease, in a Japanese population [76]. NEDD4 gene present in 15q21.3 chromosomal locus, is involve in up regulation of collagen type 1 and fibronectin, that result in extracellular matrix formation [24].

An independent case-control study was conducted to find correlation between SNPS i: e rs2118610, rs873549, rs2271289, rs1511412) and phenotypes of keloid cases in Chinese Han population. This study revealed that inheritance patterns of four SNPs (particularly SNP rs2271289) were dominant in severe keloid cases, in comparison with mild cases and control groups. Similar pattern of association of SNP rs2271289 with keloid cases, appeared in family with no case history of keloids as well as in groups having multiple keloid sites. These associations revealed that SNP rs2271289 is a strong contributing factor and a likely candidate in keloid pathology [114].

Association of FOXL2 gene, keloid and SNP rs1511412 have also been identified in Japanese population [76], but this association wasn't significant in the Chinese Han population [116] may be due to low frequency of this variant. Another SNP rs1511412 showed significant association with FOXL2 gene and keloid cases, which appeared as genetic risk factor for keloid development in various ethnic groups of Asian population [64].

A comprehensive study of familial keloids, based on genetic and clinical parameters, was conducted in mostly African Americans, White, Japanese, and African Caribbean families. Individuals affected with keloids exhibited a variable pattern of expression within the families, for example some family members had minor keloids on earlobes and other had large body areas highly affected with severe keloids. In same family, seven members were identified as unaffected but obligate carriers for keloid phenotype. The genetic analysis revealed an autosomal dominant inheritance pattern along with variable phenotypic expression [71].

Gene Expression

Gene regulation and unique genetic components have also been studied in keloid dermal fibroblasts (KDF). Studies revealed up-/downregulated expression of various genes (◘Table 8.1). The specific genes and their differentially regulated expression may have direct implications toward understanding the keloid development [25].

MicroRNAs (miRNA)

MicroRNAs are 21–23 nucleotide molecules, targeting the 3'UTR of mRNA and microRNA deregulation may indicate a potential need for clinical intervention [2]. Role of various miRNAs has been established for activation of fibroblasts. A study reported 32 microRNAs differentially expressed in keloid tissues [63], in which total 23 miRNAs (e.g. miR-4269, miR-21, miR-382) were up-regulated and 9 miRNAs (e.g. miR-205, miR-203, miR-200b/c) were down-regulated. These miRNAs are involved in various cellular signaling networks particularly wound- healing, development of scar and collagen synthesis [39]. Various studies revealed that microRNAs play a key regulatory role in keloid fibroblasts, for instance, miR200b was found associated with abnormal proliferation in fibroblasts and miR200c was involved in radiation-induced cell apoptosis pathway [50, 55, 56, 61, 117]. These microRNAs may be considered potential candidates for therapeutic targets for keloids [33]. Three common miRNAs, has-miR-21, has-miR-199a-5p and has-miR-214 were found in some studies [69, 104, 105] among them, has-miRNA-21 exhibited variable expression [40]. Comparative expression profiles study of miRNA was further extended and found that, keloid derived fibroblasts have total nine different miRNAs as compared to the normal skin fibroblasts. Out of nine, six were up-regulated (hsv1-miR- H7, miR-320c, miR-31- 5p, miR-23b-3p, miR-152, miR-30a-5p) and three (miR-143-3p, miR-4328 and miR-145-5p) were down-regulated [54, 66]. Some of the key miRNAs that appear differentially expressed in keloid cells have been assessed in more detail the table below (◘Table 8.2).

Long noncoding RNA (lncRNA)

Long noncoding RNA, remains uncovered with respect to their association with keloid pathology. The advanced microarray technology was used first time to investigate the keloids in 2015 by Liang et al. group that demonstrated constantly up-regulated (total 1,731) and down-regulated (782) lncRNAs in keloids. In this study, a total of 55 pathways were highlighted: out of which 11 pathways were related to the upregulated transcripts and 44 with downregulated transcripts in keloids. In addition to that, it has been found that the CACNA1G-AS1, as one of the selected lncRNA, may have a potential role in keloid development [58]. The lncRNAs regulating encoding transcripts/genes are considered to participate in Wnt signaling pathway in keloids [95]. The lncRNA H19 stimulate cell proliferation in keloid fibroblasts which reversed by H19 siRNA treatment on keloid fibroblasts [113].

Small Interfering RNA (siRNA)

RNA interference is an evolutionally conserved genetic regulatory mechanism involving inhibition of target gene expression at transcriptional, or translational level, or by degrading the mRNA [101]. Advances in gene silencing [102] provide the opportunity to apply RNA interference technology to uncover the details of molecular mechanisms maintain keloid tissue growth [6]. It is found that β-catenin expression significantly increased in keloid tissue [18] and has been shown to have a role in the regulation of keloid scarring. Knockdown of

Table Differential gene/protein expression markers in keloid-derived primary fibroblasts

S. No	Cellular genetic marker	Expression studies	Level	Role in keloid fibroblasts	Sample source	Role in normal dermal fibroblasts	Reference
1	TGF-β1	mRNA Site-specific gene expression by qRT-PCR	Slightly more	Fibrosis-inducing factors Fibronectin biosynthesis Leads to overproduction of ECM	Primary keloid-derived fibro P2–P4	Proliferation, collagen Deposition and transdifferentiation	[14, 46, 60]
2	TGF-β3	mRNA	Low	Fibrosis-inducing factors	Primary keloid-derived fibro P2–P4	reduces connective tissue (collagen) deposition	[14]
3	TGF-βRII	mRNA	Low	Fibrosis-inducing factors	Primary keloid-derived fibro P2–P4	TGF-β downstream signaling	[14]
4	TGF-βRI/TGF-βRII	mRNA by real-time PCR Immunohistochemistry	High	Enhanced collagen synthesis	Primary keloid-derived fibro P2–P4	TGF-β downstream signaling	[14]
5	Versican (CS/DS–proteoglycan (PG) (VCAN)	mRNA by real-time PCR protein by dot blot, Western blot, and immunostaining	High	Excessive deposition contributes significantly to keloid volume	Keloid tissue and primary keloid-derived fibroblast	Cell adhesion, migration, proliferation, differentiation	[107]
6	Lumican (LUM)	Microarray analysis (mRNA KL Fb/mRNA normal Fb)	High	//	Primary keloid-derived Fb, passage 2 and 4	//	//
7	Aggrecan	//	//	//	//	//	//
8	Collagen a1 (X)	//	//	ECM component	//	//	//
9	Collagen a1 (II)	//	//	//	//	//	//
10	Collagen a2 (IX)	//	//	//	//	//	//
11	Collagen a1 (XI)	//	//	//	//	//	//
12	Collagen a1 (VIII)	//	//	//	//	//	//
13	Thrombospondin 1	//	//		//		//
14	Collagen a1 (XVII)	//	//	//	//	//	//
15	Collagen a3 (IX)	//	//	//	//	//	//

16	HIF1A (Hypoxia-inducible factor1, alpha)	mRNA by real-time PCR Protein by immunohistochemistry, immunofluorescence staining, Western blot	//	Transcriptional regulator, which helps the cells to adapt in the hypoxic microenvironment. Indicators are ECM accumulation and cell proliferation, invasion, and differentiation/ transformation (transition of human dermal fibroblasts to a myofibroblast-like phenotype via the TGF-β1/Smad3 pathway)	Keloid tissue and primary keloid-derived fibroblast		[68, 115]
17	Vimentin	//	//	Mesenchymal marker	//	EMT marker	//
18	Fibronectin	//	//	Mesenchymal marker	//	EMT marker	//
19	Connective tissue growth factor (CTGF)	qRT-PCR Protein by Western blot Immunohistochemistry	//	Fibrosis	// Keratinocyte-fibroblast coculture	Cell adhesion, migration, proliferation, angiogenesis	[46, 115, 49]
20	Atypical chemokine receptor 3 (ACKR3)	qRT-PCR	//	Cholesterol biosynthesis I/ II, Vasculo-/angiogenesis cancer tissue morphology	Keloid tissue and primary keloid-derived fibroblast		[46]
21	Tumor necrosis factor (TNF)	//	//	//	//		//
22	Ephrin receptor B4 (EPHB4)	//	//	//	//		//
23	Forkhead box F2 (FOXF2)	//	//	//	//		//
24	Insulin-like growth factor (IGF) binding protein 3 (IGFBP3)	//	//	Activating collagen synthesis and cell proliferation, decreasing apoptosis	//		[86]
25	Transgelin	//	//	Early detecting cell transformation marker	//	Proteins responsible for changes in cell shape and structure	//
26	Annexin A2 (ANXA2)	//	//	Marker of apoptosis	//	Apoptosis	//
27	Ribosomal protein S18	//	//	Protein synthesis	//	Protein synthesis	//

(continued)

Table

S. No	Cellular genetic marker	Expression studies	Level	Role in keloid fibroblasts	Sample source	Role in normal dermal fibroblasts	Reference
28	60 S ribosomal protein (L36a)	Clontech's Atlas™ Human cDNA Expression Array	Low	Protein synthesis	//	Protein synthesis	[25]
29	Nuclease-sensitive element DNA binding protein (NSEP)	Clontech's Atlas™ Human cDNA Expression Array	Low	Transcription	//	Transcription and regulation of essential growth control genes	[25]
30	Interleukin-6 (IL-6)	Translational study for IL-6, Pro-hybridization and ELISA	//	IL-6-induced cell proliferation	Primary keloid-derived fibroblast, passages 4 to 8	Immunoregulatory cytokine known for role in fibrotic autoimmune diseases	[106, 38]
31	Vascular endothelial growth factor (VEGF)	VEGF-ELISA kit	//	Increases granulation-tissue formation	Primary keloid-derived fibroblast passages 2	Angiogenesis	[93, 38]

Abbreviations: *KL* keloid; *Fb* fibroblasts. Symbols: //, same as above

Table Differential expression of miRNAs and their effects on keloid fibroblasts

S. No	Type of microRNA	Expression level in keloid fibroblasts	Role in keloid phenotype	Reference
1.	miR-7	Low	Induce excessive collagen expression	[31]
2.	miR-29a	Low	Collagen I and III expression regulation, TGF-β/Smad signaling pathway, fibrosis	[73, 41, 112]
3.	miR-199a	Low	Influence proliferation of keloid fibroblasts via cell cycle regulation	[104, 105, 109]
4.	miR-21	High	Stimulate fibroblast proliferation and apoptosis via P13K/AKT pathway and synthesis of extracellular matrix	[62, 75, 100]
5.	miR-196a	High	Regulates the stabilized elevated expression of COL1A1 and COL3A1 genes	[1, 48, 54]
6.	miR-152	High	It promotes keloid fibroblast proliferation and collagen synthesis	[54, 63]

β-catenin/siRNA inhibits cell proliferation and induces arrest in G0/G1 phase of cell cycle. It also induces apoptosis in fibroblasts via down-regulation of cyclin D1 and Wnt2 pathways. Keloid fibroblasts (KFs) overexpress AMF (autocrine motility factor), which acts through RhoA/ROCK1 signaling network, to enhance their cell migration and proliferation. Knocking down AMF/siRNA significantly reduces the migration as well as proliferation potential of KFs that ultimately reduces keloid size [98].

TIMP-1 and small interfering RNA regulation has an important role in keloid pathology. Generally, it is known that keloid phenotype appears as a result of disproportion between synthesis and degradation of extracellular matrix. There are two main vital components (i) Matrix metalloproteinase (ii) Tissue inhibitors of metalloproteinase, which regulate the process of synthesis degradation and remodeling of ECM. Knockdown of TIMPs (siTIMP-1 or siTIMP-2)/siRNA resulted in suppression of MMP-1/TIMP-1 and MMP-1/TIMP-2 complex molecules but upregulation of MMP-2 and increased collagen type I degradation. KFs also showed increased apoptosis and reduced cell viability [3].

The role of siRNA during TGF-β-induced regulation of of PTB (Polypyrimidine Tract-Binding Protein) in keloid pathophysiology has been demonstrated recently [43]. It is a splicing regulator and known to play an important role in tumor cell proliferation, invasion and metastasis. TGF-β1 stimulation caused over expression of PTB along with its upstream regulatory component (C-MYC) in keloid derived fibroblasts, resulting in dysregulation of alternative splicing events, leads to enhanced fibroblast proliferation and deposition of fibronectin in keloid. PTB/siRNA knockdown shift the alternative splicing of RTN4 and USP, and caused significant reduction in fibroblasts proliferation and deposition of COL3A1 and FN1, that resulting in the fast regression of keloid tissues.

Silencing the Smad2 (Sma and *Drosophila* mothers against decapentaplegic homolog 2) downregulate the TGF-β-induced synthesis of procollagen, in keloid derived fibroblasts [35]. The role of siRNA during Smad3 (Sma and *Drosophila* mothers against decapentaplegic homolog 3)-induced TGF-β signaling in keloid pathogenesis has been studied. Smad3 is recently characterized as an intracellular effector of TGF-β signaling pathway. TGF-β participate as key component in fibrotic pathology by stimulating keloid fibroblasts to synthesize extracellular matrix excessively, including collagen I and III. The knockdown of Smad3/siRNA expression caused significantly and uniquely decrease in types I and III procollagen level. Thus Smad3 is thought to play a significant role in the TGF-β-induced keloid fibrosis [101].

Keloid derived fibroblasts over expressed NLRC5 (NOD-like receptor family CARD domain containing 5) belongs to the family of nucleotide-binding domain and leucine-rich repeat. It has been shown that silencing of NLRC5 results inhibition of proliferation and expression of ECM in keloid derived fibroblasts via inhibition of TGF-β1/Smad signaling network, suggesting potential therapeutic target keloids [67]. Increased expression of Stat3 (signal transducer and activator of transcription 3) was also found in keloid tissue. Stat3 is a latent transcription factor activated under the stimulation of various growth factors and cytokines during wound-healing process. Short interfering RNA inhibited its expression and subsequent phosphorylation and resulted in reduction of collagen synthesis, cell proliferation and migration in keloid derived fibroblasts, hence suggesting another therapeutic candidate for the treatment of keloids [59].

Keloid fibroblasts characteristically showed overexpression of collagen and PAI-1. Short interfering RNA targeted treatment results in reduction the collagen deposition, which showed that PAI-1-targeted siRNA interference may offer therapeutic alternative in keloid formation [99]. Another study showed that silencing of PAI-1 caused significant reduction in keloid volume up to 28% in fourth week. It also decreased the synthesis of collagen I and III and resulted in shrinkage of keloid tissue mass [96].

VEGF (vascular endothelial growth factor) plays vital roles in the regulation of inflammation and angiogenesis during wound-healing process. The role of vector-based RNAi (shRNA) for inhibition of VEGF expression in keloid fibroblasts has been studied. siRNA sequences (clone of three potential short interfering RNA sequences) were used to silence the VEGF gene in keloid fibroblasts that resulted in significantly inhibited VEGF gene expression and fibroblasts growth. In addition, the expression of plasminogen activator inhibitor-1 (PAI-1) was also downregulated. This study provides the insight about the modulation of VEGF production as a potential therapeutic strategy for keloid [111].

Silencing by HIF-1α siRNA in keratinocytes resulted in decreased expression levels of fibronectin and vimentin, whereas ZO-1 and E-cadherin expression levels were restored. This indicated that HIF-1α stimulation can regulate the respective mesenchymal changes, caused by hypoxia in the keloid derived keratinocytes during keloid development [68].

Knockdown of PAI-2, Hsp27, α2β1-integrin/siRNA also cause significant reduction in ECM deposition, cell anchorage, and mobility in keloid derived fibroblasts [94]. Hsp70/siRNA and Hsp47-shRNA knockdown decreased collagen synthesis in keloid derived fibroblasts [20, 90]. hTERT gene regulates telomere length homeostasis and influences cell cycle of fibroblasts. Knockdown of hTERT-siRNA in keloid fibroblasts was shown to reduce telomere length and fibroblast growth [87].

The role of siRNA in apoptosis of keloid fibroblasts has also been investigated. Keloids exhibited increased reactive oxygen species (ROS) production and disrupted apoptosis mechanisms. ROS plays an important role in the induction of apoptosis under pathological conditions. Cellular defense mechanisms against oxidative stress and apoptosis are regulated by nuclear factor erythroid 2-related factor 2 (Nrf2) through activation of B-cell lymphoma 2 (Bcl-2) protein. Transfection of fibroblasts with the Nrf2-specific siRNA resulted in increased apoptosis and decreased cell viability [53]. NRG1/ErbB2/Src/PTK2 signaling pathway in fibroblast migration and the role of siRNA have been investigated in keloid development. Keloid fibroblasts exhibit upregulation of the polypeptide growth factor neuregulin-1 (NRG1) and receptor tyrosine-protein kinase erbB-2 (ErbB2) oncogene that contributes to altered cytokine expression profiles, increased Src and protein tyrosine kinase 2 (PTK2/FAK) gene expression, and migration in keloid fibroblast. siRNA knockdown of ErbB2 gene resulted in reduced migration and Src/PTK2 expression but didn't affect the NRG/ErbB2/Src/PTK2 network, revealing the possibility that this network may affect migrating potential of keloid fibroblasts indirectly [47]. Therefore, siRNA silencing on various targeted mechanisms such as Smad2,3-TGF-β, HIF-1α-EMT, PAI-1-VEGF production, and NRG1/ErbB2/Src/PTK2 signaling pathway in keloid pathogenesis, proposes that their production can be modulated by using siRNA based regulation, and this strategy seems promising candidate for keloid therapeutics.

Microarray Analysis

Various advanced molecular biology techniques such as PCR, cDNA approaches, cloning, whole genome sequencing provides the huge platform to investigate the differentially regulated genes in term of microarray analysis from variety of biological samples [70]. Functional genomic provides a tool to probe and monitor the genetic interactions [27]. Complex pattern of genotypic differences and respective multiple fibrosis-related pathways in keloid fibroblasts have been studied by microarray approach. Comparative Affymetrix-based microarray analysis was carried out on keloid fibroblast RNA. Approximately 500 genes were found differentially regulated out of total the total 38,000 genes observed. Interestingly, study also revealed that increase in expression of various IGF-binding protein and related protein in comparison with set of protein related to Wnt signaling pathway, who exhibited decrease in expression [91]. Total 2,215 differentially expressed genes (DEGs) have been found in comparative analysis of after and before normal wound, and surprisingly total 3,161 DEGs have been identified in keloid-prone individuals. Among those genes, only 513 genes were related to normal individuals, total set of 1,449 genes were found specifically related to keloid phenotype. Moreover, hierarchical distribution of differentially expressed keloid-specific genes resulted into two distinct clusters. Further probing into keloid-specific pathways revealed 24 pathways linked with differentially activated genes. Most importantly, some other vital signaling pathways like NOTCH, MAPKs, TLRs and insulin regulation, have also been found altered during post-wounding analysis in keloid prone individuals. Furthermore, Genetic association network analysis revealed, divergent gene expression profile of key genes that contribute in cytokines signaling pathways [79, 83].

Epigenetics

Study of inheritable characteristics of genome that doesn't affect the genetic sequences but only gene function, comes under the term of epigenetics. It is also known to contribute significantly in regulation of various gene expressions. Recently, there is further extension to this terminology that is epigenetic modification, which is currently being applied to get comprehension of molecular aspects of keloid pathology. This study revealed that there are some evidences pointing the involvement of epigenetic changes/modifications triggering the constant activation of fibroblasts in keloid [30]. These epigenetic alterations include changes in microRNAs, DNA methylation as well as histone modifications. These three event are well known crucial events that involve in early cellular growth, differentiation and development, hence these aspects of molecular features have also been included as an important candidate for investigations to understand their role/associations in keloid pathology [28]. Recent studies are coming up with findings about the epigenetic mechanisms that may contribute in keloid formation [42].

Methylation

DNA methylation is the well-known aspect of epigenetic modification [103]. It has been hypothesized that DNA methylation is responsible to maintain the myofibroblats transformation of fibroblasts during the process of fibrosis in wound healing events, this modification set the basis for deviation from normal wound-healing mechanism. Gene expression profile acquired by myofibroblasts is significantly differ from fibroblasts [81, 97]. Therefore it is crucial to understand respective epigenetic modifications that resulted in acquiring highly differentiated gene expression profile in my myofibroblasts that will help to trace the respective network leading to fibrotic phenotype in keloids [77]. Previous research study found that keloid fibroblasts showed alternations in DNA methylation [84]. Involvement and significance of epigenetic modification in keloid pathology has been revealed in recent study, that showed reversal of expression profile in TGF-β1, phosphor-smad2, 3 (down-regulation) and smad7 (up-regulation) by the treatment of 5-aza-dC (5-aza-2 deoxycytidine), which is an inhibitor of DNA methyltransferase [118].

Expression of DNA methyltransferase 1 (DNMT1) was found 100% elevated in keloid as compared to the fibroblast (8%) from normal skin samples [32], suggesting its involvement in keloid scar formation. Furthermore, different DNA methylation patterns have also been studied in keloid vs normal cells and tissue and analyzed via large scale genome profiling using advanced approach (Infinium Human Methylation 450 BeadChip), results explained that 152 unique genes showed total 192 different methylation patterns in promoter region CpGs. Moreover respective gene network analysis, revealed four common hierarchical regulatory networks, consisting of four key regulators, (i) PENK (ii) PRKG2, (iii) pryoxamide (iv) tributyrin, and total 19 intermediate regulatory molecules. This analysis highlighted the involvement of regulatory networks in keloid phenotype development [36, 45] and with the development of this study approach in recent research since last five years, methylome of keloid have been characterized as most hypo-methylated rather than hyper-methylated [45].

List of hyper-methylated genes includes CACNB2, ACTR3C, PAQR4, SLCO2B1, C1orf109, LRRC61, AHDC1, FYCO1, CMKLR1 and CCDC34 as compared to hypo-methylated group of genes, which are GHDC, DENND1C, MX2, ANKRD11, SCML4, GALNT3, IFFO1, WIPF1, PPP1R13L and CFH. Recently, further analysis was carried out using bioinformatics approach by applying Ingenuity Pathway Analysis (IPA) software on data set, obtained from keloid samples, revealed some key pathways shows significant association with keloids. These pathways include (i) histidine degradation VI (ii) metastasis signaling pathway of colorectal cancer (iii) phospholipase C signaling (iv) P2Y purinergic receptor signaling and (v) Gai signaling pathway [44]. Keloid fibroblasts having multiple genes with differential methylation, exhibited significant difference in expression profile of genes related to fibrosis such as IGFBP5 (IGF/IGF-binding protein 5), JAG1 (Jagged 1), SFRP1 (secreted frizzled-related protein1), MMP3 (matrix mettallopeptidase 3), CTGF (connective tissue growth factor) and DPT (dermatopontin) [84]. These finding support the statement about the involvement of DNA methylation in keloid formation, but needs further extension of research studies to explore respective key changes/modification that leads subsequent stages of development resulted in keloid pathogenesis [36, 44, 45].

Histone Modifications

Histone modifications include changes in distal N-amino acids specifically, phosphorylation at Threonine or Serine, ubiquitination at Arginine or Lysine and acetylation at Lysine amino acid. There are some enzyme such as histone deacetylases (HDACs) and acetyltransferases (HATs), which are involve in these modifications, and result in altered gene expression profile [7]. Interestingly, it has been noted that histone deacetylases over expressed in keloid tissue. This over expression pattern has also been observed under TGF-β1 induced stimulation in normal fibroblasts and murine Swiss 3T3 fibroblasts [34]. *In vitro* research study showed that treating the keloid fibroblasts with HDAC inhibitor resulted in decreased production of collagen [92]. Inhibition of histone acetyltransferases caused anti-fibrotic affects, increased expression of p300 (which is a cofactor, essential for acetylase activity) in fibroblasts (isolated from scleroderma patients samples) [37].

These studies suggest that both DNA methylation and histone modification are crucial to cause differential gene expression profile, exhibited by keloid fibroblasts, furthermore, as such, any sustainable modification responsible to deliver epigenetic changes, can leads towards phenotypic alteration of keloid fibroblasts. This scenario recommending that inhibitors of histone modification can be an important candidate to consider with therapeutic point of view for management of keloid pathology [5, 80, 84].

Mutations

Role of mutations was investigated in a study conducted in keloid cases from a Caucasian population (95 cases). Large scale genome wide analysis in the exon (1–7) and promoter regions showed presence of some novel mutations in Caucasian population [13]. But up till now, none of the gene mutations have been found associated with keloid cases [88]. One *in vitro* study reported a p53 mutation that was found in keloid fibroblasts from cultured cells [26], that may suggest the role of acquired inheritable gene changes in keloid cells [88].

Copy Number Variation

Copy number variations (CNVs) are known to be associated with various human disorders including skin diseases. Research study conducted in keloid cases from Caucasian population revealed that CNVs found at 11q11, 8p23.1, 19p13.1, 22q13.1, 17q12, and 2q14.3, specifically 6p21.32 (that contain HLA-DRB5 region) are associated with keloid pathology [89].

FISH (Fluorescence In Situ Hybridization)

Keloid derived fibroblasts exhibited differential phenotypic and genotypic expression as compared to neighboring normal skin fibroblasts. Real-time RT-PCR and proteomics tools (2-DAGE, immunoblot analysis, and immunohistochemistry) have been used to investigate these differentially expressed specific set of genes and proteins in keloid derived fibroblasts. Proteomic analysis revealed that there are sixteen different spots which differentiate keloid fibroblasts from normal fibroblasts, among all, Hsp70 was most up-regulated protein in keloid derived fibroblasts. These results were also validated by immunohistochemical and western blot analysis conducted on keloid vs normal skin tissue. This study indicated that Hsp70 overexpression may be associated with keloid pathology and its inhibition can be studied for therapeutic purpose [52].

Conclusions

Keloids are benign dermal tumors that develop as a result of a dysregulated cutaneous wound-healing process. Several research findings support the idea that there is an association between various genetic elements such as linkage, autosomal-dominant, oligo-genic or additive inheritance in families and keloid development, predominantly in people of African and Asian descent. In addition to that, differential gene expression studies in families and keloid fibroblasts indicate heterogeneous genetic events, revealing complexity of underlying genetic basis of keloids. Therefore, it's quite obvious that single gene phenomena is not a possible causative factor for keloid formation. To address this complexity, a likely scenario may involve the understanding of genetic pathway interactions including environmental factors, healing mechanisms, wound matrix degradation, and immunologic response.

Take-Home Messages

1. Keloid is a complex skin pathology with varied susceptibilities and ethnicities. This disease is a clinical challenge because it lacks effective treatment and often recurs after excision.
2. Well-defined comprehensive mode of inheritance is still not known because of insufficient genetic investigations.
3. HLA system represents the highest level of diversity of any functional genetic association with keloid disease.
4. Recent advanced approaches like high-throughput microarray facilitating the genetics and epigenetic investigations may be helpful in understanding the underlying complex basis of keloid formation.
5. There could be a possibility to identifying potential candidate set of genetic markers for diagnostic or prognostic purpose.
6. There is need to uncover the specific biological mechanism and respective signaling networks of keloid fibroblasts.

Acknowledgments This study was supported by the National Research Foundation and the South African Medical Research Council grants.

References

1. Adhyatmika A, Putri KS, Beljaars L, Melgert BN. The elusive antifibrotic macrophage. Front Med. 2015;2:81.
2. Ambros V. The functions of animal micrornas. Nature. 2004;431:350–5.
3. Aoki M, Miyake K, Ogawa R, Dohi T, Akaishi S, Hyakusoku H, Shimada T. siRNA knockdown of tissue inhibitor of Metalloproteinase-1 in keloid fibroblasts leads to degradation of collagen type I. J Invest Dermatol. 2014;134:818–26.
4. Ashcroft KJ, Syed F, Arscott G, Bayat A. Assessment of the influence of HLA class I and class II loci on the prevalence of keloid disease in Jamaican afro-Caribbeans. Tissue Antigens. 2011;78(5):390–6.
5. Awakura Y, Nakamura E, Ito N, Kamoto T, Ogawa O. Methylation-associated silencing of SFRP1 in renal cell carcinoma. Oncol Rep. 2008;20(5):1257–63.
6. Bagabir R, Syed F, Paus R, Bayat A. Long-term organ culture of keloid disease tissue. Exp Dermatol. 2012;21(5):376–81.
7. Bassett SA, Barnett MP. The role of dietary histone deacetylases (HDACs) inhibitors in health and disease. Nutrients. 2014;6(10):4273–301.
8. Bayat A, Arscott G, Ollier WER, Ferguson MWJ, Mc Grouther DA. Description of site specific morphology of keloid phenotypes in an Afrocaribbean population. Br J Plast Surg. 2004;57(2):122–33.
9. Bayat A, Arscott G, Ollier WER, Mc Grouther DA, Ferguson MWJ. Keloid disease: clinical relevance of single versus multiple site scars. Br J Plast Surg. 2005;58(1):28–37.
10. Bayat A, Bock O, Mrowietz U, Ollier WE, Ferguson MW. Genetic susceptibility to keloid disease and transforming growth factor beta 2 polymorphisms. Br J Plast Surg. 2002; 55(4):283–6.
11. Bayat A, Bock O, Mrowietz U, Ollier WE, Ferguson MW. Genetic susceptibility to keloid disease and hypertrophic scarring: transforming growth factor beta1 common polymorphisms and plasma levels. Plast Reconstr Surg. 2003;111(2): 535–43.. discussion 544-6
12. Bayat A, Bock O, Mrowietz U, Ollier WE, Ferguson MW. Genetic susceptibility to keloid disease: transforming growth factor beta receptor gene polymorphisms are not associated with keloid disease. Exp Dermatol. 2004;13(2):120–4.
13. Bayat A, Walter JM, Bock O, Mrowietz U, Ollier WER, Ferguson MWJ. Genetic susceptibility to keloid disease: mutation screening of the TGF-β3 gene. Br J Plast Surg. 2005;58: 914–21.
14. Bock O, Yu H, Zitron S, Bayat A, Ferguson MWJ, Mrowietz U. Studies of transforming growth factors Beta 1–3 and their receptors I and II in fibroblast of keloids and hypertrophic scars. Acta Derm Venereol. 2005;85:216–20.
15. Brown JJ, Ollier W, Arscott G, Ke X, Lamb J, Day P, Bayat A. Genetic susceptibility to keloid scarring: SMAD gene SNP frequencies in afro-Caribbeans. Exp Dermatol. 2008;17(7):610–3.
16. Brown JJ, Bayat A. Genetic susceptibility to raised dermal scarring. Br J Dermatol. 2009;161(1):8–18.
17. Brown JJ, Ollier WE, Thomson W, Bayat A. Positive association of HLA-DRB1*15 with keloid disease in Caucasians. Int J Immunogenet. 2008;35(4–5):303–7.
18. Cai Y, Zhu S, Yang W, Pan M, Wang C, Wu W. Downregulation of β-catenin blocks fibrosis via Wnt2 signaling in human keloid fibroblasts. Tumor Biol. 2017;39(6):1–8.
19. Charron D. HLA, immunogenetics, pharmacogenetics and personalized medicine. Vox Sang. 2011;100(1):163–6.
20. Chen JJ, Jin PS, Zhao S, Cen Y, Liu Y, Xu XW, Duan WQ, Wang HS. Effect of heat shock protein 47 on collagen synthesis of keloid *in vivo*. ANZ J Surg. 2011;81(6):425–30.
21. Chen Y, Gao JH, Liu XJ, Yan X, Song M. Linkage analysis of keloid susceptibility loci on chromosome 7p11 in a Chinese pedigree. Nan Fang Yi Ke Da Xue Xue Bao. 2006;26(5): 623–5. 637
22. Chen Y, Gao JH, Yan X, Song M, Liu XJ. Location of predisposing gene for one Han Chinese keloid pedigree. Chin J Plast Surg. 2007;23(2):137–40.
23. Choo SY. The HLA system: genetics, immunology, clinical testing, and clinical implications. Yonsei Med J. 2007;48(1): 11–23.
24. Chung S, Nakashima M, Zembutsu H, et al. Possible involvement of NEDD4 in keloid formation; its critical role in fibro blast proliferation and collagen production. Proc Jpn Acad Ser B Phys Biol Sci. 2011;87:563–73.
25. Cohly HHP, Scott H, Ndebele K, Jenkins JK, Angel MF. Differential gene expression of fibroblasts: keloid versus normal. Int J Mol Sci. 2002;3:1162–76.
26. De Felice B, Garbi C, Santoriello M, Santillo A, Wilson RR. Differential apoptosis markers in human keloids and hypertrophic scars fibroblasts. Mol Cell Biochem. 2009;327(1–2):191–201. https://doi.org/10.1007/s11010-009-0057-x.
27. De Felice B, Garbi C, Wilson RR, Santoriello M, Nacca M. Effect of selenocystine on gene expression profiles in human keloid fibroblasts. Genomics. 2011;97(5):265–76.
28. Dwivedi RS, Herman JG, McCaffrey TA, Raj DS. Beyond genetics: epigenetic code in chronic kidney disease. Kidney Int. 2011;79(1):23–32.
29. Dyal CM. Investigation of predictive factors in keloid fortmation. Yale Medicine Thesis Digital Library. 1989;2547. http://elischolar.library.yale.edu/ymtdl/2547.
30. Egger G, Liang G, Aparicio A, Jones PA. Epigenetics in human disease and prospects for epigenetic therapy. Nature. 2004;429(6990):457–63.
31. Etoh M, Jinnin M, Makino K, Yamane K, Nakayama W, Aoi J, Honda N, Kajihara I, Makino T, Fukushima S, Ihn H. microRNA-7 down-regulation mediates excessive collagen expression in localized scleroderma. Arch Dermatol Res. 2013;305:9–15.
32. Qipa EY, Hengshu Z. The expression of DNMT1 in pathologic scar fibroblasts and the effect of 5-aza-2-Deoxycytidine on cytokines of pathologic scar fibroblasts. Wounds. 2014;26: 139–46.

33. Feng J, Xue S, Pang Q, Rang Z, Cui F. miR-141-3p inhibits fibroblast proliferation and migration by targeting GAB1 in keloids. Biochem Biophys Res Commun. 2017;490:302–8.
34. Fitzgerald O'Connor EJ, Badshah II, Addae LY, Kundasamy P, Thanabalasingam S, Abioye D, Soldin M, Shaw TJ. Histone deacetylase 2 is upregulated in normal and keloid scars. J Invest Dermatol. 2012;132:1293–6. https://doi.org/10.1038/jid.2011.432.
35. Gao Z, Wang Z, Shi Y, Lin Z, Jiang H, Hou T, Wang Q, Yuan X, Zhao Y, Wu H, Jin Y. Modulation of collagen synthesis in keloid fibroblasts by silencing Smad2 with siRNA. Plast Reconstr Surg. 2006;118(6):1328–37.
36. Garcia-Rodriguez L, Jones L, Chen KM, Datta I, Divine G, Worsham MJ. Causal network analysis of head and neck keloid tissue identifies potential master regulators. Laryngoscope. 2016;126:E319–24.
37. Ghosh AK, Varga J. The transcriptional coactivator and acetyltransferase p300 in fibroblast biology and fibrosis. J Cell Physiol. 2007;213:663–71.
38. Giugliano G, Pasquali D, Notaro A, Brongo S, Nicoletti G, D'Andrea F, Bellastella A, Sinisi AA. Verapamil inhibits interleukin-6 and vascular endothelial growth factor production in primary cultures of keloid fibroblasts. Br J Plast Surg. 2003;56:804–9.
39. Gregory PA, Bert AG, Paterson EL, Barry SC, Tsykin A, Farshid G, Vadas MA, Khew-Goodall Y, Goodall GJ. The miR-200 family and miR-205 regulate epithelial to mesenchymal transition by targeting ZEB1 and SIP1. Nat Cell Biol. 2008;10:593–601.
40. Guo XR, Liang J, Huang RL, Lu L, Jin YD, Luo SJ, Wu ZY. Differential expression of microRNAs in human keloids. Zhongguo Zuzhi Gongcheng Yanjiu. 2012;16:9370–5.
41. He Y, Huang C, Lin X, Li J. MicroRNA-29 family, a crucial therapeutic target for fibrosis diseases. Biochimie. 2013;95:1355–9.
42. He Y, Deng Z, Alghamdi M, Lu L, Fear MW, He L. From genetics to epigenetics: new insights into keloid scarring. Cell Prolif. 2017:e12326.
43. Jiao H, Dong P, Yan L, Yang Z, Lv X, Li Q, Zong X, Fan J, Fu X, Liu X, Xiao R. TGF-β1 induces polypyrimidine tract-binding protein to alter fibroblasts proliferation and fibronectin deposition in keloid. Sci Rep. 2016;6:38033.
44. Jones LR, Greene J, Chen KM, Divine G, Chitale D, Shah V, Datta I, Worsham MJ. Biological significance of genome-wide DNA methylation profiles in keloids. Laryngoscope. 2017;127:70–8.
45. Jones LR, Young W, Divine G, Datta I, Chen KM, Ozog D, Worsham MJ. Genome-wide scan for methylation profiles in keloids. Dis Markers. 2015;943176.
46. Jumper N, Hodgkinson T, Paus R, Bayat A. Site-specific gene expression profiling as a novel strategy for unravelling keloid disease pathobiology. PLoS One. 2017;12(3):e0172955. https://doi.org/10.1371/journal.pone.0172955.
47. Jumper N, Hodgkinson T, Paus R, Bayat A. A role for Neuregulin-1 in promoting keloid fibroblast migration via ErbB2-mediated signaling. Acta Derm Venereol. 2017;97(6–7):675–84.
48. Kashiyama K, Mitsutake N, Matsuse M, Ogi T, Saenko VA, Ujifuku K, Utani A, Hirano A, Yamashita S. miR-196a downregulation increases the expression of type I and III collagens in keloid fibroblasts. J Invest Dermatol. 2012;132:1597–604.
49. Khoo YT, Ong CT, Mukhopadhyay A, Han HC, Do DV, Lim IJ, Phan TT. Upregulation of secretory connective tissue growth factor (CTGF) in keratinocyte-fibroblast coculture contributes to keloid pathogenesis. J Cell Physiol. 2006;208(2):336–43.
50. Kurashige J, Mima K, Sawada G, Takahashi Y, Eguchi H, Sugimachi K, Mori M, Yanagihara K, Yashiro M, Hirakawa K, Baba H, Mimori K. Epigenetic modulation and repression of miR-200b by cancer associated fibroblasts contribute to cancer invasion and peritoneal dissemination in gastric cancer. Carcinogenesis. 2015;36:133–41.
51. Laurentaci G, Dioguardi D. HLA antigens in keloids and hypertrophic scars. Arch Dermatol. 1977;113(12):1726.
52. Lee JH, Shin JU, Jung I, Lee H, Rah DK, Jung JY, Lee WJ. Proteomic profiling reveals upregulated protein expression of Hsp70 in keloids. Biomed Res Int. 2013;2013:1. https://doi.org/10.1155/2013/621538.
53. Lee YJ, Kwon SB, Kim CH, Cho HD, Nam HS, Lee SH, Lee MW, Nam DH, Choi CY, Cho MK. Oxidative damage and nuclear factor Erythroid 2-Related Factor 2 protein expression in normal skin and keloid tissue. Ann Dermatol. 2015;27(5).
54. Li C, Bai Y, Liu H, Zuo X, Yao H, Xu Y, Cao M. Comparative study of microRNA profiling in keloid fibroblast and annotation of differential expressed microRNAs. Acta Biochim Biophys Sin. 2013;45:692–9.
55. Li J, Chen X, Zhou Y, Xie H, Li J, Li J, Su J, Yi M, Zhu W. Risk of keloid associated with polymorphic PTEN haplotypes in the Chinese Han population. Wounds. 2014;26(1):21–7.
56. Li P, He QY, Luo CQ. Overexpression of miR-200b inhibits the cell proliferation and promotes apoptosis of human hypertrophic scar fibroblasts in vitro. J Dermatol. 2014;41:903–11.
57. Li S, Wang M. Chen Dong-ming, bi Hong-sen, Tang Y, Bao Wei-han. Immunogenetic regulation of HLA-DR, DQ, DP and CD1a positive cells in the pathogenesis of keloid and hypertrophic scar. Afr J Microbiol Res. 2012;6(43):7084–8.
58. Liang X, Ma L, Long X, Wang X. LncRNA expression profiles and validation in keloid and normal skin tissue. Int J Oncol. 2015;47:1829–38.
59. Lim CP, Phan T-T, Lim IJ, Cao X. Stat3 contributes to keloid pathogenesis via promoting collagen production, cell proliferation and migration. Oncogene. 2006;25:5416–25.
60. Liu Y, Li Y, Li N, Teng W, Wang M, Zhang Y, Xiao Z. TGF-β1 promotes scar fibroblasts proliferation and transdifferentiation via upregulating MicroRNA-21. Sci Report. 2016;6:32231.
61. Lin J, Liu C, Gao F, Mitchel RE, Zhao L, Yang Y, Lei J, Cai J. miR-200c enhances radiosensitivity of human breast cancer cells. J Cell Biochem. 2013;114:606–15.
62. Liu Y, Wang X, Yang D, Xiao Z, Chen X. MicroRNA-21 affects proliferation and apoptosis by regulating expression of PTEN in human keloid fibroblasts. Plast Reconstr Surg. 2014;134:561e–73e.
63. Liu Y, Yang DP, Xiao ZB, Zhang MB. miRNA expression profiles in keloid tissue and corresponding normal skin tissue. Aesthet Plast Surg. 2012;36:193–201.
64. Lu W, Zheng X, Liu S, Ding M, Xie J, Yao X, Zhang L, Hu B. SNP rs1511412 in FOXL2 gene as a risk factor for keloid by meta-analysis. Int J Clin Exp Med. 2015;8(2):2766–71.
65. Lu W-S, Li-Qiong C, Wang Z-X, Li Y, Wang J-F, Feng-Li X, Quan C, He S-M, Yang S, Xue-Jun Z. Association of HLA class I alleles with keloids in Chinese Han individuals. Human Immunol. 2010;71(4):418–22.
66. Luan Y, Liu Y, Liu C, Lin Q, He F, Dong X, Xiao Z. Serum miRNAs signature plays an important role in keloid disease. Curr Mol Med. 2016;16:504–14.
67. Ma HL, Zhao XF, Chen GZ, Fang RH, Zhang FR. Silencing NLRC5 inhibits extracellular matrix expression in keloid fibroblasts via inhibition of transforming growth factor-b1/Smad signaling pathway. Biomed Pharmacother. 2016;83:1016–21.

68. Ma X, Chen J, Xu B, Long X, Qin H, Zhao RC, Wang X. Keloid-derived keratinocytes acquire a fibroblast-like appearance and an enhanced invasive capacity in a hypoxic microenvironment *in vitro*. Int J Mol Med. 2015;35:1246–56. https://doi.org/10.3892/ijmm.2015.2135.
69. Makino K, Jinnin M, Hirano A, Yamane K, Eto M, Kusano T, Honda N, Kajihara I, Makino T, Sakai K, Masuguchi S, Fukushima S, Ihn H. The downregulation of microRNA let-7a contributes to the excessive expression of type I collagen in systemic and localized scleroderma. J Immunol. 2013;190: 3905–15.
70. Mantripragada KK, Buckley PG. Diaz de Ståhl T, Dumanski JP: genomic microarrays in the spotlight. Trends Genet. 2004;20:87–94.
71. Marneros AG, Norris JEC, Olsen BR, Reichenberger E. Clinical genetics of familial keloids. Arch Dermatol. 2001;137(11):1429–34.
72. Marneros AG, Norris JEC, Watanabe S, Reichenberger E, Olsen BR. Genome scans provide evidence for keloid susceptibility loci on chromosomes 2q23 and 7p11. J Invest Dermatol. 2004;122(5):1126–32.
73. Maurer B, Stanczyk J, Jungel A, Akhmetshina A, Trenkmann M, Brock M, Kowal-Bielecka O, Gay RE, Michel BA, Distler JH, Gay S, Distler O. MicroRNA-29, a key regulator of collagen expression in systemic sclerosis. Arthritis Rheum. 2010;62:1733–43.
74. McCarty SM, Syed F, Bayat A. Influence of the human leukocyte antigen complex on the development of cutaneous fibrosis: an immunogenetic perspective. Acta Derm Venereol. 2010;90:563–74.
75. Mu SZ, Sun YW, Wang GD. Down-regulation of miR-21 inhibits the HSF cells proliferation and the PI3K/Akt pathways via PDCD4. Chin J Aesthet Med. 2015;24:39–43.
76. Nakashima M, Chung S, Takahashi A, Kamatani N, Kawaguchi T, Tsunoda T, Hosono N, Kubo M, Nakamura Y, Zembutsu H. 2010. A genome-wide association study identifies four susceptibility loci for keloid in the Japanese population. Nat Genet. 2010;42:768–71.
77. Neary R, Watson CJ, Baugh JA. Epigenetics and the overhealing wound: the role of DNA methylation in fibrosis. Fibrogenesis and tissue repair. 2015;8:18.
78. Niessen FB, Spauwen PH, Schalkwijk J, Kon M. On the nature of hypertrophic scars and keloids: a review. Plast Reconstr Surg. 1999;104:1435–58.
79. Onoufriadis A, Hsu CK, Ainali C, Ung CY, Rashidghamat E, Yang HS, Huang HY, Niazi U, Tziotzios C, Yang JC, Nuamah R, Tang MJ, Saxena A, de Rinaldis E, McGrath JA. Time series integrative analysis of RNA sequencing and microRNA expression data reveals key biologic wound healing pathways in keloid-prone individuals. J Invest Dermatol. 2018;138(12): 2690–3.
80. Palii SS, Van Emburgh BO, Sankpal UT, Brown KD, Robertson KD. DNA methylation inhibitor 5-Aza-2′-deoxycytidine induces reversible genome-wide DNA damage that is distinctly influenced by DNA methyltransferases 1 and 3B. Mol Cell Biol. 2007;28(2):752–71.
81. Phan SH. Biology of fibroblasts and myofibroblasts. Proc Am Thorac Soc. 2008;5(3):334–7. https://doi.org/10.1513/pats.200708-146DR.
82. Rabello FB, Souza CD, Junior JAF. Update on hypertrophic scar treatment. Clinics (Sao Paulo). 2014;69:565–73.
83. Ramos ML, Gragnani A, Masako FL. Microarray as a new tool to study hypertrophic and keloid scarring. Wounds. 2009;21(2):57–63.
84. Russell SB, Russell JD, Trupin KM, Gayden AE, Opalenik SR, Nanney LB, Broquist AH, Raju L, Williams SM. Epigenetically altered wound healing in keloid fibroblasts. J Invest Dermatol. 2010;130(10):2489–96. https://doi.org/10.1038/jid.2010.162.
85. Santos-Cortez RLP, Hu Y, Sun F, Benahmed-Miniuk F, Tao J, Kanaujiya JK, Ademola S, Fadiora S, Odesina V, Nickerson DA, Bamshad MJ, Olaitan PB, Oluwatosin OM, Leal SM, Reichenberger EJ. Identification of ASAH1 as a susceptibility gene for familial keloids. Eur J Hum Genet. 2017;25(10): 1155–61.
86. Satish L, Lyons-Weiler J, Hebda PA, Wells A. Gene expression patterns in isolated keloid fibroblasts. Wound Repair Regen. 2006;14(4):463–70.
87. Shang Y, Yu D, Hao L. Liposome–adenoviral hTERT-siRNA knockdown in fibroblasts from keloids reduce telomere length and fibroblast growth. Cell Biochem Biophys. 2015;72:405–10.
88. Shih B, Bayat A. Genetics of keloid scarring. Arch Dermatol Res. 2010;302(5):319–39.
89. Shih B, Bayat A. Comparative genomic hybridization analysis of keloid tissue in Caucasians suggests possible involvement of HLA-DRB5 in disease pathogenesis. Arch Dermatol Res. 2012;304:241–9.
90. Shin JU, Lee WJ, Tran TN, Jung I, Lee JH. Hsp70 knockdown by siRNA decreased collagen production in keloid fibroblasts. Yonsei Med J. 2015;56(6):1619–26.
91. Smith JC, Boone BE, Opalenik SR, Williams SM, Russell SB. Gene profiling of keloid fibroblasts shows altered expression in multiple fibrosis-associated pathways. J Invest Dermatol. 2008;128(5):1298–310.
92. Spallotta F, Cencioni C, Straino S, Nanni S, Rosati J, Artuso S, Manni I, Colussi C, Piaggio G, Martelli F, Valente S, Mai A, Capogrossi MC, Farsetti A, Gaetano C. A nitric oxide-dependent cross-talk between class i and iii histone deacetylases accelerates skin repair. J Biol Chem. 2013;288:11004–12.
93. Steinbrech DS, Mehrara BJ, Chau D, Rowe NM, Chin G, Lee T, Saadeh PB, Gittes GK, Longaker MT. Hypoxia upregulates VEGF production in keloid fibroblasts. Ann Plast Surg. 1999;42:514–9.
94. Suarez E, Syed F, Alonso-Rasgado T, Mandal P, Bayat A. Up-regulation of tension-related proteins in keloids: knockdown of Hsp27, α2β1-Integrin, and PAI-2 shows convincing reduction of extracellular matrix production. Plastic and Reconstructive Surgery. 2013;131(2):158e–73e. https://doi.org/10.1097/PRS.0b013e3182789b2b.
95. Sun XJ, Wang Q, Guo B, Liu XY, Wang B. Identification of skin related lncRNAs as potential biomarkers that involved in Wnt pathways in keloids. Oncotarget. 2017;8:34236–44.
96. Syed F, Bagabir RA, Paus R, Bayat A. Ex vivo evaluation of antifibrotic compounds in skin scarring: EGCG and silencing of PAI-1 independently inhibit growth and induce keloid shrinkage. Lab Investig. 2013;93:946–60.
97. Tao H, Huang C, Yang JJ, Ma TT, Bian EB, Zhang L, Lv XW, Jin Y, Li J. MeCP2 controls the expression of RASAL1 in the hepatic fibrosis in rats. Toxicology. 2011;290(2–3):327–33. https://doi.org/10.1016/j.tox.2011.10.011.
98. Yi T, Jin L, Zhang W, Ya Z, Cheng Y, Zhao H. AMF siRNA treatment of keloid through inhibition signaling pathway of RhoA/ROCK1. Genes & Diseases. 2018;xx:1–8.
99. Tai-Lan T, Hwu P, Ho W, Yiu P, Chang R, Wysocki A, Benya PD. Adenoviral overexpression and small interfering RNA suppression demonstrate that plasminogen activator Inhibitor-1 produces elevated collagen accumulation in normal and keloid fibroblasts. Am J Pathol. 2008;173(5):1311–25.
100. Wang X, Liu Y, Chen X, Zhang M, Xiao Z. Impact of MiR-21 on the expression of FasL in the presence of TGF-beta1. Aesthet Surg J. 2013;33:1186–98.
101. Wang Z, Gao Z, Shi Y, Sun Y, Lin Z, Jiang H, Hou T, Wang Q, Yuan X, Zhu X, Wu H, Jin Y. Inhibition of Smad3 expression

decreases collagen synthesis in keloid disease fibroblasts. J Plast Reconstr Aesthet Surg. 2007;60(11):1193–9.
102. Watts JK, Corey DR. Silencing disease genes in the laboratory and the clinic. J Pathol. 2011;226(2):365–79.
103. Weisenberger DJ, Velicescu M, Cheng JC, Gonzales FA, Liang G, Jones PA. Role of the DNA methyltransferase variant DNMT3b3 in DNA methylation. Mol Cancer Res. 2004;2: 62–72.
104. Wu ZY, Lu L, Guo XR, Zhang PH. Identification of differently expressed microRNAs in keloid and pilot study on biological function of miR-199a-5p. Zhonghua Zheng Xing Wai Ke Za Zhi. 2013;29:279–84.
105. Wu ZY, Lu L, Liang J, Guo XR, Zhang PH, Luo SJ. Keloid microRNA expression analysis and the influence of miR-199a-5p on the proliferation of keloid fibroblasts. Genet Mol Res. 2014;13:2727–38.
106. Xue H, McCauley RL, Zhang W. Elevated interleukin-6 expression in keloid fibroblasts. J Surg Res. 2000;89:74–7.
107. Yagi Y, Muroga E, Naitoh M, Isogai Z, Matsui S, Ikehara S, Suzuki S, Miyachi Y, Utani A. An *ex vivo* model employing keloid-derived cell–seeded collagen sponges for therapy development. J Investig Dermatol. 2013;133:386–93.
108. Yan X, Gao JH, Chen Y, Song M, Liu XJ. Preliminary linkage analysis and mapping of keloid susceptibility locus in a Chinese pedigree. Chinese J Plast Surg. 2007;23(1):32–5.
109. Yang X, Lei S, Long J, Liu X, Wu Q. MicroRNA-199a-5p inhibits tumor proliferation in melanoma by mediating HIF-1alpha. Mol Med Rep. 2016;13:5241–7.
110. Zhang G, Jiang J, Luo S, Tang S, Liang J, Yao P. Analyses of CDC2L1 gene mutations in keloid tissue. Clin Exp Dermatol. 2012;37:277–83.
111. Zhang GY, Yi CG, Li X, Zheng Y, Niu ZG, Xia W, Meng Z, Meng CY, Guo SZ. Inhibition of vascular endothelial growth factor expression in keloid fibroblasts by vector-mediated vascular endothelial growth factor shRNA: a therapeutic potential strategy for keloid. Arch Dermatol Res. 2008;300(4):177–84.
112. Zhang GY, Wu LC, Liao T, Chen GC, Chen YH, Zhao YX, Chen SY, Wang AY, Lin K, Lin DM, Yang JQ, Gao WY, Li QF. A novel regulatory function for miR-29a in keloid fibrogenesis. Clin Exp Dermatol. 2016;41:341–5.
113. Zhang J, Liu CY, Wan Y, Peng L, Li WF, Qiu JX. Long noncoding RNA H19 promotes the proliferation of fibroblasts in keloid scarring. Oncol Lett. 2016;12:2835–9.
114. Zhao Y, Liu SL, Xie J, Ding MQ, Lu MZ, Zhang LF, Yao XH, Hu B, Lu WS, Zheng XD. NEDD4 single nucleotide polymorphism rs2271289 is associated with keloids in Chinese Han population. Am J Transl Res. 2016;8(2):544–55.
115. Zhao B, Guan H, Liu J-Q, Zheng Z, Zhou Q, Zhang J, Su L-L, Hu D-H. Hypoxia drives the transition of human dermal fibroblasts to a myofibroblast-like phenotype via the TGF-β1/Smad3 pathway. Int J Mol Med. 2017;39(1):153–9. https://doi.org/10.3892/ijmm.2016.2816.
116. Zhu F, Wu B, Li P, Wang J, Tang H, Liu Y, Zuo X, Cheng H, Ding Y, Wang W, Zhai Y, Qian F, Wang W, Yuan X, Wang J, Ha W, Hou J, Zhou F, Wang Y, Gao J, Sheng Y, Sun L, Liu J, Yang S, Zhang X. Association study confirmed susceptibility loci with keloid in the Chinese Han population. PLoS One. 2013;8(5):e62377.
117. Zhu HY, Bai WD, Li C, Zheng Z, Guan H, Liu JQ, Yang XK, Han SC, Gao JX, Wang HT, Hu DH. Knockdown of lncRNA-ATB suppresses autocrine secretion of TGF-beta2 by targeting ZNF217 via miR-200c in keloid fibroblasts. Sci Rep. 2016;6:24728.
118. Zou QP, Yang E, Zhang HS. Effect of the methylation enzyme inhibitors of 5-aza-2- deoxycytidine on the TGF-beta/smad signal transduction pathway in human keloid fibroblasts. Chinese J Plast Surg. 2013;29:285–9.

20

Treatment of Immature Scars: Manual Massages

Docteur N. Frasson

Contents

Background

Scar massages are used to improve skin qualities in terms of flexibility, adhesions, pruritus, and pain. The specific techniques are not always mastered by all the therapists. Indeed pathological scars can appear following strong massage movements or too long sessions during the inflammation stage. The techniques must be controlled and take into account the inflammation, the appearance, and the localization of the scar.

Introduction

Care of the burn skin and scars requires specific treatments to reduce and control the inflammation stage and its consequences [1, 2]. Adapted rehabilitation technique restores flexibility and limits esthetic and functional sequelae. The treatment will progress and be adapted throughout the scar maturation process. Several specific manual massages are part of the treatment but have to be applied respecting the inflammation, the fragility, and the localization of the scar [3, 4, 5].

Indications of Manual Massages

Manual massages allow to improve cutaneous mobility compared with the deep plan and its elasticity. They are indicated on burn scars but also in case of traumatic or surgical scars [6].

They can be started as soon as the scar tissue is epidermized and solid and allows to support specific manual techniques. The massages are contraindicated when the tissue is thin and hyper-inflammatory. When the skin is fragile and presents a vitropression test less than 1.2 seconds, the massages will be realized at first around the scar [7, 8].

Description of the Techniques

Morice Orthodermic Stretching

Orthodermic stretchings such as they were described by René Morice are compatible with an inflammatory skin. Indeed the technique can be summarized by a fixed pulpaire pressure associated with a moderated stretching supported in the inverse direction of the retraction. This kind of massages is frequently used on the face and dorsal side of the hand.

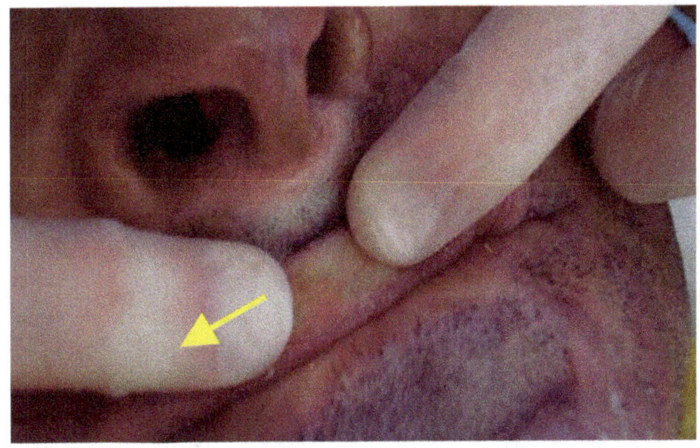

Punctual Crushing

The punctual crushing is also used during the inflammatory stage and allows to crush the edges of grafts or hypertrophic scars. The pressure is moderated, vertical, and realized with the pulp of one or several fingers. The pressure can be circular but without practicing however of friction or lifting fingers.

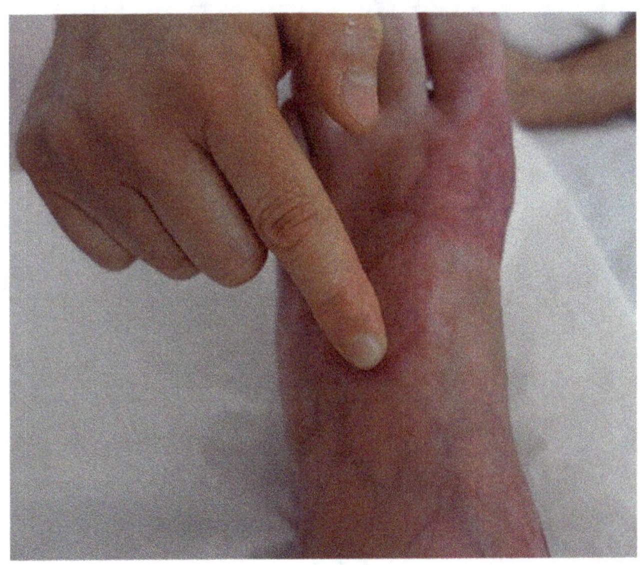

Static Fold

Statics folds are realized during the inflammation stage on a solid epidermis and when the vitropression test is close to 2 seconds. They improve various plans if sliding and have an action on the suppleness of the skin.

According to the surface or area to be treated, they are realized between two fingers or more globally between two hands. There are no movements of friction during this care.

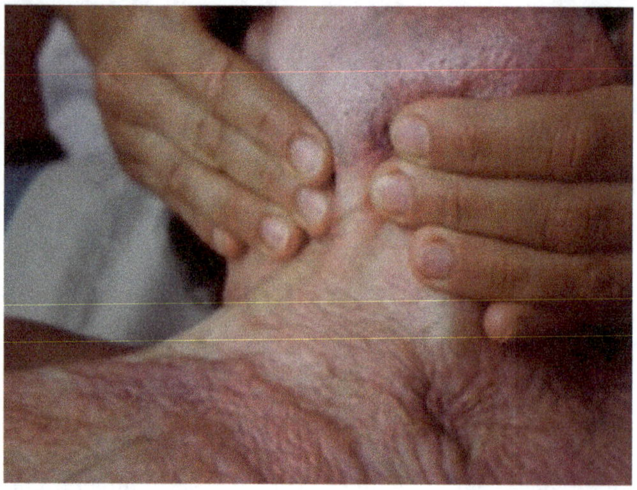

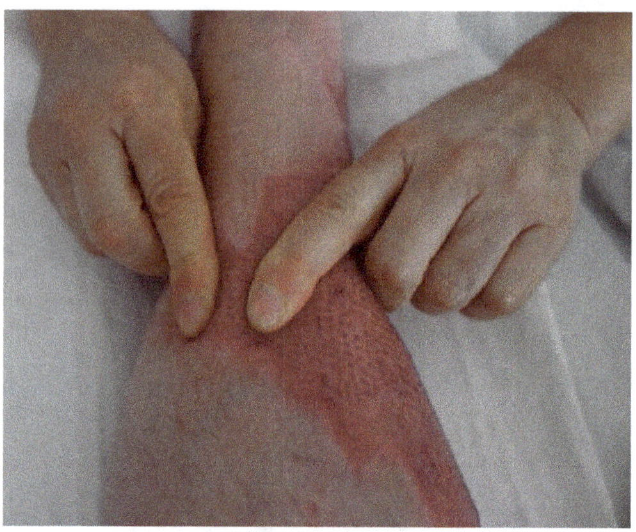

Palpate-Rolling

When the vitropression test gets closer to 3 seconds, the static fold evolves in rolled fold. This also significantly softens the deep plans and fibrosis scars. Palpate-rolling has also an interest to raise adhesions. It is crucial to observe the scar tissue before, during, and after the massage treatment.

Efficacy

The massages are widely used within the care and rehabilitation of burns and scars.

The techniques have a role in the improvement of the characteristics and evolution of the scar.

Conclusion

Treatment of skin and scar following burn injuries must be performed with caution and requires the input of the whole multidisciplinary team. It is necessary to align the treatment according to the stage of scar maturation. The inflammation of the scar is the main factor to consider to guide the therapist's treatment [9].

Bibliography

1. Anthonissen M, Daly D, Janssens T, Van den Kerckhove E. The effects of conservative treatments on burn scars: a systematic review. Burns. 2016;42(3):508–18. https://doi.org/10.1016/j.burns.2015.12.006. Epub 2016 Jan 15.
2. Gavroy JP, Poveda A, Oversteyns B, Plantier G, Rouget D, Griffe O, Teot L, Costagliola M, Ster F. Intérêt du "test de vitro pression" dans le suivi des cicatrices de brulures a partir de 50 observations. Ann Medit Burns Club. 1995;VIII(1).
3. Cho YS, Jeon JH, Hong A, Yang HT, Yim H, Cho YS, Kim DH, Hur J, Kim JH, Chun W, Lee BC, Seo CH. The effect of burn rehabilitation massage therapy on hypertrophic scar after burn: a randomized controlled trial. Burns. 2014;40(8):1513–20. https://doi.org/10.1016/j.burns.2014.02.005. Epub 2014 Mar 12.
4. Shin TM, Bordeaux JS. The role of massage in scar management: a literature review. Dermatol Surg. 2012;38(3):414–23. https://doi.org/10.1111/j.1524-4725.2011.02201.x. Epub 2011 Nov 7.
5. Roques C, Téot L, Frasson N, Meaume S. PRIMOS: an optical system that produces three-dimensional measurements of skin surfaces. J Wound Care. 2003;12(9):362–4. PMID: 14601231.
6. Ault P, Plaza A, Paratz J. Scar massage for hypertrophic burns scarring-a systematic review. Burns. 2018;44(1):24–38. https://doi.org/10.1016/j.burns.2017.05.006. Epub 2017 Jun 29.
7. Najafi Ghezeljeh T, Mohades Ardebili F, Rafii F, Manafi F. The effect of massage on anticipatory anxiety and procedural pain in patients with burn injury. World J Plast Surg. 2017;6(1):40–7.
8. Najafi Ghezeljeh T, Mohades Ardebili F, Rafii F. The effects of massage and music on pain, anxiety and relaxation in burn patients: randomized controlled clinical trial. Burns. 2017;43(5):1034–43. https://doi.org/10.1016/j.burns.2017.01.011. Epub 2017 Feb 4.
9. Finnerty CC, Jeschke MG, Branski LK, Barret JP, Dziewulski P, Herndon DN. Hypertrophic scarring: the greatest unmet challenge following burn injury. Lancet. 2016;388(10052):1427–36.

21

Epidemiology of Scars and their Consequences: Burn Scars

Margriet E. van Baar

Contents

Background

This chapter focuses on the epidemiology of burn scars and their consequences. Burn scars are the result of a pathological healing process in specific burn injuries.

The occurrence of burn injuries and resulting scars and their consequences will be discussed. This includes scar contractures and reconstructive surgery. Next, the predisposing factors for the occurrence of burn scars will be addresses. The chapter ends with the clinical implications.

Burn Injuries and Their Treatment

Burn injuries are a global public health problem. According to estimates of the WHO, burn injuries cause 180,000 deaths every year. The majority of these deaths occur in low- and middle-income countries. Two-third of these deaths occur in the WHO regions of Africa and Southeast Asia.

The nonfatal burns are a leading cause of morbidity, including long hospitalizations, disability and problems in returning to normal life. In the United States annually, 486,000 burn injuries receive medical treatment. In addition, 40,000 hospitalizations are related to burn injuries.

National burn injury incidence data are scarce. In Europe, incidence rates of hospitalized burn injuries are reported between 2 and 29 per 100,000 inhabitants; in Australia, 36 per 100,000 has been reported.

Reviews on burn injury incidence data describe a decline in the incidence rates of burn-related hospital admissions in both low- and middle-income countries. In high-income countries, a similar trend is observed.

Burn Care

In the past decades, there has been a shift in focus from mortality to morbidity in burn care in high-income countries. Recently, the European Burns Association stated in its guidelines that "the main goal of burn care is to ensure optimum resuscitation in the emergency period and then to reach re-epithelialization of injured or destroyed skin either by support of spontaneous healing or by surgical necrectomy and grafting with split thickness skin graft. Subsequent treatment is to ensure the optimum post burn quality of life". This goal only includes the minimum surgical procedure. In nowadays burn care, other surgical techniques including skin substitutes, full skin transplantations and ReCell are also applied.

In high-income countries, a trend is described towards a growing specialized burn care. In the Netherlands, the majority of these hospital admissions are seen in specialized burn centres. This is in line with the trend towards further specialization of health care in general and also because of limited travel distances in our country. In addition, it has been suggested that many patients are transferred towards tertiary care facilities because of a lack of basic skills in the assessment and care of burn wounds at community and rural hospitals.

Acute Phase

The acute treatment of burn injuries is guided by their severity, indicated by the burn size and the burn depth. Burn size is represented by the percentage of the total body surface area burned (TBSA). The burn depth is related to the dermal layers which are affected by the burn injury. Accurate diagnosis of both burn size and burn depth is crucial to start appropriate treatment at the correct level of care required. It guides the initiation of fluid resuscitation, acute escharotomy in case of circumferential deep burns and the decision for conservative or surgical wound treatment. Burn size also has an important prognostic value in predicting burn-related mortality. Both burn size and burn depth are of prognostic value for eventual burn scar pathology.

The most widely used classification for burn injuries divides burns into three categories of increasing depth: superficial partial-thickness, deep partial-thickness and full-thickness burns. Superficial partial-thickness burns involve only the epidermal layer and the superficial part of the dermis. In deep partial-thickness burns, the epidermis and the majority of the dermis are destroyed, with damage to deeper skin structures such as blood vessels, nerves and hair follicles. In full-thickness burns, all layers of the skin are destroyed, and there may also be damage to subdermal structures, such as the muscle, cartilage or bone. In these wounds, no viable epidermal appendages remain in the bottom of the wound, which makes spontaneous healing from the wound bed impossible.

In superficial partial-thickness burns, conservative treatment will be chosen to support spontaneous wound healing, which is expected within 10–14 days. In deep partial-thickness burns, surgical treatment is sometimes necessary to reach wound closure. In full-thickness burns, surgical wound closure will be necessary in the majority of wounds, except in the very small-sized ones.

Other important parts of burn care include oedema management, early mobilization and scar management.

Treatment protocols vary between burn centres, including wound dressings, early mobilization and timing of surgery. According to Dokter et al., in the Netherlands, 45% of all burn injury patients admitted to burn centres receive surgery approximately 15 days post burn. In burn centres in Australia and New Zealand, a similar proportion is operated upon (47.2%) in general within 1 week post burn (mean 6 days post burn).

Prevalence of Burn Scars and Their Consequences

Definition of Scars

The consequences of burns can be severe, affecting multiple domains. The focus in this chapter is on the prevalence of pathological physical scar formation and its consequences.

Burn scars can cause aesthetic and functional problems, resulting in limitations in activities of daily living, the return to normal social roles and impacted quality of life. The psychological consequences will be further elucidated elsewhere in this book.

Early studies on pathological scarring in burn wounds have distinguished between hypertrophic scars and contractures (Magliacani (1997) in [1]).

Hypertrophic scars are a dominant type of pathological scar formation after burns. Nowadays, hypertrophic scarring is described as "the greatest unmet challenge after burn injury."

Hypertrophic scars are generally elevated, firm and erythematous. They can also tend to be pruritic and tender. By definition, they are limited to the site of the original wound and grow in size by pushing out the scar margins. Hypertrophic scarring is known to decrease with time.

Next to hypertrophic scars, contractures are another important type of pathological scar formation after burns. A contracture is defined as the pathological result of excessive scarring and ongoing scar contraction that results in loss of range of motion (ROM) over joint areas. Scar contractures may limit daily functioning and as a result affect health-related quality of life after burns.

Modern scar assessment addresses a broader range of scar features from both the patients' perspective and the perspective of the health-care professional. Scar quality from a patient perspective depends on the presence or absence of several visual, tactile and sensational features [2]. For research purposes, an ideal scar evaluation protocol should include both subjective and objective measurements. These different perspectives will result in different scar assessment tools and different scar outcomes. Results indicate the level of scar morbidity and not the mere presence or absence of scar pathology.

Examples of frequently used scar assessment scales are the Vancouver Scar Scale and the Patient and Observer Scar Assessment Scale (POSAS; see ▶ www.posas.org).

A final approximation of burn scarring is the occurrence of reconstructive surgery after burns. The need for reconstructive surgery after burn injuries can be viewed upon as an indicator for problematic scar development, requiring a surgical intervention to relieve scar morbidity.

Prevalence of Hypertrophic Scarring

The estimates of prevalence of scarring vary widely. Prevalences of hypertrophic scarring between 8% and 67% are reported [3]. These data are all related to burn centre populations in high-income countries.

One of the first reports was written by Deitch et al. in 1983, based on a combined retrospective and prospective study in a mixed population of children and adults. They reported hypertrophic scars after conservative wound healing in 30% of their patients with a dark skin and in 15% of their Caucasian/White patients at 9 to 18 months post burn. Hypertrophic scars were documented in case of increased thickness or elevation of the burn wound; changes in colour or pigmentation alone were not classified as hypertrophy.

Two decades later, Bombardo reported a prevalence of 67% of hypertrophic scars in a dominantly Caucasian sample of patients after major burns. Again, data were based on retrospective chart analysis in patients after major burns, examining the mentioning of the word hypertrophic in the charts. No description was provided on the timing of the scar assessments.

More recently, estimates of prevalence of hypertrophic scars are derived on assessments using validated instruments. The Vancouver Scar Scale is traditionally a well-known scale to evaluate burn scars. In 2017, Wallace et al. assessed the prevalence of hypertrophic scars, using the Modified Vancouver Scar Scale. Raised hypertrophic scarring over 1 mm was reported in 7.8% of the patients treated in a Western Australian burns unit up to 1 year post burn [4].

Prevalence of Contractures

Although contractures are a dominant feature after burn injuries, data on prevalence of burn scar contractures are scarce. In a recent review by Oosterwijk [5] et al., only 10 relevant studies were available for inclusion. The prevalence at discharge was 38–54% and decreased with an increasing time post burns.

The included studies indicated an elevated risk for contractures in deep or surgically treated burn injuries, in females and children. In addition, contractures seemed to occur more frequently in the upper extremity joints, specifically in the shoulder and elbows.

Assessment of scar contractures was based on range of motion measurement in six studies; in four studies, the method of scar contracture assessment was not described. In addition, study design, study period, study population and timing of scar contracture assessment varied largely. Consequently, the authors concluded that "prevalence of scar contractures after burn is insufficiently reported and varies considerably between studies." This impedes the analysis of determinants of scar contractures and possible interventions [5].

Recently, Schouten et al. assessed scar contractures in a prospective cohort study using passive ROM assessments up to 12 months. Scar contractures one year post burn were only found in operated burned joints. Scar contractures at discharge in non-operated joints all returned back to normal in 6 to 9 months. Again, scar contractures were more often seen in the upper part of the body, especially in the shoulder [6].

Scar Quality Assessment

In contrast to the assessment of scar hypertrophy or scar contractures, scar quality assessment addresses a broader assessment of scar-related characteristics, including colour, thickness, relief, pliability, pain and pruritus. The Patient Scar Assessment Scale and the Patient and Observer Scar Assessment Scale (POSAS), for example, consist of the two six-item numeric scales reflecting the patient's perspective and the observer's perspective. This is in contrast to another frequently used scale, the Vancouver Scar Scale, which reflects the observer perspective only and has some methodological difficulties, especially concerning the item "pigmentation."

The POSAS was introduced in 2004. Both the self-reported mean patient POSAS and the observer POSAS are based on scores on six individual scar characteristics. These scar characteristics are scored on a numerical 10-point scale, in which 1 represents a scar comparable with "normal skin" whereas 10 represents the "worst scar imaginable."

Using the POSAS, substantial scar morbidity is reported, even several years after the burn injury. In patients after mild to intermediate burn injuries, mean self-reported patient POSAS scores varied between 1.8 and 2.9 more than 2 years post [7]. In a similar sample 5 years post burn, these patient POSAS scores were even higher, reflecting more scar morbidity. The mean patient POSAS was 3.0, and 7% had a POSAS score above 4 (on a scale from 1 to 10) on all six scar characteristics.

In patients after severe burns (with a mean TBSA of 24.0%), scar morbidity was higher, with a patient POSAS of 4.5 (SD 2.0) [8].

Prevalence of Reconstructive Surgery

The need for reconstructive surgery after burn injuries can be viewed upon as an indicator for problematic scar development, requiring a surgical intervention to relieve scar morbidity. Of course, the possibilities to perform reconstructive surgery will influence the occurrence of reconstructive surgery.

Recent studies in patients after a burn centre admission in the Netherlands showed that 13.0% of these patients received reconstructive surgery in a ten-year follow-up period after burn injuries. In patients with head and neck burns, the prevalence of reconstructive surgery was 8.9% [9]. Vlies et al. reported a prevalence of 15% in patients after hand burns. These prevalences are lower than the one reported in the early 1990s by Prasad et al. (19.9%). This can probably be related not only to improvements in acute burn care between the 1970–1985 and 1990 but also to the more frequent use of non-surgical therapies in the rehabilitation phase, like silicones and laser therapy. Another explanation for these differences may be the higher burn size in the study of Prasad with a mean TBSA of 16.4% and 5.8% full-thickness burns, compared to our sample (9.8 and 3.4%). Also follow-up time differed; patients in the study of Prasad were followed for a variable period of 5 to 20 years.

Another Dutch study by Hoogewerf et al. in patients after head and neck burns described a prevalence of 5.3% reconstructive surgery. This prevalence is lower than the one found in the 10-year follow-up period, probably because of the shorter follow-up period of 2–7 years post burn.

Maturation Pattern

In general, hypertrophic scars develop in the first months after the burn injury. Then, scar hypertrophy is described

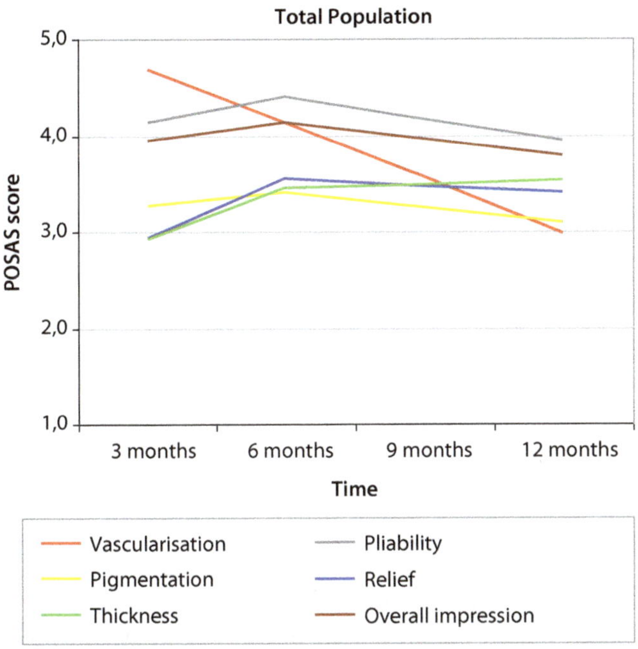

Fig. Maturation pattern after burn injuries, assessed with observer scales of POSAS (Van der Wal et al., personal communication; see also Wound Repair Regen. 2012;20:676–87)

to increase up to 6 months. At 12 months, there is a tendency to regress, according to several studies [2].

Individual scar characteristics have an individual maturation pattern. Vascularization shows a continuous decrease from 3 months post burn onwards, and relief and thickness show increased scar morbidity during at least the first year post injury (Fig. 5.1).

Factors Predicting Scar Outcome After Burns

Several studies investigated the predictors of pathological scar formation after burn injuries.

Some groups of predictors can be distinguished, including patient, injury and treatment characteristics.

Patient Characteristics

A few patient characteristics are recognized for their predictive value in pathological scar formation.

Sex: The relation between sex and scar quality is ambiguous.

There are several studies reporting a poorer scar quality in females. In Dutch studies using the Patient and Observer Scar Assessment Scale (POSAS), a poorer scar quality was reported in females two and five years after burns. Observers reported a poorer scar quality in female participants two years post burn, but the females themselves reported similar scar quality, compared to their male counterparts. However, after taking skin type and surgical treatment into account, scar quality was similar [7].

In patients five years after burns, female participants reported a similar overall patient POSAS score but a poorer overall scar opinion, compared to men. This sex differences remained, also after controlling for other relevant factors including length of hospital stay [8].

In an Australian study predicting raised scars (<1 mm) in adults, based on the Modified Vancouver Scar Scale, females had an increased risk of raised scars, also after taking into account other relevant factors [4]. In a similar study in children, no gender differences were found.

However, in earlier studies, using a variety of scar assessments, this gender difference was not observed [1].

Age: An older age has been shown to reduce the risk for pathological scarring in several studies. The risk for raised scars was reduced in patients over 45 years of age, compared to patients 30 years of age and under [2]. In a paediatric study, the youngest children (0–5 years) were at higher risk to develop raised scars [10].

Skin type: Skin type is a well-known factor influencing the scar formation and scar quality. In one of the first studies on prediction of scar quality from Deitch in 1983, scar hypertrophy was more often reported in patients with a darker skin. In recent studies, skin type is often classified using the Fitzpatrick skin type test. This score classifies skin types in six categories, from type I (palest) to type VI (deeply pigmented dark brown to darkest brown). Having skin types V or VI was associated with a poorer scar quality, based on both the patient and observer POSAS [7]. In addition, darker skin (skin types IV–VI) has an increased risk on raised scars [4]. In children, this association was not reported [10].

Injury and Treatment Characteristics

Several injury and treatment characteristics have been documented to influence scar formation and scar quality.

These include several burn severity indicators, including increased burn size (percentage of total body surface area burned (TBSA)), high %TBSA full thickness, wound complications and a longer time to wound healing.

In addition, several treatment characteristics have been described to be related to poor scar quality, including a prolonged hospital stay, type of surgery (none, ReCell, skin grafting, dermal substitute), multiple surgeries, repeated surgery in the same wound, reconstructive surgery and artificial ventilation [4, 10]. Again, all these treatment features are related to the severity of the burn injuries, complexity of wound healing and possible complications. Length of stay in these analyses is the representation or proxy for the severity of the burn injuries and the complexity of the burn care process including wound healing and possible complications.

Patient, Injury and Treatment Characteristics Combined

To identify the independent predictors of poor scar outcome, the potential predictors have to be taken into account together in one analysis, which requires adequate numbers to reach significant power of the analysis. Some examples of such studies are summarized here.

Raised scars in children up to 16 years of age, one year post burn, could be predicted by greater burn size (%TBSA), a prolonged healing time (over 14 days) and multiple surgical procedures. Patient characteristics did not contribute to this prediction of scars after burn injuries in children [10].

Raised scars in adults one year post burn could be predicted again by increasing burn size (%TBSA) and by the type of surgical intervention (as a proxy for burn depth), wound complications and prolonged hospital stay. In addition, patient predictors were found, being a young age (<30), the female gender and darker skin were for raised scars in adults [4].

Reported scar quality 2 years post burn could be predicted by one patient-related and one injury/treatment-related characteristic: a dark skin type and more than one operation in the same wound were independently related to lower long-term scar quality, 2 years after the injury [7]. Self-reported scar quality 5 years post burn was predicted by length of hospital stay. In addition, the female gender predicted the overall scar opinion. Thus, all other patient-, injury- or treatment-related potential risk factor predictors did no longer predict scar quality, after taking these predictors into account [8].

Some general remarks can be made based on these findings. Firstly, injury- and treatment-related characteristics are the main predictors of scar outcomes after burn injury. These characteristics are related to burn size (total body surface area burned) and burn depth (number or type of surgery) or the overall healing process in general (length of stay, wound healing complications). Intrinsic patient-related risk factors seem to play a role as well but are less consistent predictors of scar outcome. This includes the risk factors the female gender and also a younger age and darker skin.

An important limitation of three of the aforementioned studies is the sample size. In sample sizes up to 251 patients, only a limited number of predictors can be revealed in multivariate analysis. This was illustrated by the results of the adult study from Wallace et al.; their analyses on 616 people after burns revealed seven significant predictors [4, 10], compared to the maximum of three predictors in the other smaller-sized studies.

Clinical Relevance

Knowledge on risk factors for poor scar outcome can be used to tailor treatment, aftercare and scar prevention to these patients with a high-risk profile.

Current evidence shows that injury- and treatment-related characteristics are the main predictors of scar outcomes after burn injury. These characteristics are related to burn size (%TBSA) and burn depth (number or type of surgery) or the overall healing process in general (length of stay, wound healing complications). Intrinsic patient-related risk factors seem to play a role as well but are less consistent predictors of scar outcome. This includes the risk factors the female gender and also a younger age and darker skin.

Future studies, with greater sample sizes, will probably reveal additional predictors for scar outcome. Especially, paediatric scar outcome is not yet well studied.

Conclusion

Early studies on pathological scarring in burn wounds have distinguished between hypertrophic scars and contractures. Prevalences of hypertrophic scarring after burn injuries are reported between 8% and 67%; a recent prospective study revealed a prevalence of 8%. Data on prevalence of burn scar contractures are limited; reported prevalence at discharge varied between 38 and 54% and decreased with an increasing time post burn. Prevalence of reconstructive surgery after burn varied between 5 and 20%, up to 10 years post injury.

Factors predicting pathological scar formation after burn injuries include patient, injury and treatment characteristics. Injury- and treatment-related characteristics are the main predictors of scar outcomes after burn injury. These characteristics are related to burn size (total body surface area burned) and burn depth (number or type of surgery) or the overall healing process in general (length of stay, wound healing complications). Intrinsic patient-related risk factors seem to play a role as well but are less consistent predictors of scar outcome. This includes the risk factors the female gender and also a younger age and darker skin.

Knowledge on risk factors for poor scar outcome can be used to tailor treatment, aftercare and scar prevention to these patients with a high-risk profile.

Take-Home Messages

- Pathological scarring in burn wounds can result in hypertrophic scars and/or contractures.
- Reported prevalence of hypertrophic scarring after burn injuries varied between 8% and 67%.
- Reported prevalence of burn scar contractures varied between 38 and 54%.
- About 5 to 20% of patient after burn injuries receive reconstructive surgery, reflecting scar pathology.
- Factors predicting pathological scar formation after burn injuries include patient, injury and treatment characteristics.
- Injury- and treatment-related characteristics are the main predictors of scar outcomes after burn injury, including burn size (TBSA burned), burn depth (number of type of surgery) or the overall healing process in general (length of stay, wound healing complications).
- Intrinsic patient-related risk factors, including the female gender and also a younger age and darker skin, are less consistent predictors of scar outcome.
- Knowledge on risk factors for poor scar outcome should be used to tailor treatment, aftercare and scar prevention to these patients with a high-risk profile.

References

1. Gangemi EN, Gregori D, Berchialla P, et al. Epidemiology and risk factors for pathologic scarring after burn wounds. Arch Facial Plast Surg. 2008;10:93–102. https://doi.org/10.1001/archfaci.10.2.93.
2. van der Wal MB, Verhaegen PD, Middelkoop E, et al. A clinimetric overview of scar assessment scales. J Burn Care Res: Official Publication of the American Burn Association. 2012;33:e79–87. https://doi.org/10.1097/BCR.0b013e318239f5dd.
3. Bombaro KM, Engrav LH, Carrougher GJ, et al. What is the prevalence of hypertrophic scarring following burns? Burns. 2003;29:299–302. DOI: S0305417903000676 [pii].
4. Wallace HJ, Fear MW, Crowe MM, et al. Identification of factors predicting scar outcome after burn in adults: a prospective case–control study. Burns. 2017;43:1271–83.
5. Oosterwijk AM, Mouton LJ, Schouten H, et al. Prevalence of scar contractures after burn: a systematic review. Burns. 2017;43:41–9.
6. Schouten HJ, Nieuwenhuis MK, van Baar M E, et al. The prevalence and development of burn scar contractures. A prospective multicentre cohort study. Submitted.
7. Goei H, van der Vlies CH, Hop MJ, et al. Long-term scar quality in burns with three distinct healing potentials: a multicenter prospective cohort study. Wound Repair Regen. 2016;24:721–30.
8. Spronk I, Polinder S, Haagsma J, et al. Patient-reported scar quality of adults after burn injuries: a five-year multicenter follow-up study. Wound Repair Regen Acc.
9. Hop MJ, Langenberg LC, Hiddingh J, et al. Reconstructive surgery after burns: a 10-year follow-up study. Burns. 2014;40:1544–51. https://doi.org/10.1016/j.burns.2014.04.014.
10. Wallace HJ, Fear MW, Crowe MM, et al. Identification of factors predicting scar outcome after burn injury in children: a prospective case-control study. Burns Trauma. 2017;5:19.

22

Objective Assessment Technologies: General Guidelines for Scar Assessment

Julian Poetschke and Gerd G. Gauglitz

Contents

Background

Comprehensive scar treatment is becoming more and more readily available. Both the awareness of medical professionals regarding the impairments of severely scarred patients and their knowledge of treatment options for scars have increased significantly during recent years. Those developments have been made possible by extensive research of new treatment options and continued reevaluation of long-established ones.

However, large numbers of studies continue to rely predominantly on subjective evaluation methods like scales and questionnaires to gauge the success of their treatment. Objective scar evaluation technology, too, has shown an immense development throughout recent years, and researchers and clinicians alike can now choose from a large arsenal of options to document treatment progress and failure [1].

But while this newfound selection of tools for objective scar analysis has helped to improve research, it has also introduced new problems.

With many different manufacturers offering many different devices for analysis of a vast number of parameters, researchers are left with the dilemma to choose the right tools for their individual projects with little evidence-based recommendations available. Oftentimes, devices will not be able to measure in standardized units but will provide measurement results in the manufacturer's own proprietary format that offers little comparability with results from different research groups with different measurement tools. The process of measuring the desired parameters reliably in the oftentimes hectic environment of everyday clinical routine can be daunting too and can lead to problems with recreating measurements and making sure that repeated measurements yield comprehensible results.

In this chapter, we want to focus on the basics of objective measurement technologies that allow researchers and clinicians to find the right tools for their desired analyses, to make comprehensive plans about how to document their patients' scars in a way that can both easily and reliably be reproduced, and to understand the value and impact of the results of their measurements.

Obtaining and cultivating this knowledge can then not only lead to improving the level of evidence in scar research but also help in everyday clinical treatment scenarios where in-depth scar analysis might provide physicians with a sensitive gauge for the success or failure of their applied treatment.

Choosing the Right Tools for Each Scar

Before planning a research project or the documentation of clinical results in scar therapy based on objective assessment technology, care must be taken to identify the tools best suited for each specific undertaking. Since scar documentation as well as the consecutive sorting, assessment, and evaluation of data is considerably time-consuming, superfluous measurements should be avoided.

The first step is identifying the scar parameters that require documentation and afterward choosing the tools suitable to assess the development of the chosen parameters. When trying to assess the influence of a certain treatment option on scars, parameters most likely affected positively or negatively (e.g., side effects) should be selected.

When choosing the most suitable assessment technology, a thorough literature research should be performed to identify assessment options that have been well established and are used by other researchers as well to ensure both the suitability for the task and, later, comparability of the results between different research groups.

Ideally, comparability does not require different researchers to use identical hardware but rather that different hardware uses the same units of measurement. While this is common in ultrasound technology where most, if not all, units are able to perform measurements based on SI units, more specialized tools for profilometry or colorimetry specifically designed for application in aesthetic medicine often employ proprietary units of measurement that are difficult to compare with other researches.

While this does not necessarily mean those options are unsuited for research applications, it should be taken into consideration beforehand.

Optimizing the Measurement Process

Preparing the Surroundings

The room where measurements are conducted should be light, cool, and dry. Illumination through natural light should be minimized so that it does not influence photographic and colorimetric testing where changing outside lighting could act as a disruptive factor. The ambient temperature should neither be too warm or too cool since physiological reactions to extreme temperature (e.g., sweating, goose bumps) can influence measurements, especially regarding physiological skin parameters. Furthermore, extreme temperatures, just like humidity, could also influence the functionality and longevity of the measurement instruments. Some manufacturers even provide ambient condition sensors to monitor parameters like temperature or humidity and save the values together with the measured results. This can guarantee both superior awareness of the lab ambience as well as improve comparability of the achieved measurement results.

Configuring and Calibrating the Assessment Tools

Reliable measurements are paramount in every clinical and/or research setting. This starts with making sure that the assessment instruments are properly cared for and calibrated.

Most devices come with extensive instructions on how to calibrate them, and adhering to those recommendations is important since even small discrepancies in the measurement process can yield significantly altered results, especially with modern, highly sensitive equipment.

Instruments that have direct contact with the skin, for example, devices that measure skin elasticity, color, or physiological properties, should be cleaned regularly as sebum, hairs, and makeup can accumulate on the measuring probes and alter measurements as well as hinder successful calibration.

Photography-based systems require regular cleaning too, so that there are no specks on the lens or projector systems (e.g., PRIMOS system).

Most devices allow for a variety of parameters to be configured that can greatly influence how the measurements are conducted and what the results are going to be. Those parameters need to be defined beforehand and require standardization so that subsequent measurements can be compared. Photography-based devices that use different exposure times or white balances during measurements will result in significantly different looking images, skin elasticity values will differ greatly when on and off times of the suction probes of the Cutometer are changed, and the same is true for many other devices, too. Especially when more than one researcher is working with a certain device, care should be taken to check all the relevant parameters before measurements are performed.

Preparing the Patient

The areas to be measured should be clean and free of makeup, skin-care products, or therapeutic agents (like ointments, gels, silicon sheets).

Throughout the measurement process, patients should remain in a neutral, predefined position so as not to alter certain measurement results due to their pose. Especially during measurements regarding skin texture and relief or elasticity, identical positioning for subsequent measurements is crucial in ensuring comparability of the results. Scars that run close to or over joints are greatly affected when those joints are moved, and elasticity results, for example, might reveal drastically different results when said joints are fully flexed or extended. It can therefore help when the positioning of the patient is predefined (e.g., patient standing, arms hanging loosely on his sides) and said positioning is kept throughout all measurements (◘ Fig. 16.1).

Performing the Measurements

After all the preparations have been made, calibrations have been performed, and configurations have been checked, the measurements are performed. Here, it is important to ensure subsequent measurements are performed similarly. Camera-based systems often provide integrated overlay functions that allow the examiner to achieve identical captures during successive assessments, and some devices offer integrated software solutions to stack subsequently taken images to only measure the common areas; however sometimes, such solutions are not offered. It can therefore help to define anatomical landmarks for orientation and to fashion templates so that positioning of the measuring probe or the camera system remains constant [2].

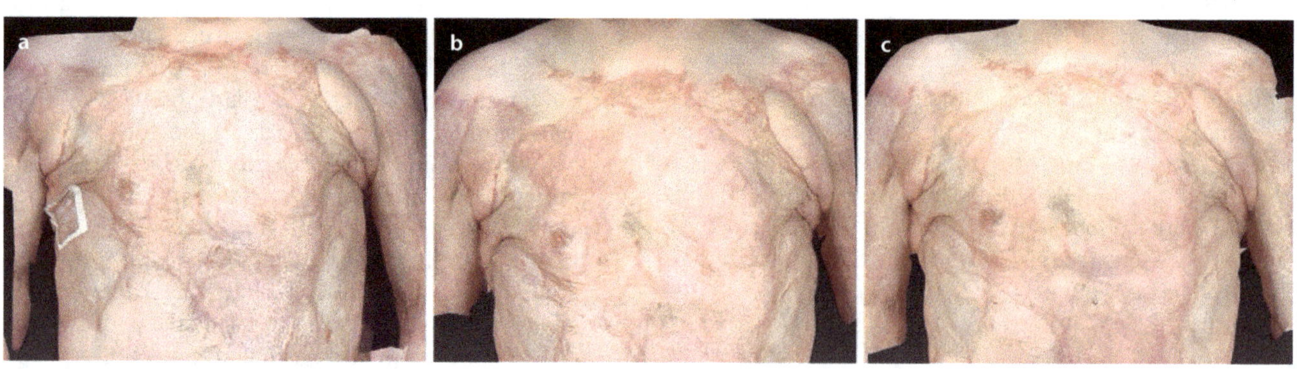

◘ **Fig.** Canfield Vectra X3 imaging before **a**, 3 months after **b**, and 6 months after **c** one session of fractional ablative laser treatment of the upper right chest. The patient had been instructed to maintain a standardized pose (standing upright, arms hanging loosely by his sides, facing forward) to ensure comparability between subsequent images

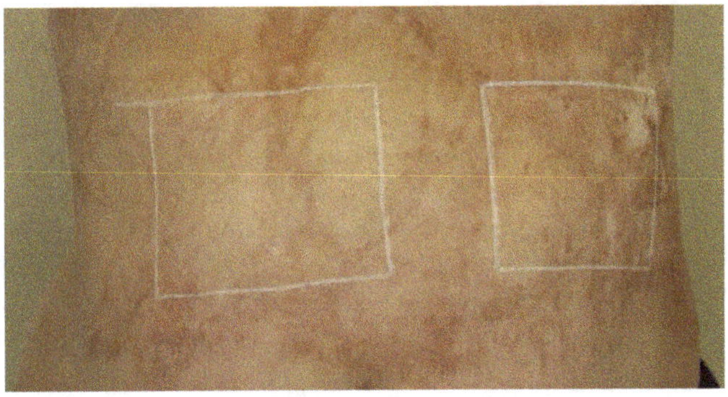

Fig. Severe burn scars on the abdomen of a female patient. Note the marked squares where one has been defined as the treat-ment and the other as the control area. By using a foil template and anatomical landmarks, those areas can be retraced for follow-up measurements which are always conducted within the marked squares to avoid confounding of the results. This course of action ensures that surface profilometry and skin elasticity measurements are always performed on the same area

Devices that measure skin elasticity or color often rely on small probes with relatively small openings through which the individual parameters are measured. This often proves challenging for the examiner since exact repositioning for a subsequent measurement often is difficult if not impossible. Furthermore, especially in widespread scarring, getting representative results from only one measurement is virtually impossible, especially if one cannot ensure that measurements are always taken at the same spot.

These problems, unfortunately, cannot be addressed satisfactorily with devices that are not able to measure the entire scarred surface, and therefore, a compromise that will allow for as great an approximation as possible is necessary. Using an increased number of measuring points in a randomized fashion is a method that has been used in current research, thus ensuring that extreme values do not dramatically alter the overall measurements and including more parts of the oftentimes inhomogeneous scar surface into the measurement [3]. There is, however, no consensus on how many measurements are necessary to adequately represent the results of a larger area. In their research, the authors have commonly used three measurements for an area of 10 cm by 10 cm when measuring skin elasticity or other parameters that rely on assessment through small probes (Fig. 16.2).

Interpreting Therapeutic Success with Objective Scar Assessment Technologies

Data Assessment and Evaluation

After the measurements, the resultant data needs to be sorted and analyzed. To present the most objective results possible, it is necessary to use the raw absolute data for further analyses. Only including relative changes makes it hard for outside observers to interpret the importance of the findings when absolute baseline values are not known. Furthermore, the level of measurement that is required for certain statistical tests is not sufficient when using relative data.

Then, tests can be performed to elucidate the statistical significance of the findings.

Clinically Important Difference

After performing statistical testing, one must consider whether the results of the measurements constitute a clinically important difference. Currently, there are no clear recommendations on what constitutes a clinically important difference in objective scar assessment in the literature. However, ideally, every modern study on scar treatment and its effects can include its own control to evaluate whether the results are clinically important.

After all, scar treatment should alleviate the patients' symptoms, improve functional impairments, and address aesthetic disfigurements. Therefore, patient-derived questionnaires like the POSAS Patient Scale or the Dermatology Life Quality Index (DLQI) can be included in the research as a control for patient satisfaction [4]. Should those questionnaires show statistically significant improvements, just like the objective assessment tools, then a clinically important difference has been achieved. While the lack of statistically significant results does not necessarily rule out a clinically important difference, it is important to consider just how sensitive modern assessment tools have become. Surface profilometry can measure changes at the micrometer scale, and other technologies boast similar sensitivities. But even if changes can be documented on such a fine scale, statistical significance of such results does not help the patients if they do not register improvements regarding their impairments.

Therefore, defining an absolute clinically important difference for objective scar assessment is neither possible nor sensible. The importance of documented improvements should always be compared to the patients' assessment of the therapeutic results to gauge the overall success.

Conclusion

Objective scar assessment has come a long way during the recent years. Today, a multitude of options for the documentation of scar treatment is available. From this variety of options, researchers and clinicians have to choose the tools best suited for their individual analysis based on the scar parameters that require documentation and the individual devices' features. Care should be taken to choose assessment technology that does not rely on proprietary assessment and evaluation formats but that is able to export results in standardized units of measurement so that comparability with other research groups and studies is ensured. Measurements should be performed in a standardized environment with well-maintained and well-calibrated tools, and conditions as well as patient positioning should not differ between measurements.

Objective scar assessment relies on using the most accurate values to represent the results which is why absolute values should always be preferred to relative values. Not only does this ensure comparability of the results, it allows for more complex statistical testing, thus ensuring improved significance of the findings.

A clinically important difference, however, cannot be derived from statistically significant findings alone. Here, the patient's perspective should be taken into consideration. As modern technology is now able to document extremely subtle changes, clinically important differences, despite significant statistical changes, can only be asserted if the patient considers them significant. This further illustrates that neither subjective nor objective scar assessment means alone should be employed. Both clinical and research protocols should include both to profit from additional information and to further characterize their findings.

Take-Home Messages

- Choosing the right objective scar assessment tools is paramount and should be based on the scar parameters that are central to the research.
- Devices that work with standardized units of measurement should be preferred to those that work with proprietary units or formats.
- Maintaining a standardized environment for the measurements both regarding the instruments (regular cleaning and calibration are required; the proper configuration should be checked before measurements are performed) and the patients (standardized posture, identical location for the measurements) is crucial.
- Absolute values should be preferred to relative values to improve the informative value and the statistical significance of the findings.
- The clinically important difference in objective scar assessment is rather a correlation between objective findings and subjective patient satisfaction, than a certain amount of improvement according to technical measurements. Modern assessment technology is oftentimes so sensitive that statistical testing reveals significant improvements before patients notice them.

References

1. Poetschke J, Schwaiger H, Gauglitz GG. Current and emerging options for documenting scars and evaluating therapeutic progress. Dermatol Surg. 2017;43 Suppl 1:S25–s36.
2. Roques C, Teot L, Frasson N, Meaume S. PRIMOS: an optical system that produces three-dimensional measurements of skin surfaces. J Wound Care. 2003;12(9):362–4.
3. Poetschke J, Dornseifer U, Clementoni MT, Reinholz M, Schwaiger H, Steckmeier S, et al. Ultrapulsed fractional ablative carbon dioxide laser treatment of hypertrophic burn scars: evaluation of an in-patient controlled, standardized treatment approach. Lasers Med Sci. 2017;32(5):1031–40.
4. Reinholz M, Poetschke J, Schwaiger H, Epple A, Ruzicka T, Gauglitz GG. The dermatology life quality index as a means to assess life quality in patients with different scar types. J Eur Acad Dermatol Venereol. 2015;29(11):2112–9.

23

Minimally Invasive Technologies for the Treatment of Hypertrophic Scars and Keloids: Intralesional Cryosurgery

Yaron Har-Shai and Lior Har-Shai

Contents

Background

A total of 100 million patients develop scars in the developed world alone each year as a result of 55 million elective operations and 25 million operations after trauma. Excessive scars form as a result of aberrations of physiologic wound healing and may develop following any insult to the deep dermis, including burn injury, lacerations, abrasions, surgery, piercings, and vaccinations. By causing pruritus, pain, and contractures, excessive scarring can dramatically affect a patient's quality of life, both physically and psychologically. Spray or contact cryosurgery is a nonsurgical therapy for the treatment of hypertrophic scars and keloids.

Cryosurgery is an effective and safe therapeutic regimen in the treatment of hypertrophic scars and keloids. Because of its major advantage of a low relapse rate, the technique, either as monotherapy or in combination, has been established as the treatment of choice for keloids and hypertrophic scars.

The cryosurgery freezing process includes four phases, which are termed "Thermal history." These phases include cooling rate, end temperature, hold time, and thawing rate. Each of these phases has an impact on the mechanism of injury on the frozen tissue. The tissue injury is induced by two synergistic arms – direct physical effects of cells freezing (intracellular ice formation) and by the vascular stasis that develops in the tissue after thawing. It is postulated that another factor in the effect on the tissue following cryosurgery is the immunologic response which is still under investigation.

Contact cryosurgery method uses metallic probes, which are circulated by a cryogen gas. This probe removes heat from the tissue and thus the tissue gradually cools. When the cryosurgical unit is activated and the probe is placed in firm contact with the tissue, an area of frozen tissue or ice ball appears, which extends radially from the cryoprobe. The lateral spread of freeze approximates the depth of freeze by a ratio of 1:1.3. Although the depth of freeze is time related, as the duration of freeze extends toward 100 seconds the lethal zone flats, that is, the deeper tissue is not affected. It has been shown that repeated contact cryosurgical sessions can exhibit a beneficial effect on keloids and hypertrophic scars and additionally prevent relapses. However, 1–20 treatment sessions using the contact cryosurgery were required to flatten those scars. In addition this method caused a high incidence of hypopigmentation. Therefore, the need for new, more potent, and quickly effective cryosurgical methods and instrumentation are warranted. Har-Shai et al. have developed the intralesional cryoneedle [1–15]. This technique exhibits an increased efficacy in the treatment of hypertrophic scars and keloids when compared with the contact method, due to the enhanced freezing area of deeply located scar tissue. In addition, fewer cryosurgical sessions are required, and less hypopigmentation is evident following the application of intralesional cryosurgery (◘ Fig. 28.1).

The Technology: Treatment Technique – CryoShape [5, 10]

With the patient lying at a supine position, the skin surface of the scar is cleansed with disinfecting solution and draped. The area of penetration into the scar and the underlying subcutaneous tissue are anesthetized locally, by a translesional approach, with Bupivacaine hydrochloride 0.5% (marcaine) [7]. Thereafter, the sterile cryoprobe (CryoShape, Life by Ice Ltd. Haifa, Israel) (◘ Fig. 28.2) is forced into the long axis, core, and mid-height of the scar in a forward rotary movement, which is parallel to the skin surface. The scar itself is grasped between the index and thumb of the other hand, until the sharp tip of the needle penetrates the opposite distal edge of the scar, thus maximizing the volume of scar tissue to be frozen. Attention is taken to prevent any penetration of the cryoneedle into the healthy surrounding skin. Sterile gauzes are placed under the proximal and distal exposed parts of the cryoprobe and care is taken to assure that the vent nostril is positioned away from the patient to prevent accidental freezing of adjacent skin or tissue (◘ Fig. 28.3).

The proximal part of the probe is connected via an elongation tube to the cryogun (CryoPro Maxi 500 cc, Cortex Technology, Hadsund, Denmark), which is filled with liquid nitrogen to three-fourth of the cryogen volume and about 15 minutes beforehand in order to allow a sufficient pressure to build-up inside it (11 psi). A full pressurized cryogen can operate continuously for 1 hour, thus two to three medium-sized keloids can be treated successively without the need to refill.

The cryogun is grasped or placed on a steady surface, which is located higher than the scar to facilitate the liquid nitrogen flow downward with no direct contact with the patient body. By activating the cryogun trigger, the pressure valve is opened and the cryogen enters the cryoneedle, thereby freezing the scar. A forced steam of the liquid nitrogen gas flows out from the vent nostril during the entire freezing process. The strength of the steam flow, which is observed by the naked eye during the entire freezing procedure, indicates an appropriate working pressure. Two ice balls appear shortly at the two cryoprobe penetration sites of the treated scar and with time they gradually spread toward each other until a complete freezing of the scar is clinically evident. The

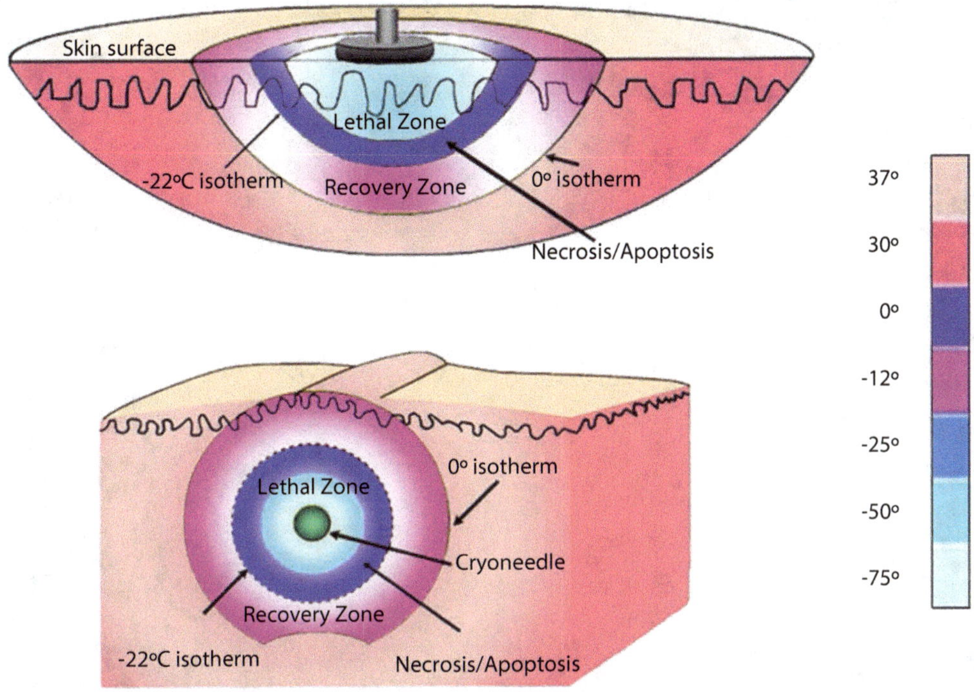

Fig. A comparison between the contact and intralesional cryosurgery methods. Upper – Contact method: Ice ball induced by the contact cryoprobe. The interface between the ice ball and unfrozen tissue represents 0 °C isotherm. The volume of tissue located between −22 °C isotherm and contact probe is the lethal zone in which cells undergo cryonecrosis. Cells situated in the warmer region between −22 °C isotherm and 0 °C isotherm (recovery zone) generally survive the freeze. The melanocytes are located within the lethal zone. Bottom – Intralesional method: Ice ball induced by the intralesional cryoneedle. The interface between the ice ball and unfrozen tissue represents 0 °C isotherm. The volume of tissue located between −22 °C isotherm and cryoneedle probe is the lethal zone in which cells undergo cryonecrosis. Cells situated in the warmer region between −22 °C isotherm and 0 °C isotherm (recovery zone) generally survive the freeze. The melanocytes are located within the recovery zone

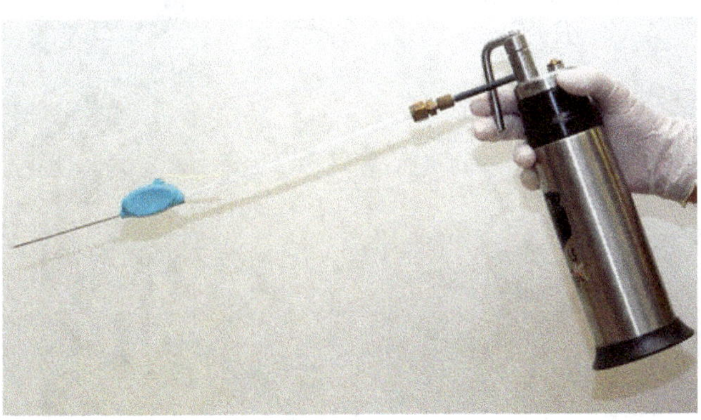

Fig. The intralesional cryosurgery system composed of the CryoShape cryoprobe which is connected to the cryogen

length of the intralesional cryosurgery process depends upon the scar volume and ranges between minutes to 3 hours without the need of time taking. Following the complete freezing of the scar, the cryogun trigger is released to stop the freezing process and the cryoneedle is left to thaw for 1–2 minutes and is withdrawn in a reverse rotary movement. After a complete thawing of the scar is clinically noticed, slight bleeding from the penetration points of the needle requires the application of a sterile dressing. If active bleeding is evident, gauzes soaked with Tranexamic Acid will end the bleeding. The patient is instructed to wash daily the treated scar and to apply an antibiotic ointment until full healing is accomplished.

In cases where the scar is longer than the cryoneedle length (10 cm) or very wide, two or three parallel needles or successive insertions of the same needle are necessary to freeze the entire keloid in one session.

When to Use Contact or Intralesional Cryosurgery?

Contact cryosurgery can be used on very small HSK with a reduced volume in which the cryoneedle cannot be inserted into. All other HSK can be treated by the intralesional cryosurgery method. In very large or giant HSK, several cryoneedles can be inserted in parallel to facilitate the freezing process.

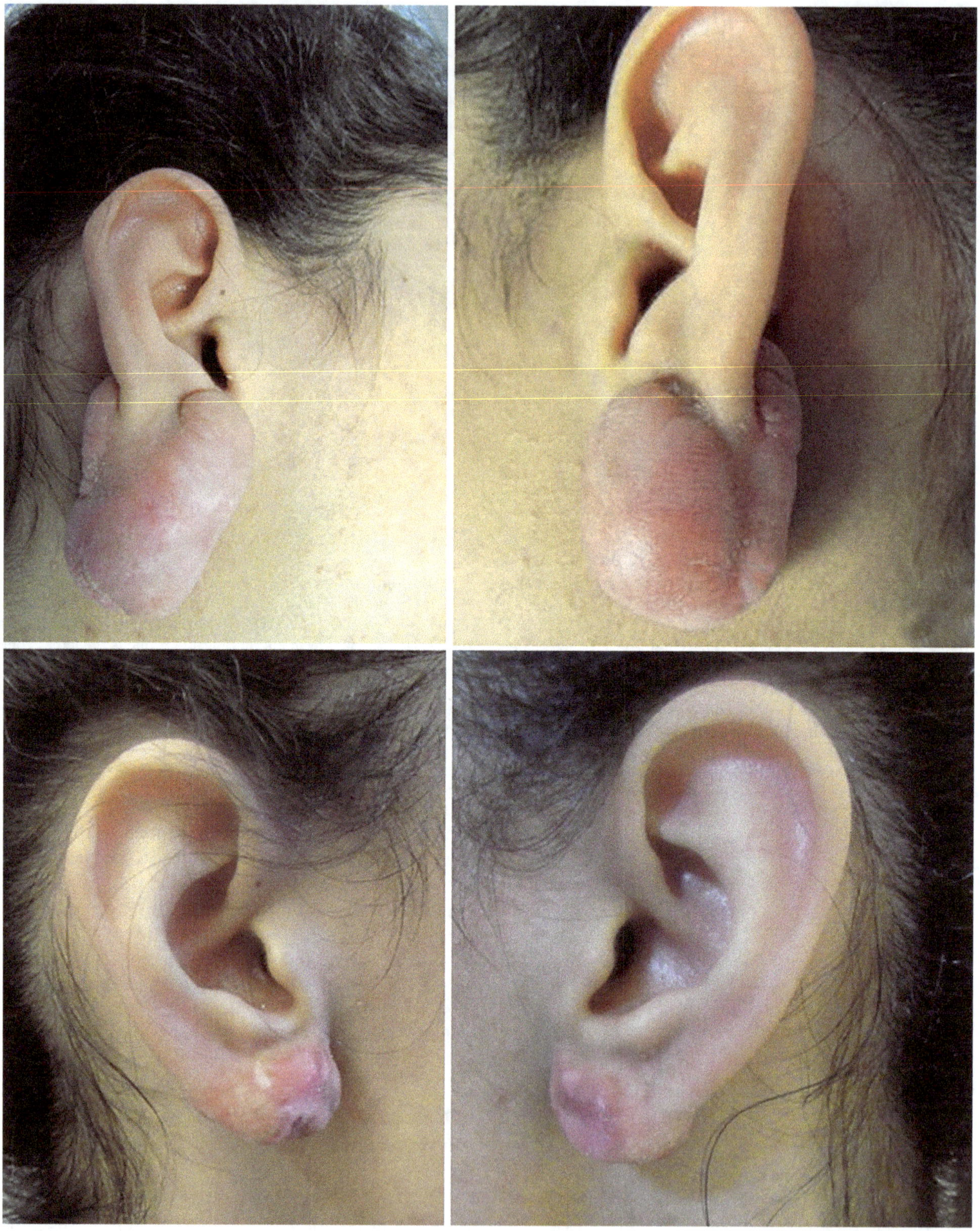

Fig. *Upper* – Preoperative view of two large keloids on the anterior and post aspects of the right and left lobules following piercing. *Lower* – Postoperative view 6 years following a single cryosession of intralesional cryosurgery demonstrating complete involution of the scars with no distortion of the lobules and without hypopigmentation or recurrence

How Many Cryosessions Are Needed for Contact or Intralesional Cryosurgery?

A total of 1–20 treatment sessions using the contact cryosurgery are required to flatten HSK scars. The interval between sessions is between 2 and 3 months.

For the intralesional method, usually a single cryosession is needed to flatten the HSK. In few cases a second cryo-treatment is needed. The interval between sessions is 6 months.

Combined Treatment

Intralesional cryosurgery can be combined with intralesional excision of the HSK [14], topical silicone gel sheeting [8], intralesional injection of steroids, and pressure garments. Following the flattening of the scars by cryosurgery, fractional CO2 lasers can be applied to further smoothen the skin surface if necessary [16].

Conclusion

This simple to operate technology can be applied as an office procedure, is safe, cost-effective, and possesses a short learning curve. This evidence-based novel intralesional cryosurgery method for the treatment of hypertrophic scars and keloids was recently intro-

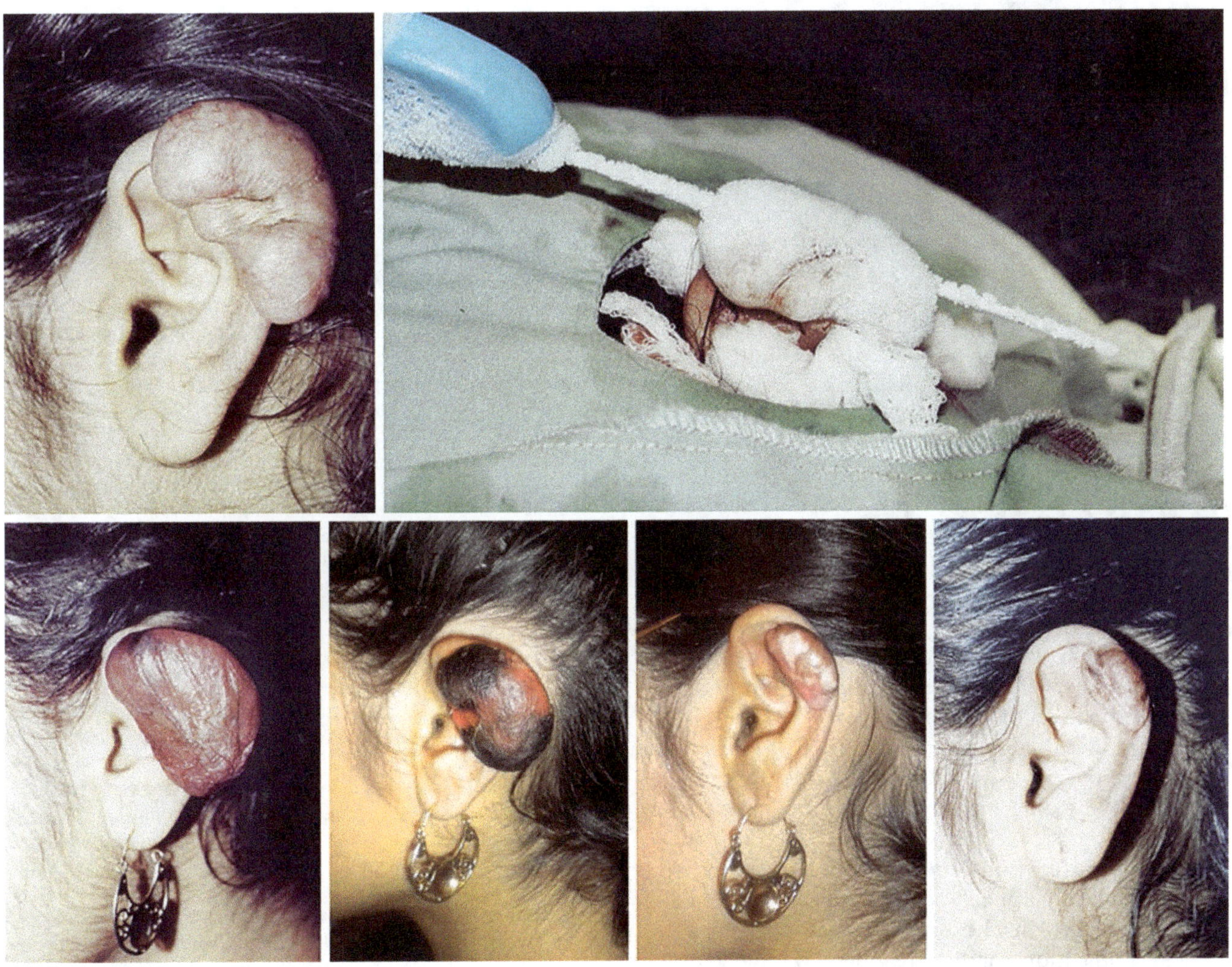

Fig. Sequential steps of the intralesional cryosurgery proce-dure and final result. *Upper left* – Preoperative view of a large keloid of the left upper ear following piercing. *Upper right* – Following penetration of the cryoneedle into the keloid, two ice balls are formed at the two penetration points of the scar. Warm gauzes are placed opposite to the treated scar (posterior aspect of the auricle) in order to prevent cryoinjury to the auricular cartilage. *Lower left to lower right* – One week following the cryo-treatment a blister is evident; 3 weeks following treatment scar necrosis is evident; 6 months following the treatment the helical keloid has reduced significantly without distortion of the lobule and with almost no hypopigmentation; 4 years following a single cryosession, the scar is flat with some extra pliable skin above it which can be excised via an intralesional approach. No recurrence is evident

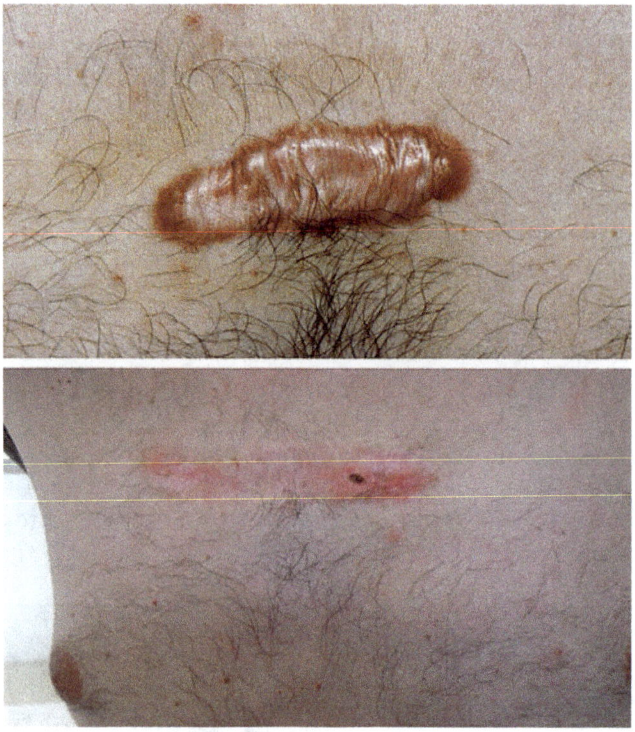

◘ Fig. *Upper* – Preoperative view of a large keloid scar on the anterior chest following acne. *Lower* – Postoperative view demonstrating a complete flattening of the scar 10 years following a single cryosession with no recurrence or hypopigmentation

duced. This method was shown to be effective in the treatment of hypertrophic scars and keloids, and has achieved significant superior clinical results when compared with the existing treatment modalities (◘ Figs. 28.3, 28.4, and 28.5). In addition, it was demonstrated [4, 10] that this method has significantly reduced the patient concern and deformity scores in a scale from 1 (no concern and deformity) to 5 (severe concern and deformity) in 11 patients in whom keloids developed following aesthetic surgery. It was concluded that intralesional cryosurgery provides the plastic surgeon with an effective instrument to treat such scars following aesthetic surgery, thus reducing the dissatisfaction of patients.

The intralesional cryosurgery methods has two main advantages over the spray or contact cryosurgery techniques. Usually only a single cryosession in needed, and it exhibits significantly less hypopigmentation due to better survival environment for the melanocytes, thus can be effectively applied on black/darker-colored skin [1–3]. These beneficial advantages have an important clinical application for the treatment of hypertrophic scars and keloids especially on the face, which is the most crucial area of concern to the patient. Furthermore, the common treatment modalities which were mentioned to treat such a scar would necessitate several treatments and a long therapeutic period while the final results are unpredictable.

In summary, the intralesional cryosurgery technique might be added to the armamentarium of treatment modalities to effectively treat keloid scars. This method is easy to use, safe, can be applied on any size and shape of scars, requires a short learning curve, consumes less liquid nitrogen, and can be applied as an office procedure.

Take-Home Message

Intralesional cryosurgery, which is an evidence-based method, is probably the best treatment for a variety of HSK (small, intermediate, large, and oversized) that achieves remarkable clinical results in a high proportion of patients with minimal hypopigmentation and usually by a single cryo-treatment.

References

1. Har-Shai Y, Amar M, Sabo E. Intralesional cryotherapy for enhancing the involution of hypertrophic scars and keloids. Plast Reconstr Surg. 2003;111:1841–52.
2. Har-Shai Y, Sabo E, Rohde E, Hyams M, Assaf C, Zouboulis CC. Intralesional cryosurgery enhances the involution of recalcitrant auricular keloids: a new clinical approach supported by experimental studies. Wound Repair Regen. 2006;14:18–27.
3. Har-Shai Y, Dujovny E, Rohde E, Zouboulis CC. Effect of skin surface temperature on skin pigmentation during contact and intralesional cryosurgery of keloids. J Eur Acad Dermatol Venereol. 2007;21:191–8. Erratum in: J Eur Acad Dermatol Venereol. 21:292, 2007.
4. Har-Shai Y, Brown W, Labbê D, Dompmartin A, Goldine I, Gil T, Mettanes I, Pallua N. Intralesional cryosurgery for the treatment of hypertrophic scars and keloid following aesthetic surgery: the results of a prospective observational study. Int J Low Extrem Wounds. 2008;7:169–75.
5. Har-Shai Y. Intralesional cryosurgery – a new and effective technology for the treatment of hypertrophic scars and keloids. Chapter II-10.1. In: Krupp S, Rennekampff H-O, Pallua N, editors. Plastische Chirurgie, Klinik und Praxis. Landsberg: Ecomed Medicin, Verlag Group; 2008. p. 1–7.
6. Har-Shai Y, Mettanes I, Genin O, Spector I, Pines M. Keloid histopathology after intralesional cryoneedle treatment. J Eur Acad Dermatol Veanerol. 2011;25(9):1027–36.
7. Mirmovich O, Gil T, Lavi I, Goldine I, Mettanes I, Har-Shai Y. Pain evaluation and control during and following the treatment of hypertrophic scars and keloids employing contact and intralesional cryosurgery – a preliminary study. J Eur Acad Dermatol Veanerol. 2012;26:440–7.
8. Stromps JP, Dunda S, Eppstein RJ, Babic D, Har-Shai Y, Pallua N. Intralesional cryosurgery combined with topical silicone gel sheeting for the treatment of refractory keloids. Dermatol Surg. 2014;40:996–1003.
9. Chopinaud M, Pham A-D, Labbê D, Verneuil L, Gourio C, Benateau H, Dompmartin A. Intralesional cryosurgery to treat keloid scars: results from a retrospective study. Dermatology. 2014;229:263–70.

10. Har-Shai Y, Har-Shai L. Intralesional cryosurgery for the treatment of upper lip keloid following deep chemical peeling. Eur J Plast Surg. 2014;37:679–82.
11. Har-Shai Y, Zouboulis CC. Intralesional cryosurgery for the treatment of hypertrophic scars and keloids. Chapter 86. In: Abramovich W, Graham G, Har-Shai Y, Strumia R, editors. Dermatological cryosurgery and cryotherapy. London: Springer; 2016. p. 453–74.
12. Roitman A, Luntz M, Har-Shai Y. Intralesional cryosurgery for the treatment of keloid scars following cochlear implant surgery and removal of cholesteatoma. Eur J Plast Surg. 2016;39:307–12.
13. O'boyle CP, Shayan-Arani H, Hamada MW. Intralesional cryotherapy for hypertrophic scars and keloids: a review. Scars Burn Heal. 2017;3:1–9.
14. Har-Shai L, Pallua N, Grasys I, Metanes I, Har-Shai Y. Intralesional excision combined with intralesional cryosurgery for the treatment of oversized and therapy-resistant keloids of the neck and ears. Eur J Plast Surg. 2018;41:233–8.
15. Zouboulis CC, Har-Shai Y, Orfanos CE. Cryosurgical treatment of keloids and hypertrophic scars. Chapter 85. In: Abramovich W, Graham G, Har-Shai Y, Strumia R, editors. Dermatological cryosurgery and cryotherapy. London: Springer; 2016. p. 413–51.
16. Har-Shai Y, Har-Shai L, Artzi O. Two-step treatment of bulky keloids on the cheeks after deep chemical peeling: intralesional cryosurgery followed by pulsed dye and ablative fractional CO2 laser. Eur J Plast Surg., published online 20 March, 2020. https://doi.org/10.1007/s00238-020-01651-x

24

Treatment of Immature Scars: Evidence-Based Techniques and Treatments

Julian Poetschke and Gerd G. Gauglitz

Contents

Background

Effective scar treatment has come a long way in recent years. Classifications allow us to differentiate between individual types of scars and allow us to propose scientifically proven therapeutic regimes to improve even severe pathological scarring. This has helped not only in improving functional and aesthetic results in the affected patients but also to ameliorate their oftentimes severely impaired quality of life.

However, efforts have long been underway to prevent pathological scarring altogether. Hopes are that through early intervention in fresh scars, excessive scarring can be limited or prevented altogether.

The use of compression garments or silicone gel sheeting has long been established to steer the scar maturation process away from excessive and proliferative scarring disorders. Flavonoids, too, have proven a promising option for the prevention of excessive scarring in recent years.

Through the advent of newer techniques for the treatment of hypertrophic scars and keloids and fresh insights into the pathophysiology of excessive scarring, new methods for scar prevention are currently making their way into routine practice.

Since fractional photothermolysis has shown its potential in mitigating proliferative scarring and aiding scar remodeling in mature scars, more and more researchers are attempting to alter these ongoing processes in fresh scars to prevent excessive scarring.

This chapter explores the different modalities for scar prevention (see ◘ Table 22.1), their mode of action, and the evidence supporting their use.

◘ **Table** Treatment modalities for immature scars, their indications, and recommendations for treatment

Treatment modality	Indication	Treatment paradigm
Pressure therapy	Gold standard for burn injuries after skin grafting or after deeper second-degree burns that have healed without surgery	Begin treatment as soon as the skin grafts are stable enough or after reepithelialization in wounds that have healed without surgery
		Garments should be worn for as close to 24 hours per day as possible for 6 to 12 months, depending on the level of scar activity
		Garments should be replaced regularly, at least every 3 months so as to ensure sufficiency
	As an adjunct after earlobe keloid excision	Pressure earrings should be worn for as close to 24 hours per day as possible after surgery to minimize the risk of keloid resurgence, starting on the day of suture removal
	Children with linear hypertrophic scarring or keloids, where intralesional treatment is not an option	Same treatment paradigm as in burn scarring. Especially in younger children, sudden growth can require frequent garment replacement
Silicone-based products	First-line therapy for linear and widespread hypertrophic scarring as well as minor keloids and first option for the prevention of hypertrophic scarring	Sheets or patches should be applied to the desired area for 12 to 24 hours per day. Treatment times can vary depending on scar activity, but 3 to 6 months of treatment should be performed
		Gels should be applied to the scarred area two to three times per day. They are better suited for mobile areas close to joints
Onion extract	Can be considered for the treatment of hypertrophic scarring or scar prevention	Treatment recommendations vary depending on the manufacturer
		Patches are commonly applied for 6 to 12 hours overnight for 3 to 6 months
Pulsed dye laser (PDL)	Can be considered for the treatment of erythematous and pruritic postsurgical scars	No clear recommendations or fixed treatment paradigms exist; however, studies indicate that up to three treatment sessions are required for favorable results

Table (Continued)

Treatment modality	Indication	Treatment paradigm
		In most studies, treatment is begun at the date of suture removal or shortly thereafter
Fractional ablative CO_2 laser	Should be considered in patients where excessive scarring is expected (after severe burns/trauma)	Expert committees recommend starting treatment one to three months after the original injury to modulate the scarring process
		Again, no carefully researched treatment paradigms exist; however, based on the data available, low-density, high-energy treatment of the deep dermis in combination with careful superficial smoothening seems favorable
	Experimentally, the laser has been used intraoperatively for scar improvement	To aid with the wound healing, this laser has been used to treat the wound margins intraoperatively before placing the sutures. One to two passes of low-density, high-energy laser treatment were performed on the wound margins
		Thus far, this research was mostly empiric and uncontrolled; thus, no recommendations regarding its use can be made, and caution should be used when considering it
Fractional nonablative Er:Glass laser	Indications for this laser are similar to those of the CO_2 laser	Treatment with the Er:Glass laser has less side effects than with the CO_2 laser; however, its treatment effects are reduced as well, thus requiring more sessions for similar results
		As with the CO_2 laser, little research on the potential for immature scar treatment has been performed, so no clear recommendations can be made

Techniques for the Treatment of Immature Scars

Pressure Therapy

Upon the discovery of the clinical effects of pressure garments on hypertrophic burn scarring by Silverstein and Larson in the late 1960s, the results of further research on the topic performed at Shriners Burns Institute in Galveston, Texas, were published in the early 1970s. This led to the onset of pressure garment therapy use to prevent hypertrophic scar formation in burn patients. Ever since, this method has become the gold standard for scar prevention in burn patients in many countries around the world. While the exact mode of action has not been fully understood, pressure garment therapy supposedly decreases capillary perfusion in the affected tissue, thus leading to localized tissue hypoxia which in turn increases the rate of fibroblast apoptosis, thus leading to a reduced production of collagen. A recent preclinical study by DeBruler et al. investigated the effects of early pressure garment application after skin grafting in burned Duroc pigs and found an increased level of matrix metalloprotease-1 (MMP1) in pigs that received pressure garment treatment within 1 week of grafting [1]. While further research on the matter is required and influences on the levels of collagen I and III or transforming growth factor 1 could not be proven, increased levels of MMP1 which is a known contributor in scar remodeling might help to explain the effects of pressure garment therapy.

Pressure garments come in the form of stockings, pants, sleeves, suits, bandages, girdles, and clip-on earrings, and for locations that are hard to reach through circularly applied pressure, special pelottes can routinely be fitted to allow for effective treatment of nearly every anatomic location. Garments should be worn for as close to 24 hours per day as possible and are usually recommended for at least 6–12 months. In patients showing scar activity after 12 months, treatment is often prolonged for up to 18 months. Being worn for such long times takes a significant toll on the garments which loosen drastically over time, thus requiring regular replacement to ensure sufficient pressure. In our experience, garment replacement is necessary at least every 3 months. To allow patients to wash their compression garments regularly, at least two complete sets should be available at any given time. In patients with physically demanding jobs, wear times might be reduced even further, and more pairs for regular changing might be required.

Pressure garment therapy is very taxing on the patient and compliance is often lacking. Especially during the summer, patients experience sweating and skin maceration, as well as strong odor. In countries without comprehensive health insurance, treatment cost is another important factor. Even in patients where only small areas of the body are affected, treatment over the course of a year will easily cost between one and two thousand euros for a small pressure garment like a glove (◘ Fig. 22.1) or a sleeve alone, whereas larger pieces or even suits for the whole body will cost low to medium five-figure sums, especially when combined with other treatment modalities.

The current consensus on the pressure applied through garments recommends between 20 and 25 mmHg, as studies have shown a higher efficacy when compared to lower-pressure garments (10–15 mmHg).

Even though pressure garment therapy has now been in clinical use for over 40 years, hard clinical data on its efficacy is largely missing, and the existing literature is quite heterogenous.

Early adopters of the technique like Larson, Kischer, and Tolhurst reported favorable results on the reduction of hypertrophic scar formation. More recently, Van den Kerckhove et al. reported positive effects on scar thickness when treating patients with garments with at least 15 mmHg of pressure, and Engrav et al. demonstrated that scars under compression were noticeably softer and thinner in their clinical study in 2010 aided by objective measuring devices. However, a large meta-analysis by Anzarut et al. in 2009 was unable to discern differences in scars treated with pressure garments and untreated scars [2]. In 2013, Atiyeh et al. came to a similar conclusion and questioned the widespread use and recommendation, especially in the light of the often poor patient compliance and the resultant cost-effectiveness of this course of treatment. Especially in burn patients, this course of treatment, however, has become the accepted standard. This makes randomized controlled trials with an untreated patient population nearly impossible on ethical grounds, thus limiting the designs of further studies investigating this treatment method.

Thus far, based upon many different studies indicating the clinical efficacy of pressure garment therapy, current guidelines for the treatment and prevention of pathological scarring recommend its use while noting the less than robust level of evidence.

Furthermore, pressure garment therapy can be considered in children with linear hypertrophic scarring or keloids, where intralesional treatment is abandoned because of side effects or the associated risk of the treatment and pressure garment therapy has empirically shown greater efficacy than in adults.

In patients that received surgical treatment for earlobe keloids, pressure earrings have been shown to greatly reduce the risk of keloid recurrence and are thus regularly recommended as an adjunct. Pressure earrings are readily available from specialized orthopedic technicians, and if keloids are excised elsewhere on the ear, like on the helix, tragus, or other parts of the ear, special splints can be custom-made.

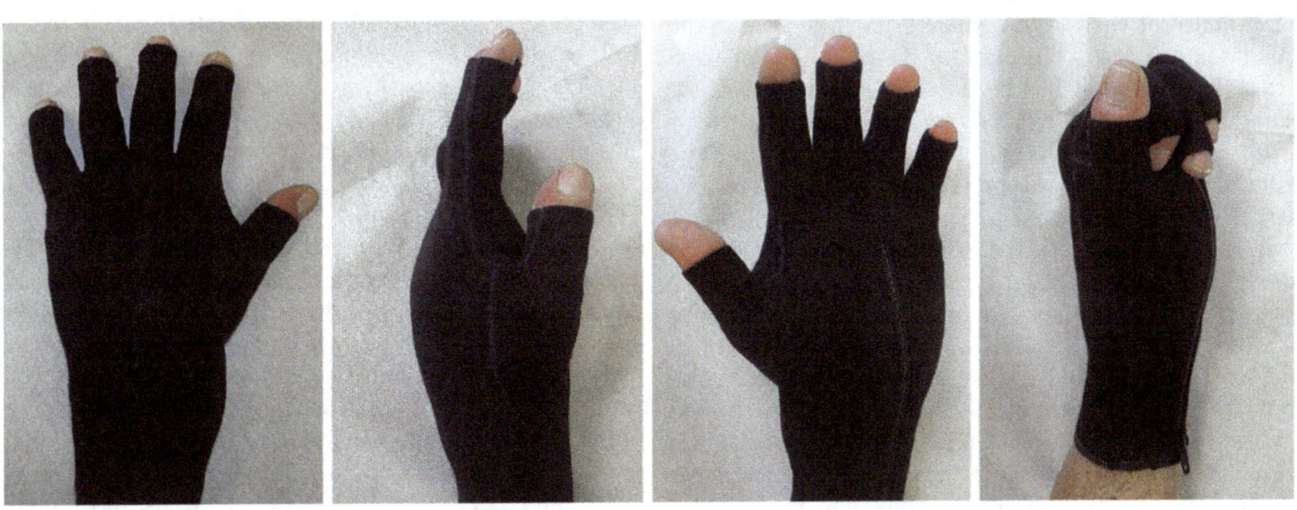

◘ **Fig.** Patient with severe burn scarring of the left hand wearing a compression glove. The glove allows full function (full finger flexion and extension) while providing full coverage

Silicone-Based Products

Silicone-based products come in a variety of forms. They are available as creams, oils, gels, or, most commonly, patches or sheets that can be applied to the affected areas. Their mode of action regarding the treatment and prevention of excessive scarring has not yet been fully understood, but it is stipulated that the occlusive effect of the silicone inhibits the transepidermal loss of water (TEWL), thus ensuring sufficient hydration of the skin. Thus far, no properties of silicone, which directly influence the process of scarring, have been discovered.

Treatment with silicone-based products can be started after complete reepithelialization of the wounds. Sheets or patches should be applied for 12–24 hours per day throughout 3–6 months. Gel- or cream-based silicone products are better suited for areas that are subject to constant motion (i.e., large joints) where wound dressings might prove unsuitable. To achieve the desired effect, applying the gel two to three times daily is recommended.

Patches and sheets come in many different forms and thicknesses. Commonly, thicker sheets last longer than thinner ones. Larger sheets can be cut into the desired size. They should be cleaned with water and special cleaning solutions that come with the product regularly and can be put back on their carrier foil for storing in between applications. Reusing a single sheet is usually possible for 6–8 weeks, before the silicone disintegrates and becomes gelatinous in its structure, whereupon a fresh sheet should be used.

Side effects or allergies to silicone-based products are rarely observed. Skin maceration through the occlusive effect is possible, whereupon patients can reduce the application time of the silicone.

Silicone has been used in the treatment of immature scars since the early 1980s, where it was first used in the Adelaide Children's Hospital for the treatment of burn scars. Ever since, it has become one of the pillars for early scar intervention. Different prevention and treatment studies have reported outcomes documenting the efficacy of silicone for preventing scar hypertrophy. Cruz-Korchin compared patients after bilateral mammoplasty, after which the scars on one breast were dressed with silicone sheets for 12 hours a day for 2 months while the other remained without preventative treatment. Results demonstrated scar hypertrophy in 60% of the untreated breasts after 2 months, whereas only 25% of the scars in the treatment group showed hypertrophy. Ahn et al., in 1991, could demonstrate that surgical incisions treated with silicone gel bandages showed less proclivity for hypertrophy than an untreated control.

In 2001, Gold et al. showed that patients suffering from abnormal scarring showed significantly less hypertrophic scarring when treated with silicone gel sheeting after skin surgery compared to an untreated group of patients.

However, a variety of studies have failed to document significant effects regarding scar prevention of treatment through silicone-based products. In 1998, Niessen et al. failed to show positive effects regarding scar prevention through silicone gel sheeting and even reported a higher rate of hypertrophic scar development than in their control group treated with nonocclusive micropore in their breast reduction scar model.

Cochrane Reviews in 2006 and 2013 noted the generally poor quality of prevention and treatment studies analyzing the effects of silicone regarding pathological scarring [3]. While seemingly reducing the risk of abnormal scarring in high-risk patients and improving scar parameters such as color and softness in existing scars, significant bias was a main critique point in most studies.

Nevertheless, silicone gel sheeting is recommended as a first-line therapy for linear and widespread hypertrophic scarring, as well as minor keloids in national and international guidelines on the management of pathological scarring, and has furthermore been noted as an important option for the prevention of excessive scarring.

Onion Extract

Products that contain onion extract have seen increasing popularity for the treatment of immature scars in recent years. They are available as creams or patches and commonly include adjuncts such as allantoin or heparin. Onion extract contains quercetin, a flavonoid that has anti-oxidative and anti-inflammatory properties. Experimental research has suggested that quercetin influences transforming growth factor beta 1 and 2 and SMAD signaling pathways, thus inhibiting fibroblast proliferation and collagen synthesis. In cell cultures, it has also been shown to induce matrix metalloproteinase-1 expression, thus influencing extracellular matrix remodeling.

Scar treatment is begun after complete reepithelialization of the wound is complete. Onion extract patches are commonly used overnight, where they are applied for 6–12 hours over the course of 12–24 weeks, though no clear recommendations regarding the length of treatment exist to date. Gels are often applied multiple times throughout the day for weeks or months, according to manufacturer recommendations, though there is a variance between different formulations and manufacturers.

Regarding the efficacy of onion-extract-based products, different studies documented significant potential regarding the prevention of pathological scarring. Draelos et al. reported a significantly improved appearance of fresh surgical scars treated with onion extract gel when compared with a control group in two different studies in 2008 and 2012. Parameters positively influenced through the treatment included scar softness, redness, texture, and global appearance. In 2006, Ho et al. evaluated the effects of onion extract gel on scarring after Q-switched Nd:YAG laser tattoo removal in a Chinese patient population and reported significantly less scarring in the treatment group than in the control group.

In 2018, a randomized controlled study by Prager et al. on 125 subjects with fresh postsurgical scars that were treated with an overnight patch containing onion extract, allantoin, and heparin demonstrated significantly better rated scars by both patients and investigators after 12 and 24 weeks of treatment when compared to the control group [4]. Overall treatment comfort was good, and no safety concerns were identified.

Some studies have, however, come up with less positive conclusions. Chung et al. investigated the effects of an onion extract gel when compared with a petrolatum emollient on fresh surgical scars and found no difference between the treatments. Ocampo-Candini et al. published a randomized controlled trial documenting the development of Pfannenstiel scars after cesarean section under treatment with onion extract gel and found no significant improvement over their untreated control group when comparing POSAS scores.

Overall, this relatively new treatment option requires further intense scientific evaluation to improve the level of evidence regarding its efficacy. Due to the promising data that has been collected thus far, current guidelines support the consideration of onion-extract-based formulations for the treatment of hypertrophic scarring as well as the prevention of excessive scarring after surgery.

Pulsed Dye Laser (PDL)

The pulsed dye laser is a nonablative laser with a wavelength of 585 or 595 nm. Its target chromophore is oxygenized hemoglobin, and application of the laser will therefore lead to coagulation of capillaries, thus inducing tissue hypoxemia. In scar tissue, this effect will induce a reduction of profibrotic processes and stimulate scar remodeling.

Alster et al. reported significant therapeutic benefits of the PDL for the treatment of keloids in 1995; however, other research groups failed to replicate their findings with some even showing high numbers of recurrence. Further clinical research, however, has established the laser potential for the treatment of erythematous and pruritic scars, for which it is routinely considered. Recently, however, more and more authors have started treating fresh postsurgical scars with the PDL to elucidate whether this can favorably alter the process of scar maturation. McGraw et al. were the first to publish a study on the prevention of hypertrophic scarring with the PDL in 1999. They found that early treatment within the first few weeks after trauma or surgery resulted in a faster resolution of scar stiffness and erythema, as well as a decreased frequency of hypertrophic scarring. Furthermore, they noted an improved scar quality due to the good color match with the healthy skin. In 2003, Nouri et al. published similar findings. In their study, they included 11 patients with 12 postoperative linear scars that were divided into a treated and an untreated half. Overall, three sessions of 585 nm PDL treatment at monthly intervals were performed, whereupon the cosmetic appearance of the treated scars was reportedly significantly better, when analyzed by a blinded examiner using the Vancouver Scar Scale. In 2006, however, Alam et al. found no significant difference in their randomized controlled trial, where fresh postsurgical scars were treated with one pass of PDL treatment upon suture removal. They noted that 6 weeks after treatment, both groups had improved while the result of neither group was superior. In 2011, Kim et al. examined the effect of three sessions of PDL treatment followed by three sessions of fractional ablative erbium:YAG laser treatment on fresh thyroidectomy scars and noticed favorable effects after PDL treatment with 83% of patients expressing satisfaction with the result. Er:YAG treatment further improved the observed results [5].

To date, further studies on the potential of the PDL as an option in the treatment of fresh postsurgical scars to quicken scar maturation and to prevent scar hypertrophy exist. However, most studies lack a long-term follow-up that encompasses the entirety of the natural length of scar maturation (12–18 months), thus inhibiting judgment about whether the final results are superior to an untreated control or simply accelerate the process. Therefore, so far, no clear recommendations on the use of the PDL for scar prevention can be made, while the current literature indicates that positive results at the cost of low rates of side effects can be achieved.

Fractional Ablative Carbon Dioxide (CO_2) Laser

While the 10,800 nm carbon dioxide (CO_2) laser has been around for decades, the recent development of fractional lasers has led to a significant expansion of its therapeutic range.

In fractional units, the laser beam is divided into an array of smaller columns, leaving untreated skin islets in between. The divided laser columns ablate tissue and can reach depths of up to 4 mm newer models, with maybe their most important effects taking place in the dermis. Through the heating of the surrounding tissue, fractional CO_2 laser treatment activates heat-shock proteins which in turn stimulate antifibrotic factors such as transforming growth factor beta 3 (TGF-β3) and matrix metalloproteinases, thus stimulating scar remodeling. Additionally, through classic tissue ablation, scar surface irregularities can effectively be smoothened through use of the CO_2 laser.

After the discovery of these effects through experimental research, different clinical studies have since used the fractional CO_2 laser to treat mature burn scars. Recent studies found that a single treatment can improve scar softness and surface irregularities by up to 30% all the while positively influencing patient quality of life. While further research is warranted, current guidelines for the treatment of excessive scarring are recommending the CO_2 laser for treatment in severe widespread hypertrophic scarring.

Side effects of the treatment commonly include swelling and oozing of the wounds throughout the first days after treatment, as well as erythema, which commonly recede within 1–2 weeks after treatment. In the author's experience, when treating severe scarring with higher fluences, posttreatment hyperpigmentation often occurs but tapers off after 4–6 months after treatment.

Since the fractional CO2 laser has seen great success in the treatment of mature widespread scarring and experimental studies suggest that this laser is able to normalize the oftentimes greatly disturbed architecture of the dermal matrix, research is under way to establish the CO2 laser's abilities regarding excessive scar prevention through the treatment of immature scars.

In 2011, Ozog et al. examined the intraoperative use of the fractional CO_2 laser. Before wound closure, one-half of the wound margins were treated with one to two passes of Active FX (Lumenis Ultrapulse, Santa Clara, California, USA), before the wound was closed. Upon the final evaluation of the scars after 2–3 months post surgery, both patients and examiners rated the laser-treated scar halves superior to the untreated halves [6]. Jung et al., also in 2011, treated immature thyroidectomy scars 2–3 weeks after surgery with a fractional CO_2 laser. Patients were treated with two passes, 50 mJ of energy and 100 microbeams/cm^2 with a coverage of 12.7%. Analysis of the treatment effect after 3 months revealed significantly improved Vancouver Scar Scale scores, as well as significantly improved values measured with a skin durometer [7]. However, no comparison with an untreated control group was performed. In 2013, Lee et al. performed a split-scar study on 15 three-week-old scars. Two laser passes were delivered at 80 mJ with a density of 100 microbeams/cm^2 achieving a total coverage of 15.6%. During the final observation, 3 months after treatment, a significant improvement of Vancouver Scar Scale values superior to those made in the control group was found. Especially, scar pliability and thickness improvements were larger than those in the control group, while vascularity and pigmentation did not differ considerably.

Overall, more research on the fractional CO_2 laser's abilities regarding scar prevention is required. While initial research shows promising results and the molecular defects thus far discovered suggest that early intervention could lead to a normalization of the dermal architecture in scar tissue, many issues remain to be elucidated. To exclude natural scar regression, which is an important factor in hypertrophic scarring, as a factor, long-term follow-up of over 12–18 months is required, as well as including a control group.

Nevertheless, expert committees suggest that early treatment, 1–3 months after the original injury, should be considered, especially when excessive scarring is expected. Thus far, no study researching early laser intervention found evidence of increased scarring or other severe side effects, thus supporting the safety the laser is known for in mature scar treatment.

Nonablative Erbium Glass (Er:Glass) Laser

The 1550 nm erbium glass (Er:Glass) laser is a nonablative fractional laser. It does not remove tissue but merely applies heat in a controlled way and leaves the epidermis intact. Through the application of heat in the dermis, its effect there is similar to those of the carbon dioxide laser, albeit at a reduced rate of side effects. Since treatment with the Er:Glass laser does not leave wounds, downtime is greatly reduced. Patients commonly experience light swelling and posttreatment erythema for a few days.

Regarding its efficacy for early scar intervention, thus far, few studies exist. Tierney et al. compared PDL and Er:Glass laser treatment in 2-month-old scars after Mohs surgery in 2009. The study was performed in a split-scar fashion, and patients were blinded as to what side was being treated with which laser. Every scar received four treatment sessions at four-week intervals, and follow-up was performed 1 month after the last treatment session. Overall, patients preferred the results of the Er:Glass-laser-treated scars (83% of patients). Regarding the scar parameters, pigmentation, scar thickness, and overall aesthetic outcome were all superior in the Er:Glass group [8].

In 2014, Ha et al. compared the effects of PDL treatment to Er:Glass laser treatment in a split-scar study on 2–3-week-old thyroidectomy scars. Overall, both groups saw significantly improved scar ratings 6 months after treatment. Patients reported that they found the PDL treated scars less apparent; however, pliability appeared superior in the Er:Glass-laser-treated scars [9]. In their 2014 study, Shin et al. performed another split-scar study, this time comparing ablative fractional CO_2 laser treatment to Er:Glass laser treatment. After three treatment sessions in 2-month intervals, follow-up examinations 3 months after the last laser session revealed significant improvement of the scarring in both groups without statistically significant differences between the groups overall. However, the CO_2 laser group showed greater improvement of scar hardness, while the Er:Glass-laser-treated scars proved superior regarding their color [10].

Overall, current research has shown promise regarding the Er:Glass laser's efficacy for early scar intervention. However, thus far, few clinical studies are available, thus requiring further research on the matter. As with other laser modalities for the treatment of immature scars, further studies should focus on longer follow-up times as well as larger group samples to further improve the level of evidence.

Conclusion

Efforts to prevent pathological scarring have been underway for many decades. One of the most established methods is pressure garment therapy, which has been used in the prevention of widespread hypertrophic burn scarring since the early 1970s. Years of use have seen this modality become the gold standard, and thus, pressure garments are routinely prescribed for most burn patients in the developed world. However, upon further inspection of the evidence, hard clinical data on the efficacy of pressure garment therapy is only scarcely available. Furthermore, patient discomfort is often high, leading to infrequent treatment compliance. Other options for the treatment of immature scarring are tolerated better. Silicone gel sheeting is often applied throughout the night, and its continued use has been shown to improve scar pliability and height in connection with little to no side effects. Clinical evidence, however, is not as explicit as frequent mentions in national and international guidelines for the treatment and prevention of pathological scarring might infer. Similar in their application to silicone-based products, onion-extract-based gels, creams, and patches have appeared on the market in recent years. Often combined with further active ingredients like allantoin and heparin, they are specifically marketed for use in fresh scars, where they show promise in alleviating scar redness and firmness as well as improving further scar parameters. While additional research will determine the future role of this treatment modality, the low side-effect profile and the appearance of natural ingredients appeal to many patients. In the treatment of mature scars, and increasingly so in the treatment of fresh scars, lasers cannot be ignored. While PDL treatment has been around for years and its use in immature scars to alleviate pruritus and erythema has been well researched and documented, researchers are more and more focusing on fractional lasers. Their effects on dermal matrix remodeling through the stimulation of heat-shock proteins and the resultant effects on transforming growth factor beta isotypes and the concentration of matrix metalloproteases have resulted in researchers trying to employ these effects to modulate the active scar process in favor of remodeling rather than excessive fibrosis. While initial research, both for the ablative CO_2 laser and for the nonablative Er:Glass laser, has shown promising results, most recent studies lack sufficient follow-up observation time. To assess whether clinically measured effects are caused through treatment and not through natural scar regression over time, scar maturation must be waited for to make a final conclusion. To date, this presents the largest problems with most research on immature scars. Overall, however, patients today can rely on a variety of promising options for the prevention of excessive scarring. While not every patient requires a robust prevention regimen after surgical intervention, care should be taken to identify patients at risk for excessive scarring and to tailor a treatment algorithm according to their needs. After all, preventing a hypertrophic scar or keloid from forming saves patients from months or years of strenuous symptoms and treatment. Furthermore, today, most algorithms for the prevention of excessive scarring are well tolerated and go along with minimal treatment discomfort and side effects.

Take-Home Messages

- Pressure garment therapy is the gold standard for the prevention of widespread scarring, e.g., after burns. Even though it has been in use since the early 1970s, evidence for its efficacy is largely empiric. Additionally, side effects of pressure garment therapy often lead to low compliance which affects the treatment efficacy.
- Silicone gel sheeting has proven effective in softening scars, and its use shows little to no side effects. Its mode of action, however, remains largely unknown, and recent meta-analyses question its efficacy.

- Onion-extract-based products are available as creams and patches. Early research has shown promise regarding the prevention of pathological scarring, but further research is needed to further elucidate its role in the treatment of immature scars.
- PDL treatment has been found to improve pruritus, erythema, and stiffness in fresh postsurgical scars; however, the overall level of evidence for immature scar treatment is low.
- Fractional CO_2 laser treatment has been shown to affect dermal matrix remodeling and is therefore increasingly used to modulate immature scars. While initial studies show promise and scar pliability and height seem to improve through treatment, long-term follow-up is crucial in future studies to further strengthen the clinical evidence for this therapeutic option.
- Fractional nonablative Er:Glass laser treatment employs a similar mode of action, much like the CO_2 laser, but does not ablate tissue. Thus, downtime and side effects are greatly reduced.
- Scar prevention is imperative in patients with a history of pathological scarring to avoid severe functional, aesthetic, and psychosocial impairments.
- Most modern methods for scar prevention have a minimal likelihood of severe side effects, and treatment discomfort is commonly very low.

References

1. DeBruler DM, Baumann ME, Blackstone BN, Zbinden JC, McFarland KL, Bailey JK, et al. Role of early application of pressure garments following burn injury and autografting. Plas Reconstr Surg. 2019;143(2):310e–21e.
2. Anzarut A, Olson J, Singh P, Rowe BH, Tredget EE. The effectiveness of pressure garment therapy for the prevention of abnormal scarring after burn injury: a meta-analysis. J Plast Reconstr Aesthet Surg. 2009;62(1):77–84.
3. O'Brien L, Jones DJ. Silicone gel sheeting for preventing and treating hypertrophic and keloid scars. Cochrane Database Syst Rev. 2013(9):Cd003826.
4. Prager W, Gauglitz GG. Effectiveness and safety of an overnight patch containing Allium cepa extract and Allantoin for post-dermatologic surgery scars. Aesthet Plast Surg. 2018;42(4):1144–50.
5. Kim HS, Kim BJ, Lee JY, Kim HO, Park YM. Effect of the 595-nm pulsed dye laser and ablative 2940-nm Er:YAG fractional laser on fresh surgical scars: an uncontrolled pilot study. J Cosmet Laser Ther. 2011;13(4):176–9.
6. Ozog DM, Moy RL. A randomized split-scar study of intraoperative treatment of surgical wound edges to minimize scarring. Arch Dermatol. 2011;147(9):1108–10.
7. Jung JY, Jeong JJ, Roh HJ, Cho SH, Chung KY, Lee WJ, et al. Early postoperative treatment of thyroidectomy scars using a fractional carbon dioxide laser. Dermatol Surg. 2011;37(2):217–23.
8. Tierney E, Mahmoud BH, Srivastava D, Ozog D, Kouba DJ. Treatment of surgical scars with nonablative fractional laser versus pulsed dye laser: a randomized controlled trial. Dermatol Surg. 2009;35(8):1172–80.
9. Ha JM, Kim HS, Cho EB, Park GH, Park EJ, Kim KH, et al. Comparison of the effectiveness of nonablative fractional laser versus pulsed-dye laser in thyroidectomy scar prevention. Ann Dermatol. 2014;26(5):615–20.
10. Shin JU, Gantsetseg D, Jung JY, Jung I, Shin S, Lee JH. Comparison of non-ablative and ablative fractional laser treatments in a postoperative scar study. Lasers Surg Med. 2014;46(10):741–9.

25

Objective Assessment Techniques: Physiological Parameters in Scar Assessment

Peter Moortgat, Mieke Anthonissen, Ulrike Van Daele, Jill Meirte, Tine Vanhullebusch, and Koen Maertens

Contents

Background

With advances in medicine, we are able to modulate wound healing and scarring. In order to assess new and often costly treatments, the need for objective scar measurement tools has become increasingly important. A combination of subjective and objective measures should be the aim of every researcher. In daily practice, time is a limiting factor, and the choice for objective measurements should always incorporate feasibility and cost. Objective assessments provide a quantitative measurement of the scar. Quantitative assessment of scars requires devices to measure their physical and physiological properties. These properties include, but are not limited to, the following:

Physical parameters:

- Color
- Thickness
- Elasticity or pliability
- Texture
- Surface
- Tissue anisotropy

Physiological parameters:

- Skin hydration
- Transcutaneous oxygen level
- Tactile sensitivity

In this chapter, an overview of the assessment tools to evaluate physiological scar parameters will be given. Physiological scar parameters are scar characteristics relevant to pathological scarring which cannot be seen with the bare eye. This also means that they can only be assessed with objective assessment tools. This overview lacks skin characteristics which are measured with digital imaging systems. These assessment tools will be discussed in a separate chapter.

Skin Hydration

Skin hydration is defined as the water content of the epidermis and the dermis. Approximately 20% of water present in our body is accumulated in the skin. Of this amount, 60–70% is located in the dermis, and 15–30% is retained in the stratum corneum (SC). Functionally, the amount of water in the skin can be divided into free and bound water. In healthy skin, most of the water are bound to macromolecules. The ability of the skin to retain water is primarily related to the SC, which plays the role of the outer skin barrier, protecting the skin from water loss. The SC consists of cells called corneocytes and various lipids (fats) between them. The retention of water in the SC is dependent mainly on the presence of natural hygroscopic agents within the corneocytes and the SC intercellular lipids orderly arranged to form a barrier to trans-epidermal water loss [1]. The corneocytes are often compared to bricks and the intercellular lipids to mortar, an appropriate metaphor for a layer of skin that serves as a barrier. The corneocytes are dead cells without nuclei. They contain various substances that hold water. For our skin to feel smooth and supple, the SC has to be at least 10% water; ideally, it is 20–30%. The SC can absorb as much as five to six times its own weight and increase its volume threefold when soaked in water. But it is not simply the water content that matters. Water has an effect on the enzymes that control orderly shedding of corneocytes, a process dermatologists call desquamation. Without water, the corneocytes accumulate, so the skin becomes flaky instead of peeling off nicely, and the SC gets disorganized and full of cracks instead of being tightly packed.

The glycosaminoglycan (GAG) polymer hyaluronan (HA, hyaluronic acid) forms a scaffold on which proteoglycans and matrix proteins are organized. These supramolecular structures are able to entrap water and ions to provide the skin with hydration. HA occurs in both the dermis and epidermis, with the dermis containing the greater proportion. HA present in the epidermis may play a role in a epidermal barrier function and SC hydration [1]. The lack of interaction between water and surrounding molecules contributes to dry appearance of the skin. Water content can vary depending on varying factors as skin site, skin depth, body mass index, age, sex, diurnal hour, seasons, and climates.

Skin Hydration in the Epidermis

The epidermal thickness is variable. It had been reported to be between 40 and 240 μm thick, depending on the measuring area and method used. Water originates in the deeper epidermal layers and moves upward to hydrate cells in the outermost skin layer, the stratum corneum (SC). Aquaporins (AQPs), cell membrane-bound water channels present in the epidermis, are essential hydration-regulating elements controlling cellular water and glycerol transport. Glycerol, thus present in the outer epidermal layers, binds and holds water, important for maintaining optimal skin hydration. The epidermis contains two different levels of water, separated by the interface between the stratum granulosum (SG) and the SC. The largest gradient of water in the epidermis occurs in the underlying layers of the SG (viable epidermis), while the SC water content is 4–5 times lower [2]. This gradient isolates the SC from the body, helping to conserve important solutes and water within the viable epidermis. The presence of a water gradient at the deeper part of the SC triggers important keratinocyte functions such as the production of natural moisturizing factors (NMF). Dehydration of the upper skin layers increases when the SC water is lost more quickly than that which is received from the lower layers of the skin (viable epidermis and dermis), thus affecting the natural flow of water. Water originates in the deeper epidermal layers and moves upward to hydrate cells in the SC, eventually being lost to evaporation. Then, an evaporation barrier is needed to maintain body water homeostasis. The SC functions as the main evaporation barrier [2, 3].

Dermal Water Content

The dermis is between 1 and 4 mm thick, and it consists mainly of connective tissue. Dermis thickens as it binds more water. In the dermis, the collagen fibers, the interstitial space GAGs, and the proteoglycans can absorb large quantities of water, which leads to youthful skin. With skin fibrosis, the collagen fiber network is stretched by external mechanical forces, reduces its absorption capacity and water retention, and can lead to prolonged inflammation. Dermal hydration is highly related to the content and distribution of GAGs. The GAGs most often present in the human skin are hyaluronic acid (not attached to a protein core) and the proteoglycan family of chondroitin sulfates (GAGs attached to a protein core). GAGs bind up to 1000 times their volume in water [4]. GAGs in photodamaged or scarred skin are abnormally deposited in the papillary dermis, rather than diffusely scattered as in young skin. This aberrant localization interferes with normal water binding by GAGs, despite their increased quantity [4].

How to Measure Skin Hydration?

Many approaches exist to measure skin water content. One single method is often not enough to capture all the relevant information. Trans-epidermal water loss, stratum corneum water content, and dermal water content are equally important and related to each other.

The skin acts as a barrier against the water evaporation from the internal tissue. The water content in the skin preserves the softness and the smoothness of the skin surface. Diffusion of condensed water through the stratum corneum (SC) occurs and is highly elevated in pathological situations such as scaring; this can be measured by trans-epidermal water loss (TEWL). The results of these measurements are a good indicator of the recovery of the skin barrier and are a useful indicator of the scar maturation process [5]. TEWL is strongly related with the moisture content of the skin and can be measured with open- or closed-chamber systems [6]. The open chambers are the oldest but still most widely used.

Trans-Epidermal Water Loss: Measuring Principle

Trans-epidermal water loss represents the outward permeation of condensed water through the stratum corneum by means of diffusion [7]. TEWL can be measured by using an open-chamber method or closed-chamber method. Open chambers are open to the surrounding atmosphere and are therefore easily influenced by external air convection and turbulence. Closed-chamber methods have been designed more recently, the measuring chamber is enclosed from the surrounding atmosphere, and measurements are therefore not influenced by external air convection and turbulence.

TEWL can be calculated by measuring the water vapor pressure (VP) gradient at the skin surface. In the open-chamber method, the VP gradient is calculated by measuring the difference in VP between two distinct points aligned perpendicularly to the skin surface (see ◘ Fig. 18.1). VP is calculated as the product of relative humidity (RH) and saturated VP; this is dependent on temperature. RH is measured using capacitive sensors; temperature is measured with fast thermistors located in the cylindrical measuring chamber with open ends [7–11].

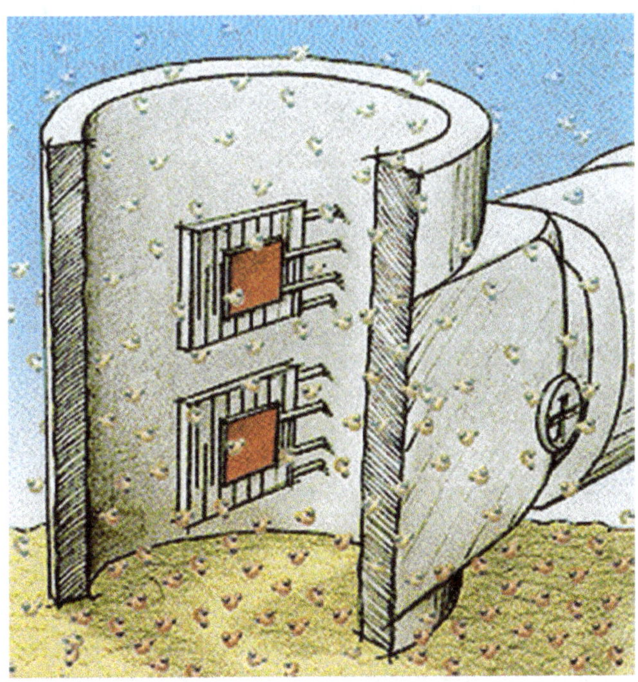

◘ **Fig.** TEWL measured by using an open-chamber method. Reused with permission from Courage + Khazaka electronic GmbH.

Open-Chamber Method

To date, the open-chamber method is still considered the most reliable method to measure water evaporation in scarred skin. Open-chamber systems measure water evaporation rate based on diffusion principles [9, 11]. The vapor density gradient is measured indirectly by two pairs of sensors (temperature and relative humidity) inside a hollow cylinder [7, 11]. The resulting data are analyzed by a microprocessor. Measurement values are given in g/m^2/h. The physiological water vapor mantle surrounding the human skin is a gradient of water with a thickness of about 10 mm. The two sensors of the evaporimeter probe are typically placed 3 and 6 mm above the skin surface. Open-chamber evaporimeters have limitations in practical use and should ideally be used in a climatized room with control of convection, temperature, and humidity [9, 10]. Used outside a climatized room, special attention should be given to air convection, room temperature, and ambient humidity [9].

The most widely used systems are the Tewameter® TM300 (Courage+Khazaka, Cologne, Germany) and the DermaLab® (Cortex, Hadsund, Denmark). Both are available as stand-alone devices or as a probe attached to a Multi Probe Adapter System like the Scarbase Duo™ (Courage+Khazaka, Cologne, Germany) and the DermaLab Combo® (Cortex, Hadsund, Denmark).

Both the Tewameter® (◘ Fig. 18.2) and the DermaLab USB® TEWL (◘ Fig. 18.3) showed good to excellent reliability and validity with rather high minimal clinically important difference (MCID) [12, 13]. The MCID is the smallest change in an outcome that a patient or a clinician would identify as important. An overview of the results is set out in ◘ Table 18.1.

Semi-Open-Chamber Method

Recordings with open-chamber evaporimeters are not intrusive to the 10 mm physiological water vapor mantle over the skin and due to its specificity sensitive to ambient airflow. Open-chamber instruments perform best under standardized ambient conditions with an air protection shield or box controlling the ambient air conditions, as described in standards [9, 10]. Closed-chamber methods are insensitive to ambient air but, unfortunately, directly intrusive to the water vapor mantle. Accumulation of water vapor in the chamber during the measurement instantly and directly influences the diffusion of water out of the skin. Thus, closed chambers interfere with the physiological skin barrier and thus cannot record physiological TEWL directly. For the same reason, measurements may only be made as an initial estimate and not continuously. In the DermaLab system (Cortex Technology, Hadsund, Denmark), a special grid serving as a semi-open windshield has been incorporated directly in the top of the open probe of this instrument. This grid is open and allows evaporation of water out of the probe chamber and at the same time protects the sensors in the probe against ambient

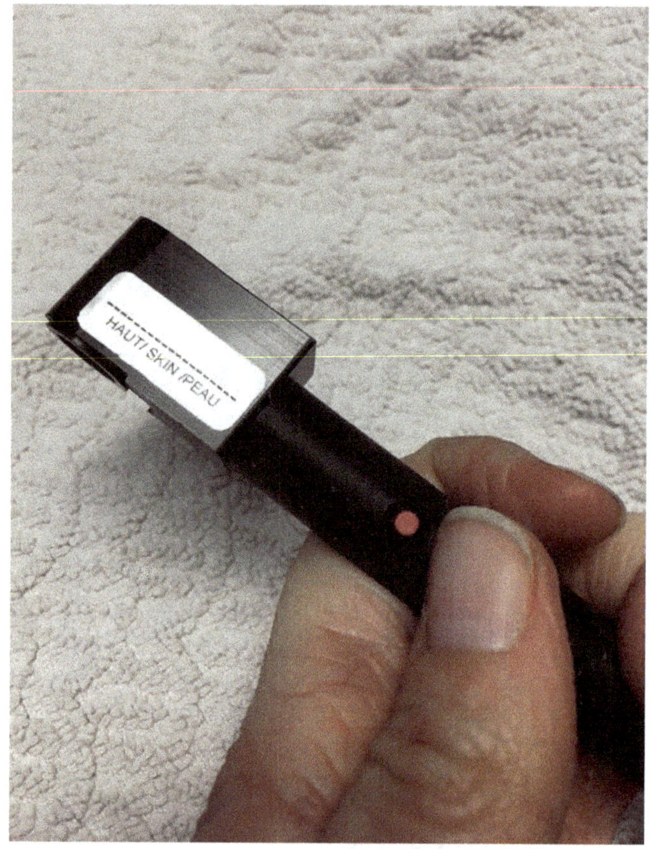

◘ **Fig.** The probe of the Tewameter® TM300. Reused with permission from Oscare. © All rights reserved

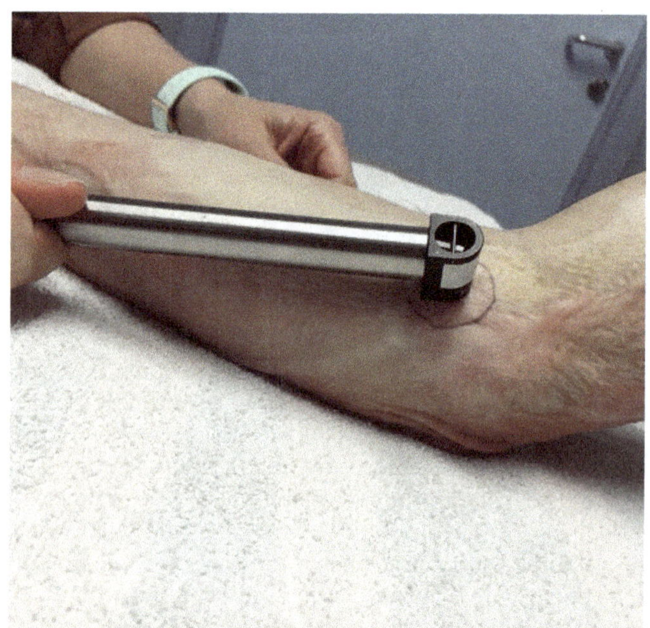

◘ **Fig.** DermaLab® USB TEWL-probe. Reused with permis-sion from Oscare. © All rights reserved

Table Comparison of reliability, validity, and MCID for trans-epidermal water loss assessment on scars

Device	Intrarater reliability (ICC)	Interrater reliability (ICC)	Validity	MCID
Tewameter® [13]	0.95	0.96	Good correlation with DermaLab® TEWL ($r = 0.93$)[b]	12%
DermaLab® TEWL [12]	0.86–0.88	0.78–0.93	DermaLab® TEWL is able to distinguish normal skin from spontaneously healed scars ($p = 0.036$)	17%

air convections. The system can be considered respectful to the water vapor mantle.

Closed-Chamber Method

Two types of closed-chamber methods are available – a condenser chamber method and an unventilated-closed-chamber method. With the unventilated-chamber method, the measuring cylinder is closed off at the top. When placed on the skin, water vapor from the skin collects in the chamber, and with time, the humidity in the chamber increases slowly at first, and thereafter linearly. Flux density (amount of water diffusing through the SC per unit distance and time) is calculated from the change in RH and temperature over time. Due to the accumulation of water vapor and humidity in the chamber, these instruments cannot be used for continuous measurements. Overall, the measurement time of unventilated-closed-chamber instruments is very short (<10 seconds). Various skin barrier impairment studies revealed that the open-chamber devices are more sensitive or discriminative and are able to detect significantly smaller differences than the closed-chamber devices [14]. The VapoMeter (Delfin Technologies Ltd., Kuopio, Finland) is an example of a unventilated-closed-chamber system [15]. The VapoMeter is simple in principle; a humidity sensor in the closed chamber measures the gradual buildup of humidity. On its commercialization, it was postulated that TEWL measurements were not affected by ambient or body-induced airflows.

Stratum Corneum Hydration Level: Measuring Principle

Hydration of the skin surface is a good indicator of epidermal function. Hydration is directly proportional to retention of electrical charge and is therefore often measured by dielectric capacitance or the conductance of the superficial skin layers [11]. Technical aspects such as type of probe surface, degree of direct galvanic contact with the skin, distance between the electrodes, and depth of measurement all vary when comparing the different technologies. Due to the higher TEWL, scar sites are dryer than control sites and seem to become dryer as they mature. Water content is very important in the evaluation of biophysical properties of scars. Evidence suggests that a sufficient amount of water in the stratum corneum (SC) keeps the skin soft and flexible and ensures that the skin appears smooth and healthy. The water holding capacity of the SC also influences its barrier function and mechanical properties [16]. Measurements of hydration are often influenced by environmental factors [7].

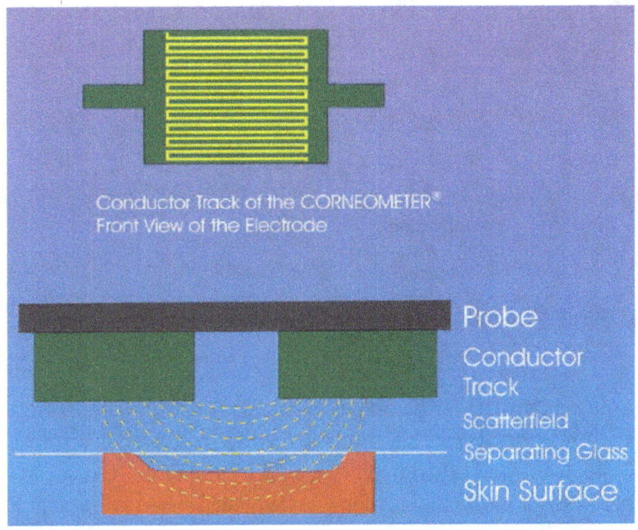

Fig. The measurement principle of the Corneometer® CM825 is based on the capacitance method. Reused with permission from Courage + Khazaka electronic GmbH. © All rights reserved

The Corneometer CM 825® (Courage+Khazaka, Cologne, Germany) is based on the capacitance method. It is a well-known and efficient instrument in measuring hydration of the SC. In the past, the measuring probe of the Corneometer used an analog signal, but now, digital technology is used, resulting in higher stability and less interferences [17].

The Skicon instruments (I.B.S. Co., Hamama-T), based on the conductance method, are also widely used. A modern version of the Skicon (Skicon-200EX®) has been developed with a new concentric interdigital probe.

Corneometer CM825®

The measuring principle is based on the capacitance method (see Fig. 18.4). Technical description of this type of instrument and its use has been published by

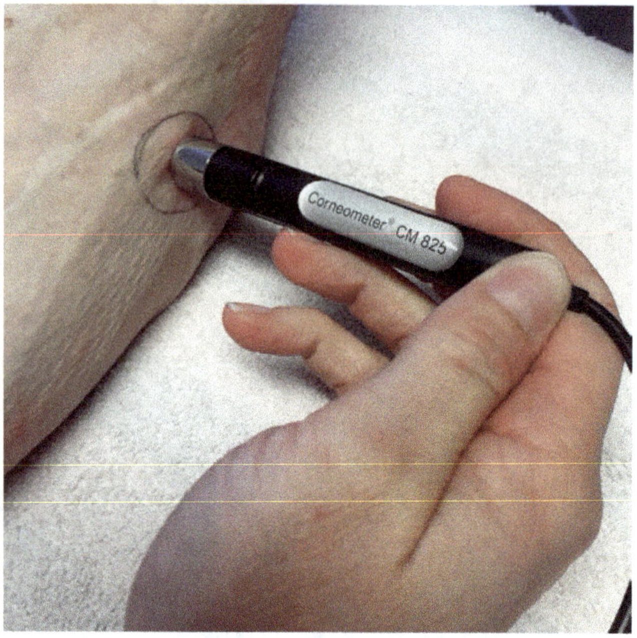

Fig. Probe of the Corneometer® CM825 device. (©Oscare)

many authors. Both probes (analog and digital) contain an interdigital grid of gold electrodes, covered by a low dielectric vitrified material (see Fig. 18.5). A resonating system in the instrument detects the frequency shift of the oscillating system related to the capacitance (and hence hydration) of the biomaterial in contact with the probe. Unlike the Skicon instruments, there is no direct galvanic contact between the electrodes of the Corneometer and the skin surface. To enable a constant pressure of the probe on the skin surface, a spring system is incorporated. According to the manufacturer, the pressure of the old analog probe is in the range of 1.1–1.8 N; the new digital probe operates at a lower pressure (about 1 N or less). The Corneometer is factory calibrated using an in vitro method. Corneometer® results obtained with different instruments in different laboratories can be pooled if a pretest validation demonstrates concordance between instrument.

Anthonissen et al. investigated the reliability of the Corneometer and concluded that the instrument can be used in clinical trials but only under very strict conditions with standardized test protocol, preferably in combination with the evaluation of other physiological parameters [18]. The results revealed excellent ICC values (ICCintra = 0.985; ICCinter = 0.984) with relatively low within-subject coefficient of variation (WSCV) (WSCVintra = 6.3%; WSCVinter = 10.6%) for, respectively, intra- and inter-observer reliability. However, the Bland–Altman plot showed that more than 5% of differences were expected to exceed 4 a.u., the limit of what has been defined as a clinically acceptable difference. Results for day-by-day variability showed good ICC value (ICCday-by-day = 0.849) and higher WSCV (WSCVday-by-day = 20.5%).

Skicon-200EX

The Skicon instruments manufactured by I.B.S. Co. are based on the conductance principle. These instruments measure the conductance (μS) of a single high-frequency current at 3.5 MHz. The measuring probe consists of 75 μm large concentric interdigital electrodes with a gap of 200 μm between the electrodes. The total probe surface is 0.8 cm^2. The probe makes use of a spring system ensuring a constant pressure force of 0.78 N when applied to the skin. The electrode makes direct galvanic contact with the skin surface. The device is calibrated in vitro using various external calibration standards in the range of 2–2000 μS conductance [19].

General Recommendations for Skin Hydration Measurements

The applied probe pressure has a large influence on hydration measurements. Despite the existence of a spring to ensure constant probe pressure, Clarys et al. have demonstrated that the measured hydration levels increase with higher probe pressures. This phenomenon is exacerbated on dryer skin (e.g., scar tissue). It is therefore advisable to use complete compression of the spring when applying the probe on the skin surface. Use a precision balance to practice obtaining more or less identical values. Finally, try to transpose this to the in vivo application of the probe on the skin surface [20].

Digital capacitance probes are very sensitive for evaluating dry/very dry skin conditions (e.g., scars), while digital conductance probes are more suited for evaluating very high levels of hydration [17].

Skin hydration has a positive correlation with ambient temperature and humidity; it is strongly affected by these two environmental parameters [7].

Results of TEWL or skin hydration measurements should be reported as differences or percent change rather than absolute values. This approach partially eliminates influencing factors.

In order to obtain reliable results for skin hydration, it is advisable to minimize, as far as possible, the influences of endogenous, exogenous, environmental, and instrument or measurement-related factors [7].

For the Corneometer®, the MCID is 7% on healthy skin and 4% on scars [18].

Dermal Water Content Measurement

Confocal Raman Spectroscopy

Raman spectroscopy is a spectroscopic technique used to observe vibrational, rotational, and other low-frequency modes in a system. Raman spectroscopy is commonly used in chemistry to provide a structural fingerprint by which molecules can be identified. Confocal Raman spectroscopy can directly measure the water content from the skin surface down to the upper epidermis with high depth resolution (5 μm) [21]. Moreover, it produces a more absolute measurement value than other methods. Using confocal Raman spectroscopy, the water content is calculated from the ratio of integrated Raman signals for water and protein. The proportionality constant is estimated from the Raman spectra of various solutions of proteins in the water. Nakagawa et al. concluded that in vivo measurement of the dermal water content with confocal Raman spectroscopy was highly reliable [22]. The benefit of using confocal Raman spectroscopy is that the depth increment between measurement points can be freely adjusted. The most widely used depth resolution of the confocal Raman spectroscopy is 5 μm. With confocal Raman spectroscopy, the smaller the region of interest, the higher the depth resolution.

Near-Infrared Spectroscopy

Near-infrared spectroscopy (NIRS) is a spectroscopic method that uses the near-infrared region of the electromagnetic spectrum (from 780 nm to 2500 nm). NIRS is based on molecular overtone and combination vibrations. One advantage is that NIRS can typically penetrate much further into a sample than mid-infrared radiation. NIRS is not a particularly sensitive technique, but it can be very useful in probing bulk material with little or no sample preparation [23].

The molecular overtone and combination bands seen in the near-IR are typically very broad, leading to complex spectra; it can be difficult to assign specific features to specific chemical components. Multivariate calibration techniques (e.g., principal components analysis, partial least squares, or artificial neural networks) are often employed to extract the desired chemical information. Careful development of a set of calibration samples and application of multivariate calibration techniques is essential for near-infrared analytical methods. NIRS can measure overall skin water content as well as of the various components constituting the skin, i.e., the stratum corneum, epidermis, and dermis. This technique has the ability to directly determine the changes in the various types of water (free, bulk, and protein-bound water), which are present in the various skin layers.

Another interesting advantage is that this technique does not require direct contact with the skin and can easily be integrated in smartphones. This technique also allows to determine the thickness of separate skin layers [24]. However, its lack of sensitivity and frequent integration of algorithms raises doubts about its reliability, which still needs to be investigated in scar tissue.

Transcutaneous Oxygen Tension

Scar maturation has been related to transcutaneous oxygen tension that can be measured with electrodes on the skin. Heat is induced to the electrode and causes oxygen and CO_2 to diffuse through the skin. In hypertrophic scar, PO_2 is lower than in healthy skin. An increase over time was correlated with clinical improvement. Upregulated levels of transcutaneous oxygen tension in treated scars correlated well with a downregulation of scar thickness assessed both clinically and by ultrasound. It is hypothesized that low levels of transcutaneous oxygen pressure ($tcpO_2$) in evolving scars result from low oxygen diffusibility through scar tissue rather than from rapid metabolic consumption of oxygen by scar tissue [25].

Tactile Sensitivity

Tactile sensitivity of the skin can be divided in two parts. Discriminative touch is a sensory modality that allows a subject to sense and localize touch. Non-discriminative touch is a sensory modality that allows the subject to sense that something has touched them, without being able to localize where they were touched. Scars are frequently accompanied with sensory deficits often remaining present months or even years after injury.

Tactile sensitivity of the skin can be measured by esthesiometers. There are different types of esthesiometers depending on their particular function. The simplest is a manual tool with adjustable points similar to a caliper. It can determine how short a distance between two impressions on the skin can be distinguished.

Another type of manual esthesiometer is used to test lower thresholds of touch or pain. The tool uses nylon monofilaments with varying calibrated diameters (see ◘ Fig. 18.6). The force needed to cause the monofilament to "buckle" determines the tactile reading (see ◘ Fig. 18.7). The filaments are calibrated by force applied, rather than by gram/mm^2 pressure ratings because sensation follows force (when the stimulated area is small).

The most commonly used is the Semmes-Weinstein Aesthesiometer and its variant the Weinstein Enhanced Sensory Test (WEST) that determines the touch perception threshold (TPT). Meirte et al. concluded that the Semmes-Weinstein monofilament test is a feasible and reliable outcome measure to evaluate TPT in burn scars, showing excellent intrarater and interrater reliability (ICC >0.90) [26].

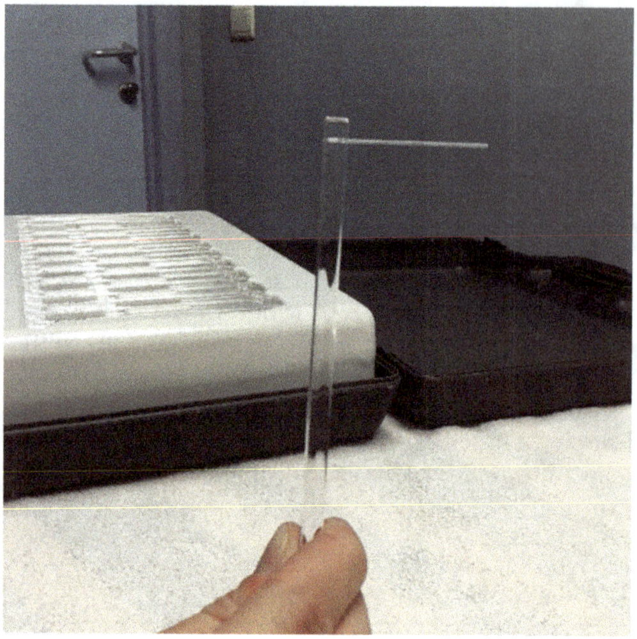

Fig. The Semmes-Weinstein Aesthesiometer® uses nylon monofilaments. (©Oscare)

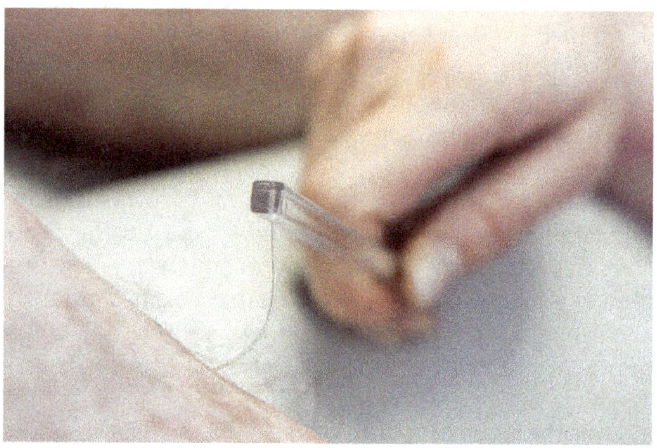

Fig. The force needed to cause the monofilament to "buckle" determines the tactile reading. (©Oscare)

Take-Home Messages

- The stratum corneum acts as an evaporation barrier to maintain body water homeostasis.
- In the epidermis, water originates from the deeper layers.
- In scars, the absorption capacity and water retention are reduced and may contribute to prolonged inflammation.
- In scars, TEWL is higher than in normal skin.
- One single method to measure skin water content is not enough to capture all the relevant information.
- The open-chamber method is the most widely used to measure TEWL.
- The dielectric capacitance method is the most reliable method to measure SC hydration level in scars.
- Confocal Raman spectroscopy is a reliable technique to measure dermal water content.
- The Semmes-Weinstein Aesthesiometer is a reliable tool to assess tactile sensitivity in scars.

Bibliography

1. Verdier-Sévrain S, Bonté F. Skin hydration: a review on its molecular mechanisms. J Cosmet Dermatol. 2007;6:75–82.
2. Warner RR, Myers MC, Taylor DA. Electron probe analysis of human skin: determination of the water concentration profile. J Invest Dermatol. 1988;90:218–24.
3. Bielfeldt S, Schoder V, Ely U, van der Pol A, de Sterke J, Wilhelm K-P. Assessment of human stratum corneum thickness and its barrier properties by *in-vivo* confocal Raman spectroscopy. Int J Cosmet Sci. 2009;31:479–80.
4. Waller JM, Maibach HI. Age and skin structure and function, a quantitative approach (II): protein, glycosaminoglycan, water, and lipid content and structure. Skin Res Technol. 2006;12:145–54.
5. Rodrigues LM, Magro JM, Contreiras Pinto P, Mouzinho M, Almeida A. Non-invasive assessment of wound-healing pathophysiology by transcutaneous indicators. Ann. Burns Fire Disasters; 2004.
6. Brusselaers N, Pirayesh A, Hoeksema H, Verbelen J, Blot S, Monstrey S. Burn scar assessment: a systematic review of objective scar assessment tools. Burns. 2010;36:1157–64.
7. du Plessis J, Stefaniak A, Eloff F, et al. International guidelines for the in vivo assessment of skin properties in non-clinical settings: Part 2. Transepidermal water loss and skin hydration. Skin Res Technol. 2013;19:265–78.
8. Imhof B. TEWL & the skin barrier. London; 2005.
9. Pinnagoda J, Tupker RA, Agner T, Serup J. Guidelines for transepidermal water loss (TEWL) measurement. A report from the Standardization Group of the European Society of Contact Dermatitis. Contact Dermatitis. 1990;22:164–78.
10. Rogiers V. EEMCO guidance for the assessment of transepidermal water loss in cosmetic sciences. Skin Pharmacol Appl Skin Physiol. 14:117–28.
11. Agache P, Humbert P. Measuring the skin: non-invasive investigations, physiology, normal constants: Springer; 2004.
12. Anthonissen M, Daly D, Fieuws S, Massagé P, Van Brussel M, Vranckx J, Van den Kerckhove E. Measurement of elasticity and transepidermal water loss rate of burn scars with the Dermalab(®). Burns. 2013;39:420–8.
13. Fell M, Meirte J, Anthonissen M, Maertens K, Pleat J, Moortgat P. The Scarbase Duo(®): intra-rater and inter-rater reliability and validity of a compact dual scar assessment tool. Burns. 2016;42:336–44.
14. De Paepe K, Houben E, Adam R, Wiesemann F, Rogiers V. Validation of the VapoMeter, a closed unventilated chamber system to assess transepidermal water loss vs. the open chamber Tewameter. Skin Res Technol. 2005;11:61–9.
15. Nuutinen J, Alanen E, Autio P, Lahtinen M-R, Harvima I, Lahtinen T. A closed unventilated chamber for the measurement of transepidermal water loss. Skin Res Technol. 2003;9:85–9.

16. Zhai H, Maibach HI. Occlusion vs. skin barrier function. Skin Res Technol. 2002;8:1–6.
17. Clarys P, Clijsen R, Taeymans J, Barel AO. Hydration measurements of the stratum corneum: comparison between the capacitance method (digital version of the Corneometer CM 825®) and the impedance method (Skicon-200EX®). Skin Res Technol. 2012;18:316–23.
18. Anthonissen M, Daly D, Peeters R, Van Brussel M, Fieuws S, Moortgat P, Flour M, Van den Kerckhove E. Reliability of repeated measurements on post-burn scars with Corneometer CM 825. Skin Res Technol. 2015; https://doi.org/10.1111/srt.12193.
19. O'goshi K, Serup J. Skin conductance; validation of Skicon-200EX compared to the original model, Skicon-100. Skin Res Technol. 2007;13:13–8.
20. Clarys P, Clijsen R, Barel AO. Influence of probe application pressure on in vitro and in vivo capacitance (Corneometer CM 825(®)) and conductance (Skicon 200 EX(®)) measurements. Skin Res Technol. 2011;17:445–50.
21. Caspers PJ, Lucassen GW, Puppels GJ. Combined in vivo confocal Raman spectroscopy and confocal microscopy of human skin. Biophys J. 2003;85:572–80.
22. Nakagawa N, Matsumoto M, Sakai S. In vivo measurement of the water content in the dermis by confocal Raman spectroscopy. Skin Res Technol. 2010;16:137–41.
23. Fresta Rosario Pignatello M, Puglisi G. Near-infrared spectroscopy: a new advance in direct measurement of moisture in skin; 1995.
24. Miyamae Y, Kawabata M, Yamakawa Y, Tsuchiya J, Ozaki Y. Non-invasive estimation of skin thickness by near infrared diffuse reflection spectroscopy—separate determination of epidermis and dermis thickness. J Near Infrared Spectrosc. 2012;20:617–22.
25. Berry RB, Tan T, Cooke ED, Gaylarde PM, Bowcock S, Lamberty BG, Hackett ME. Transcutaneous oxygen tension as an index of maturity in hyper-trophic scars treated by compression. Br J Plast Surg. 1985;38(2):163–73.
26. Meirte J, Moortgat P, Truijen S, Maertens K, Lafaire C, De Cuyper L, Hubens G, Van Daele U. Interrater and intrarater reliability of the Semmes Weinstein aesthesiometer to assess touch pressure threshold in burn scars. Burns. 2015; https://doi.org/10.1016/j.burns.2015.01.003.

26

Silicone Gel for Scar Prevention

Thomas A. Mustoe

Contents

History

Silicone gel was first discovered to be useful in the treatment of scars by Perkins in Australia and New Zealand when observations were made empirically that scars improved when silicone was used as part of a dressing. The observations although anecdotal were impressive enough that use spread to the UK, and at the University of Strathclyde in Glasgow, Scotland, a biomedical engineering student, Karen Quinn, undertook a series of studies for her PhD thesis to determine the mechanism of action and published a paper in burns [1]. She determined that neither heat nor pressure nor silicone absorption or chemical effects were responsible for its effects in studies done together with surgeon from the Plastic Surgery Unit at Canniesburn (Professor Reid). By chance, I was visiting the Canniesburn Hospital for 2 weeks and had the opportunity to observe the use of silicone gel, which was made by Dow Corning. They were already sponsoring some of my studies at Washington University School of Medicine, and I suggested a controlled clinical study which had not yet been done. The effects on immature hypertrophic scars were in some cases dramatic with each patient serving as their own control. We subsequently did a follow-up study on using silicone on very early scars to prevent hypertrophy with equally encouraging results. Although there was some skepticism, in part due to a lack of a clear mechanism of action, subsequent studies by several other investigators confirmed the efficacy. I will detail some of these studies later in this chapter.

The Role of the Epithelium in Scar Formation

Hypertrophic scars are due to an excess of collagen deposition which is almost entirely from fibroblasts. The role of excess inflammation, myofibroblasts, and other fibroblasts phenotypically that produce excess collagen, tension, and genetic factors all play a role in hypertrophic scar formation. Given that silicone is not absorbed into the skin and covers intact epithelium, the beneficial effects must be indirect through effects on the epithelium.

The epithelium serves an important barrier function. Water loss through the epithelium is limited by a functional stratum corneum, and disturbances in barrier function are associated in many dermatologic conditions with increased inflammation instigated by inflammatory growth factors and other inflammatory mediators produced by epidermal cells. Epithelial mesenchymal cell cross talk is well known.

Delay in Epithelization

When barrier function is disrupted by tissue injury, restoration of the stratum corneum lags behind epithelization which is initially only one cell layer thick as epithelium rapidly migrates over an open wound, followed by stratification, followed eventually by a multilayered stratum corneum. However, there is evidence that the immature stratum corneum does not become fully functional as a water barrier for weeks to months. During that time, there is a stimulus to restore homeostatic barrier function by increased epithelial proliferation, as manifested by increases in thickness, alterations in differentiation markers in the immature differentiating epithelium, and increased inflammatory mediator synthesis [2].

In cell culture, prevention of water loss by a liquid or high-humidity environment results in a reduction in soluble inflammatory mediators and consequently a reduction in collagen synthesis in a coculture setup with fibroblasts [3, 4]. In vivo, in models in rabbits, rats, and mice, prevention of water loss from an epithelium with an immature, deficient stratum corneum results in increase in inflammatory mediators similar to those utilizing human cells in an in vitro system [5]. There are multiple highly upregulated factors including IL-1, IL-8, and Cox-2. In total, over 1000 genes are either upregulated or downregulated in an environment where transepidermal water loss (TEWL) is limited by a semiocclusive dressing versus no covering [6].

Humans are almost unique in their tendency to heal with excessive or hypertrophic scarring. In part this is due to the "tight-skinned" characteristic of the human skin which is tightly adherent to the underlying muscle layer due to the lack of a panniculus carnosus. Thus, human wounds heal only part by wound contracture, with both a delay in epithelization and also tension forces due to the constraints on skin contraction by adherence to the underlying deeper tissues. The rabbit ear [7] mimics human skin in being firmly adherent to the underlying cartilage which splints the wound and minimizes contracture. Healing is almost entirely due to epithelization, and with wounds larger than 6 mm in diameter, healing is delayed beyond 2 weeks which in humans is the critical delay in healing sufficient to increase the risk of hypertrophic scars. In addition, during the healing process, the fibroblasts in the granulation tissue are under tension because the contractile forces generated by the myofibroblasts are counteracted by the resistance to contraction by the stiff underlying cartilage. Wounds on the rabbit ear heal with scar elevation (◼ Fig. 23.1) which both from gross visual appearance, and also histologically closely mimic human hypertrophic scars. Larger wounds with epithelization delayed beyond 2 weeks have

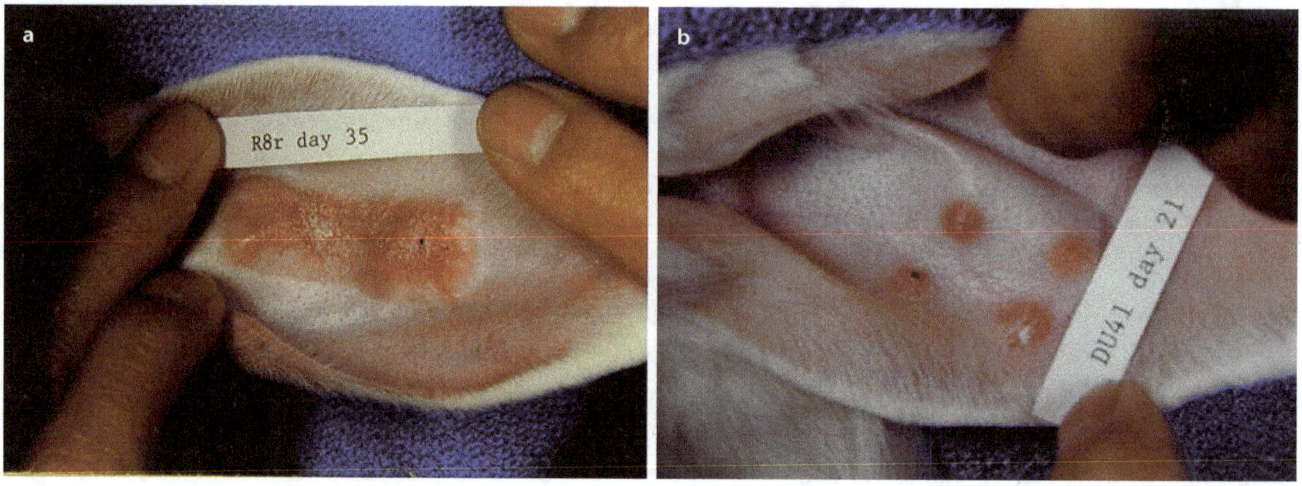

Fig. **a** A large scar in the rabbit ear created by full- thickness removal of the skin followed by healing without dressings. **b** By creating small 6–8 mm in diameter full-thickness wounds with a circular punch, healing is complete in about 2 weeks and the scar is elevated allowing quantification. This rabbit ear model has been used for all of our experimental studies

greater scar elevation, and like humans, older rabbits heal with flatter scars. The scars respond to interventions like local steroid and injections and blockers of fibrosis including TGFB antibodies and antisense to CTGF, in which both growth factors induce collagen synthesis and are upregulated in fibrotic processes. Silicone gel sheets and silicone cream both reduce scarring, and other semi-occlusive agents such as paper tape, polyurethane films, cyanoacrylates, or stoma adhesive are also effective which implicates occlusion as the working mechanism of silicone gel, when combined with negative data ruling out absorption (chemical process) or heat or pressure.

We have used this model to investigate the working mechanism of silicone gel or other occlusive dressings in a series of experiments. In our model, silicone gel resulted in decreased inflammatory cytokines including IL-1, TNF, IL-8, and Cox-2 among others. The net effect of increased hydration is a decrease in osmolarity and several extracellular fluid ions including calcium, sodium, and chloride. By controlling otherwise for potential ions and osmolarity, we found that Na concentration was the critical factor controlling signaling for the inflammatory cytokines affected by hydration. We also found that changes in extracellular Na concentration resulted in changes in transmembrane Na flux which is mediated chiefly by the Na channel ENaC. Briefly, an increase in Na concentration due to increased TEWL caused by a deficient epithelial barrier results in activation of ENaC which controls levels of COX-2 resulting in increased prostaglandins [3].

The question remained of how increases in Na concentration are sensed resulting in activation of ENaC. We looked for changes in all of the candidate Na channels in epitheilia cells that could conceivably respond to changes in Na concentration and found only one channel, Nax, had a significant response. Nax is a member of the voltage-gated Na channels but lacks the extracellular domain responsive for voltage gating. It's function previously has been unclear. NaX has been found to be Na concentration sensor in the central nervous system, but its function and presence in other organs and cell types had not been extensively studied. With a series of knockdown experiments in vitro, we established that NaX controls the entire signal transduction signaling seen with changes in Na concentration and hydration in vitro in epithelial cells and also skin explants. Utilizing our model of hypertrophic scarring in the rabbit ear, we found treatment with antisense to NaX results in a very significant reduction in scarring, similar or greater to the effects of silicone gel. Furthermore blocking downstream signals including Cox-2, IL-B, and the S-100 proteins also reduced scarring. Blocking ENaC with a clinically used pharmacologic agent, amiloride, also resulted in decreased scarring. Experiments to elucidate the signal transduction pathways further have established that NaX responds or senses high salt with activation of a serine protease, prostasin, which activates ENaC. The importance of NaX in controlling changes in the epithelium includes profound changes in epithelial differentiation, cell migration, and cell proliferation in knockdown experiments in vitro [4].

In summary the application of silicone gel to an acute scar with a deficient epithelial water barrier due to an immature stratum corneum results in decreased water loss (TEWL). This prevents the increase in Na concentration which otherwise results in an NaX-mediated complex signal transduction pathway which includes downstream activation of ENaC as well as hundreds of other genes, mirroring the kind of broad changes in gene expression found to be controlled by many cytokines such as TGFB. Other occlusive treatments are also effective, but the degree of occlusion is important (complete occlusion results in excessive hydration with impacts on surface bacterial levels as well as undesirable physical changes in the epithelium).

Clinical Studies

The first controlled clinical study to demonstrate efficacy of silicone gel utilized silicone gel sheets applied to portions of immature hypertrophic scars due to burns, trauma, or surgery, in an effort to treat immature hypertrophic scars (◘ Fig. 23.2). Treatment went on for 3 months with application of the gel for 12 hours. We found that 24-hour treatment led to maceration and was poorly tolerated. One of the challenges was to quantify the improvement in scarring. Although photographic evidence is essential, rating scar severity remains challenging and is ultimately nonquantitative. In an effort to have a completely objective and quantitative method of measuring scar severity, we turned to measuring the scar stiffness. Scars are stiffer (less elastic) than normal skin, and as scars improve they become more pliable or more elastic. Utilizing an extensometer which measures the amount of stretch when the skin is subjected to a given force, we were able to calculate Young's modulus and get an objective measure of scar stiffness. We first used an extensometer to measure the stiffness of burn scars and found that older scars were more elastic and there was a very good correlation with age of burn scar to stiffness of the scar over several years [8]. In our scar study, we found a highly statistically significant reduction in stiffness that reached closed to its maximum after 2 months of treatment, with only minor changes by extending treatment for 3 months [9]. Furthermore, the improvement was sustained after treatment was terminated. At the same time, there were a substantial reduction in scar erythema and flattening of the scar clinically which was obvious on photographs. We saw no response in a keloid and much more impressive results in immature scars, with minor effects or no effect on mature scars (scars older than 1 year without erythema).

In a follow-up study (◘ Fig. 23.3), we wanted to see if we could prevent the development of hypertrophic scars by beginning treatment early on surgical incisional scars. Again, a portion of the incision was treated with an adjacent area untreated [10]. We again utilized photography but wanted to quantify the scar volumes for an objective quantitative measure. Dental alginate was used to make a negative impression which was then converted to a positive impression using dental plaster in similar fashion to the way dentists take dental impressions for models used in a variety of dental and oral surgical procedures. The positive molds there then burred down to a totally flat surface and volumes calculated by measuring the difference in weights. Treated areas of the scars were found to have significantly less volumes as long as the untreated scar developed some hypertrophy. Not surprisingly, in scars that healed favorably, minimal or no differences were seen.

Initially, although these studies received considerable attention, even in the popular press, there was some skepticism by many clinicians, due in part to the lack of mechanism. Over the subsequent years, many studies have confirmed the observations we made relying on subjective evaluation of scar severity using a variety of scar severity scales such as the Vancouver Scar Scale and Patient and Observer Scar Assessment Scale (POSAS). In 2002, an international group developed an evidence-based analysis to develop guidelines for treatment [11] and found that there was strong evidence for the use of

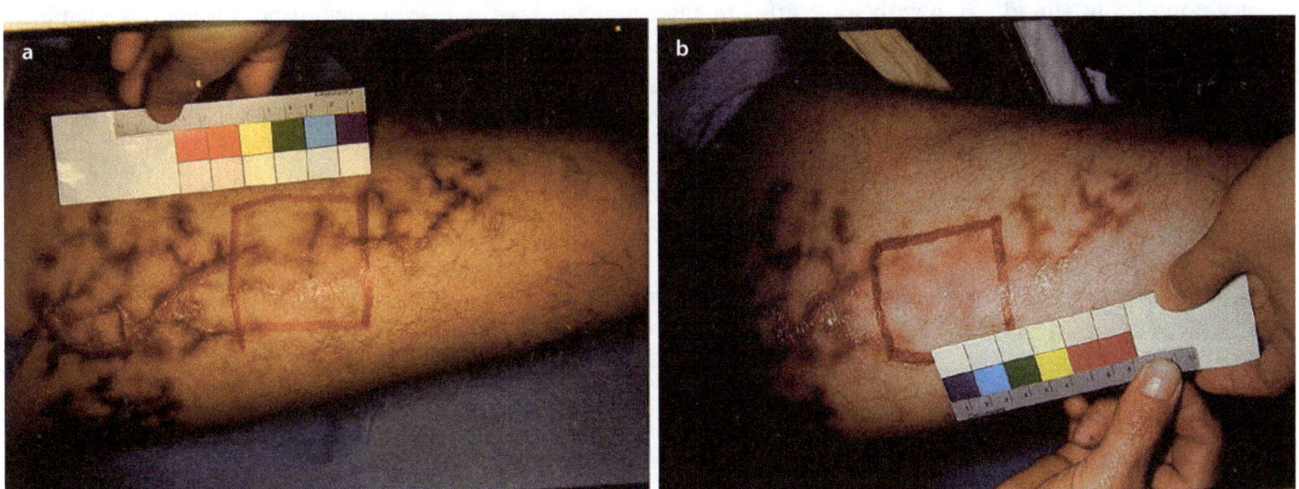

◘ **Fig. a** Partial-thickness immature hypertrophic burn scar. The square marks the planned treatment area with silicone gel. **b** After 2 months of treatment, the treated area is flatter, more pliable, and less pink

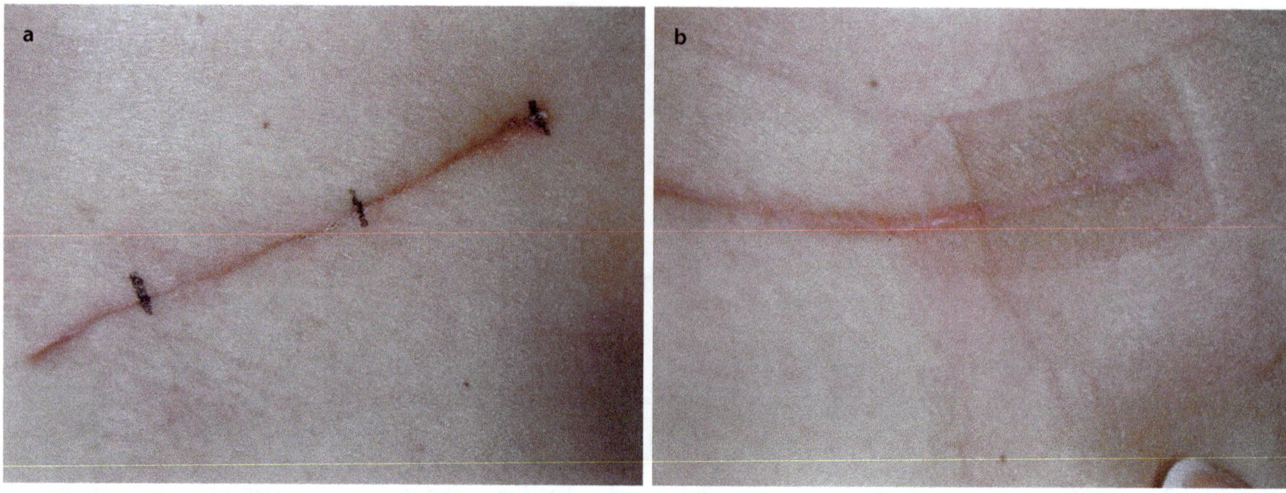

Fig. **a** A fresh surgical incision prior to treatment. One area of the scar is going to be treated preventively with the other portion of the scar serving as comparison. **b** After 2 months, the untreated scar is slightly elevated and pink in color. The area of the scar treated with silicone gel sheeting is flatter and less pink in color

silicone gel both for the treatment and prevention of hypertrophic scars.

Since 2002, many more studies have been published on silicone gel with supportive data. Most of these studies were not prospective randomized trials and by the nature of the treatment virtually impossible to blind. The Cochrane group did an analysis and noted the deficiencies of the studies and made the conclusion that solid evidence for silicone gel was lacking but failed to recognize the strengths of our early studies in which the patients served as their own control and quantitative objective data was collected.

Sheets Versus Creams

There are some limitations to silicone gel sheets. They are not completely self-adhering with some attachment method such as a covering bandage, although clothing can be used in some situations (such as a bra) to aid in fixation. In tropical climates with high humidity, the scar can develop a "heat" rash due to excessive moisture underneath the gel. The gel sheeting can pick up dirt and perspiration which makes cleaning or using new sheets essential. As a practical matter, patients have difficulty wearing the sheets 24 hours/day. Our original studies suggested that using the sheets to cover the scars needed to be utilized at least 12 hours/day to be effective.

Silicone gel creams have been alternative products that address many of the limitations of silicone gel sheeting. They can be used in tropical climates more easily, do not require any additional adherence methodology, and are easier to apply 24 hours/day with twice-daily applications. The question arises whether they are as effective. One potential limitation is the chance that the cream will be rubbed off. Some silicone creams dry in place and are less likely to rub off.

We have addressed the question of efficacy of silicone gel creams in our rabbit ear animal model of hypertrophic scarring and have found the cream to be as effective as sheeting in multiple studies. All of our studies investigating the mechanism of silicone gel that we referred to earlier utilized silicone gel cream because of its ease of use.

Multiple well-done clinical studies have been done over the last 15 years that have confirmed efficacy of silicone gel. In Asian patients who are particularly high risk for hypertrophic scars, Chan [12] performed a randomized, double-blind controlled study in 50 Asian patients with a sternotomy wound following coronary bypass surgery or cardiac valvular surgery. They found that silicone gel significantly reduced multiple scar attributes including visual parameter pigmentation, vascularity, pliability, height, as well as symptoms of pain and itchiness compared with control wounds ($p \leq 0.02$ for all). No treatment-related adverse effects were reported. To date, no comparison studies have directly compared the efficacy of sheeting to silicone gel cream. Due to the very thin film formed by silicone gel cream and the uncertainty of how effectively it remains in place when subjected to rubbing by clothing or movement, it is quite possible or even likely that sheeting might be more effective, but in practice this may be offset by the ease in 24 hours/day use.

Recently a meta-analysis of all prospective randomized controlled trials as well as additional controlled studies between 1990 and 2014 found a total of 11 studies that qualified involving 864 patient scars in which the silicone gel was used to prevent scars. They found a highly positive result from silicone gel or silicone gel sheeting particularly in patients at high risk, but even when all patient were included, the results were statistically significant ($p < 0.02$) [13].

In summary, silicone gel sheeting has an almost 40-year history, with widespread clinical use for 20 years. Our laboratory and others have found a compelling mechanism based on the semiocclusive properties of silicone gel, which normalize transepidermal water loss in scars with a deficient stratum corneum barrier function, and via the Na channels ENaC and Nax regulated.

Bibliography

1. Quinn KJ, Evans JH, Courtney JM, Gaylor JD, Reid WH. Nonpressure treatment of hypertrophic scars. Burns Incl Therm Inj. 1985;12:102–8.
2. O' Shaughnessey K, Roy N, Mustoe TA. Homeostasis of the epidermal barrier layer: a theory of how occlusion decreases hypertrophic scarring. Wound Repair Regen. 2009;17:700–8.
3. Xu W, Hong SJ, Zeitchek M, Cooper G, Jia S, Ping X, Quresh HA, Zhong A, Porterfield MD, Galiano RD, Surmeier DJ, Mustoe TA. Hydration status regulates sodium flux and inflammatory pathways through epithelial sodium channel (ENaC) in skin. J Invest Dermatol. 2015;135(3):796–806.
4. Xu W, Hong SJ, Zhong A, Xie P, Jia S, Xie Z, Zeitchek M, Niknam-Bienia S, Zhao J, Porterfield DM, Surmeier DJ, Leung KP, Galiano RD, Mustoe TA. Sodium channel Na_x is a regulator in epithelial sodium homeostasis. Sci Transl Med. 2015;7(312):312ra177.
5. Gallant-Behm CL, Du P, Lin S, Marucha PT, DiPietro LA, Mustoe TA. Epithelial regulation of mesenchymal tissue behavior. J Investigative Dermatology. 2011;131:892–9. Pubmed ID 21228814.
6. Xu W, Jia S, Xie P, Zhong A, Galiano RD, Mustoe TA, Hong SJ. The expression of Proinflammatory genes in epidermal keratinocytes is regulated by hydration status. J Invest Dermatol. 2013;134:1044–55.
7. Morris DD, Zhao LL, Bolton L, Roth SI, Ladin DA, Mustoe TA. Acute and chronic models for excessive dermal scarring: quantitative studies. Plast Reconstr Surg. 1997;100:674–81.
8. Bartell TH, Monafo WW, Mustoe TA. Noninvasive in vivo quantification of elastic properties of hypertrophic scar: hand held elastometry. J Burn Care Rehabil. 1988;9:657–60.
9. Ahn ST, Monafo W, Mustoe TA. Topical silicone gel: a new treatment for hypertrophic scars. Surgery. 1989;106:781–7.
10. Ahn ST, Monafo WW, Mustoe TA. Topical silicone gel for the prevention and treatment of hypertrophic scar. Arch Surg. 1991;126:499–504.
11. Mustoe TA, Cooter R, Gold M, Hobbs R, Ramelet AA, Shakespeare P, Stella M, Teot L, Wood F, Ziegler U. International clinical guidelines for scar management. Plastic and Reconstr Surg. 2002;110:560–72.
12. Chan KY, Lau CL, Adeeb SM, Somasundaram S, Nasir-Zahari M. A randomized, placebo-controlled, double-blind, prospective clinical trial of silicone gel in prevention of hypertrophic scar development in median sternotomy wound. Plast Reconstr Surg. 2005;116(4):1013–20.
13. Hsu K-C, Luan C-W, Tsai Y-W. Review of silicone gel sheeting and silicone gel for the prevention of hypertrophic scars and keloids wounds. 2017;29:154–8.

27

Minimally Invasive Technologies for Treatment of HTS and Keloids: Low-Dose 5-Fluorouracil

Wei Liu, Xiaoli Wu, Zheng Gao, and Lingling Xia

Contents

Introduction

Hypertrophic Scar and Keloid Information

Keloid is the most difficult pathological scar to treat and cure and it is characterized with uncontrolled growth, invasion into normal skin, and expansion beyond the original wound boundary with severe pain and itching [1]. In addition, high recurrence rate after various therapies is a common feature of keloids. These characters similar to those of tumors render keloids more like a "benign skin tumor" rather than a fibrotic tissue per se. Because of this, anticancer therapies such as chemotherapy and radiotherapy have been applied to keloid treatment.

HTS is another type of pathological scar, characterized with the deposition of excessive amounts of collagen matrix along with significant angiogenic process, which eventually leads to a raised and red scar with severe tissue contracture and painful and itching symptoms. HTS eventually resolves by itself after tissue maturation. Nevertheless, this process can take 1–2 years or even longer with disturbing symptoms and functional disability, which needs to be intervened for improving symptoms and preventing patients from disability. With this perspective, anticancer therapy approaches such as chemotherapy and radiotherapy might be also applied [2, 3].

Chemotherapy for Keloids and Hypertrophic Scar

Intralesional injection is a routine procedure for keloid treatment, and steroid injection alone could lead to recurrence rate higher than 50% [2], indicating the necessity of involving others drugs as a combined drug treatment. Chemotherapy for keloid was tried as early as 1989 [1]. The common drugs for keloid chemotherapy include 5-FU, Bleomycin, and Mitomycin C, etc. [2, 3]. The usual delivery way is intralesional injection of chemotherapy drug alone or combined injection of both chemo-agents and steroids.

In recent years, chemotherapy on HTS has been tried either as intralesional injection or combined with post-laser therapy with positive results [3]. Because of its self-resolving nature, chemotherapy for HTS remains an exploratory area for its balanced value between the efficacy and the side effect. Therefore, most studies of pathological scar chemotherapy focus on keloids and it will be the focus of this chapter as well.

5-FU and Its Combined Use of Steroids

Among the various chemotherapy agents, 5-FU, a pyrimidine analog with antimetabolite activity, might be the most commonly used drug for keloid chemotherapy. Dr. Fitzpatrick R.E. started intralesional injection of 5-FU for both keloid and HTS since 1989 using the concentration of 50 mg/ml with positive results [1]. Later, Gupta and Kalra [4] and Nanda and Reddy [5] also reported their 5-FU applications in keloid treatment with a dose of 50 mg/ml, and the intralesional injection was administered weekly, lasting for 12–16 weeks with positive results. With this dose, pain is the most common side effect and ulceration could occur as high as 21.4% [5].

5-FU intralesional injection was listed as an emerging therapy for keloid and HTS in "International clinical recommendation on scar management" [2], but was listed as a formal therapeutic option for HTS and keloid with monthly injection interval in "Updated international clinical recommendations on scar management: Part 2 – algorithms for scar prevention and treatment" [3]. In addition, a combined use of 5-FU with steroids not only enhanced the therapeutic efficacy, but also reduced pain suffering post-injection [1]. In the literature, high-dose (40–50 mg/ml) 5-FU injection is usually combined with steroid at a volume ratio varying from 9:1 [1] to 7.5:2.5 [6].

According to published literatures [1–6], 5-FU is a safe drug with no obvious side effect for the use in a relatively short time period (such as 2–6 months). However, whether it can be safely used for a long term at the reported dose (40–50 mg/ml) remains unclear because the accumulated effect of chemotherapy agents would be a concern if they are continuously used for a long time.

The Rational of Using Low-Dose 5-FU Injection for Keloid Treatment

To address the potential concern of 5-FU's side effects, our group proposed the application of low dose 5-FU for keloid treatment because of the following reasons:

1. Keloid necrosis caused by high dose 5-FU injection should be avoided simply because any new wound will accelerate keloid development and worsen the clinical situation. Inactivating keloid cells and remodeling keloid tissue rather than destroying keloid tissue are the correct strategy for keloid therapy with intralesional injection.

2. A sustainable and long-term therapy (2–3 years) is usually required for keloid treatment in order to completely cure keloids and prevent their recurrence. To do so, a low dose of chemotherapy agent is necessary not only for safety concern, but also for proper working mechanism of tissue remodeling.
3. Low-dose 5-FU will be sensitive enough for inducing endothelial cell apoptosis/death and destroying neovascular structure during keloid development, and will also be enough to inhibit fibroblast activities such as proliferation, invasion, and matrix production.
4. This therapeutic model provides good basis for other conjunctive therapies including surgery, laser, and steroid injection to remove or to flatten keloid tissue by partial keloid destruction or tissue remodeling. It also avoids host production of risk factors that will trigger keloid development and recurrence, in which growth factors and neovascularization play significant roles.

Background

After careful literature review and exploratory testing, concentrations ranging from 1.5 to 5 mg/ml were decided as the low dose of 5-FU for clinical use with at least monthly injection interval in order to avoid any significant systemic side effect and local side effect such as adverse effect on hemopoietic system and severe pain and tissue ulceration. According to our clinical experience in treating more than 10,000 cases during the past 18 years of clinical practice, this method has been proved safe for patients with a therapeutic time period ranging from 2 to 5 years or even longer, and no severe side effect has ever been observed thus far. In addition, this dose also has the effective rate of more than 97.14% in term of relieving pain and itching symptom, softening and flattening keloid scar, and the recurrence rate is significantly decreased after long term therapy [7]. However, drug resistance to 5-FU was observed in some patients, and for these patients a bit higher doses could also be applied but were always limited to less than 9 mg/ml concentration to avoid significant side effects.

Importantly, low-dose 5-FU injection aims to disrupt or destroy neovascularity of keloid tissue and inhibit fibroblast proliferation, rather than to destroy keloid tissue; thus low-dose 5-FU will not be able to majorly flatten or soften keloid tissues, in which abundant collagen and other matrices need to be degraded with steroid's effect. Therefore, combined injection with steroid is needed in order to flatten and soften keloid tissue. Nevertheless, injected low-dose 5-FU is able to timely demolish neovascularity induced by steroid injection, and thus render treated keloids to become relatively malnourished post-drug injection and thus less possible to reoccur.

Meanwhile, reduced vascularity also allows the longer stay of the injected drug inside keloids due to the reduced drug absorption via tissue capillaries, and thus enhance the drug efficacy and reduce the side effects. The case 1 demonstrates how this strategy could be applied to treat keloid tissue with intralesional injection of combined 5-FU and steroid at a low dose in order to gradually remodel the keloid into normal-looking skin [8].

Clinical Protocol of Low-Dose 5-FU Injection Therapy

The protocol for intralesional injection of low-dose drugs includes the injection of 5-FU alone or 5-FU combined with steroid. In general, the combined injection of 5-FU and triamcinolone acetonide will be a preferred method, unless the keloid scar is heavily vascularized, which will need 5-FU injection first to demolish tissue vascularity before steroid injection. The key points of this protocol include the following:

1. *Drug preparation*: Triamcinolone acetonide should be mixed with 2% lidocaine, and then 5-FU stock solution can be further mixed with them to maintain the concentrations of 5-FU between 1.5 and 5 mg/ml and steroid between 3 and 9 mg/ml. Low concentrations of both drugs will enable better control of the side effects such as severe pain, tissue ulceration, and atrophy as well as the drug-induced angiogenesis. Also, the volume ratio between the drug and lidocaine should be 3–5:1 in order to reduce the pain suffering during and after the drug injection. As a routine, the concentrations should always start from relatively high (5-FU: 3–4 mg/ml; triamcinolone acetonide at 8–9 mg/ml) and gradually reduced as below described.
2. *Injection procedure:* To avoid pain, 1 ml syringe with 26–27G needles is generally recommended for the injection and multi-entrance manner should be applied. Briefly, each injection should deliver about 0.2 ml volume and then change the injection sites to make sure for even distribution of the drugs. When performing, the keloid tissue should be held between two fingers with pressure in order to prevent drug from oozing into surrounding normal skin. In addition, before injection, blood withdrawal should be tested to avoid direct drug injection into a blood vessel. When injecting, the drug should be pushed hard into the tissue in order to create a pressure in the tissue between the fingers and whiten the injected tissue, this manner will make sure that the injected drugs will deeply infiltrate inside the keloids, but not to noninjected region, and thus to enhance the efficacy and reduce the side effect.

3. *Adjustment of drug concentrations and injectional interval*: Here, an important concept is that this procedure does not try to destroy keloid, but rather to remodel the keloid tissue gradually via inactivating keloid fibroblast and degrading keloid matrices. Therefore, the drug concentration should be adjusted according to the status of treated keloids. The followings are the general principles:
   A. Steroid concentration should be gradually reduced when keloids become softened and flattened as overdoses of steroid will cause tissue atrophy. In addition, sudden withdraw of steroid is well known for causing reoccurrence of other steroid-treated diseases, such as autoimmune disease, and thus the principle of gradual steroid withdrawal should also be applied to keloid treatment.
   B. 5-FU concentration should be reduced when tissue angiogenesis is significantly inhibited or keloid is significantly inactivated with improved symptoms. Vice versa, a higher concentration of 5-FU should be used when significantly enhanced angiogenesis is observed or keloid remains highly activated and less responsive to the drug treatment.
   C. Adjustment of drug injection interval: With the progress of drug treatment, injection interval should also be gradually prolonged as a way of gradual withdrawal of steroid and 5-FU, and thus to better prevent keloid recurrence. In general, initial drug injection will be administered every 4 weeks for a few months. Afterwards, the injection can be adjusted for every 6 weeks to 10 weeks for several months, and finally adjusted to every 12 weeks with further reduced drug concentrations for several repeats. According to our experiences, most keloid will be resolved eventually without a high recurrence rate.
   D. Long-term therapy for localized nodule: As shown in case 1, localized nodule is often observed as the last part of noncured keloid or as the first sign of reoccurred keloid, which needs to be continuously injected with an interval of every 6 to 12 weeks until a final resolution (also see case 3).

Low-Dose 5-FU-Based Injection Therapy for HTS and Keloids

The best candidate for low dose 5-FU injection is the keloid type that usually exhibits relatively soft and flatten but red color with significant signs of inflammation such as severe pain, itching, erythema, and rapid invasion into normal skin (◘ Fig. 30.1a). Keloid types that are more like tumors, such as cauliflower-shaped solid tissue with relative dark color, fit better for surgical therapy (◘ Fig. 30.1b), but 5-FU-based injection can be well employed as well for preventing keloid relapse after surgical removal.

In general, single or multiple keloids with small sizes (diameter less than 2 cm) and located at various parts of the body are the best candidates for drug injection treatment.

Large-sized keloids will not be ideal candidates for drug treatment by intralesional injection because of potential side effects of both 5-FU and steroids.

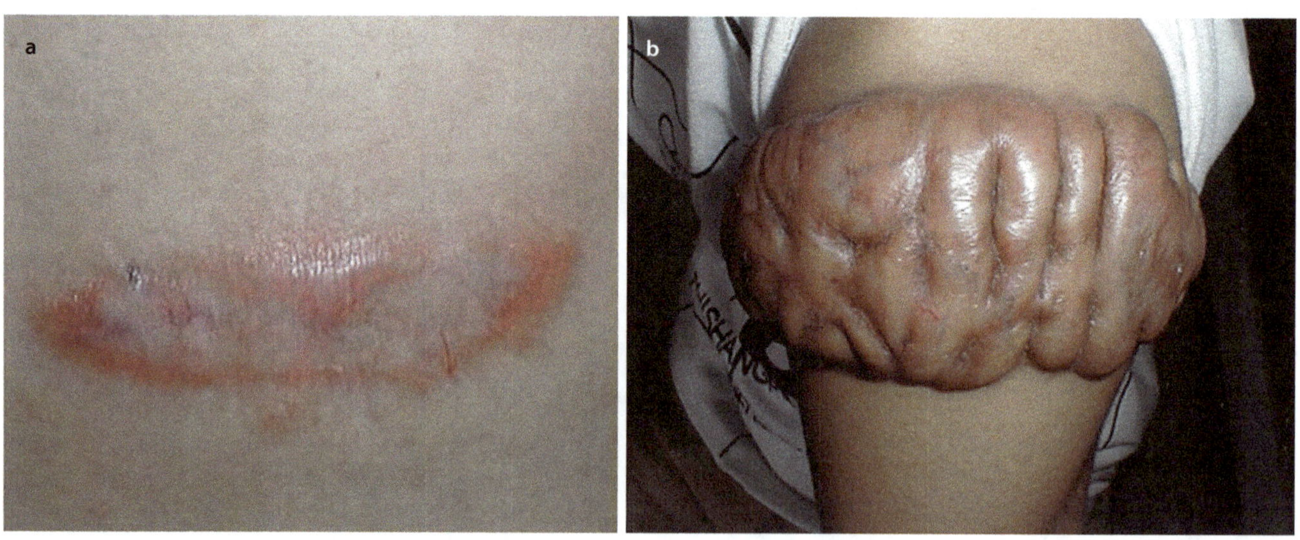

◘ **Fig.** Keloids are generally divided into two types: **a** inflammatory type; **b** tumor-like type

Important Concepts of Keloid Curing and Relapse Rate for Low-Dose 5-FU-Based Therapy

Insufficient treatment might be the most important reason for not being able to cure a keloid and preventing its reoccurrence

A softened and flattened keloid along with disappearance of the symptom does not necessarily indicate that a keloid is cured and the treatment is completed. Rather, the keloid is in a temporary inactivated stage under the drug pressure. Like cancer therapy, drug treatment can remove most of disease cells but there will always be a portion of cells (residue cells) that survive after chemotherapy and become quiescent and drug resistant [9, 10]. Once the drug pressure is relieved, these cells become reactivated and enter an active stage with rapid proliferation and production of matrices, growth factors, and angiogenic factors, and eventually lead to a reoccurred keloid.

To prevent this from happening, a continuous drug pressure should be applied to any of these residue cells to inactivate or remove them once they become activated. In the literature, most studies report the successful treatment of keloid with the criteria of flattening and softening of the treated keloid along with disappeared symptoms of pain, itching, and erythema as judged by Vancouver Score or Patient and Observer Scar Assessment Scale (POSAS). But the cessation of drug injection improperly will likely lead to keloid to reoccur simply because these treatments did not really remove or remodel the residual quiescent keloid cells into normal skin cell phenotype. This might be the key reason why high recurrence rate remains after keloid injection therapy, to which less attention has been paid in the literature.

In our group, it has been observed that 2–3 years are usually required for completely curing keloids by 5-FU and steroid injection in most cases. More importantly, preventive drug injection at a later stage aiming to prevent reoccurrence is essential and is performed by gradual drug withdrawal via reduced doses and prolonged injection intervals. As shown in case 3, there was a large-sized keloid in a woman's abdominal region, and a total of 6.5 years were spent to completely cure the keloid via combined injection of both 5-FU and steroids at a low concentration. During this process, the first 3 years were spent on treatment of the keloid, whereas the last 3 years were spent on preventive therapy to timely treat the reoccurred keloid nodules.

5-FU-Based Injection Therapy for Recurrence Prevention of Surgically Removed Keloids

Although low-dose 5-FU injection has been proven effective for primary keloid treatment and reoccurrence control, the efficiency would be too low to be an ideal method. As described earlier, the conversion of a keloid tissue into a normal-like skin will be a long-term process. On the contrast, preventing the conversion of normal wound cells into keloid cells would be much easier, in which 5-FU could play an important role.

Surgical excision has now become the first-line keloid treatment in our group because it is an efficient way of keloid treatment. In particular, keloids with a size larger than 2 cm in diameter and possible for primary closure after surgery are the best indication for surgical therapy. Most importantly, the use of low-dose 5-FU injection along with other procedures enables us to prevent the development of new keloids in a surgically created wound. Therefore, the "treatment model" of injection therapy will be shifted to the "prevention model" of surgical treatment, and 1-year time period will be usually long enough to achieve satisfactory results in most keloid patients as shown in cases 4 and 5.

There are three key issues that are essential for the success in this surgical procedure, including (1) anti-tension procedures by proper multilayer suturing and anti-tension device application; (2) wound irrigation with combined 5-FU and steroids during the surgical procedure; (3) post-surgery radiotherapy and combined 5-FU injection. The procedures are described in the following sections.

Surgical Procedure for Keloid Excision

Briefly, after local anesthesia with 2% lidocaine injection, the keloid will be surgically excised followed by multilayer suturing (including fascia and dermal and epidermal layers). 5-FU wound irrigation was reported valuable for preventing keloid recurrence from surgical procedure [11]. Thus, wound irrigation with combined 5-FU (about 3 mg/ml) and triamcinolone acetonide (about 8 mg/ml) should be performed, and excessive drug liquid should be extruded out of the wound before its closure. With the clinical experience over 3,000 cases, no failure of wound healing has even been observed when a wound was irrigated at this dose.

After wound closure, tension-reduction device such as "zipline" should be applied immediately to guarantee a tension-free zone in the wound area. Afterwards, the patients should receive irradiation on the wound within 24 hours post-surgery with a dose of 4–5 grays once a day for a total of 4 days using electron beam as the irradiation source.

Postsurgical Monitoring and Preventive Injection of 5-FU

After the procedure, the patients are advised to visit the clinic monthly to closely monitor the status of surgical site and silicone gel is generally needed for application on the wound site. In most cases, the above procedure is enough to keep the sutured wound quiescent and non-activated, and the wound tissue will maintain erythema-free and symptom-free for pain and itching (see case 4). If this maintains with no further signs of recurrence, the tension-reduction device can be removed after continuous wearing for at least 6 months.

For high-risk patients, including those who have previous history of postsurgical reoccurrence, multiple keloids, or previous recurrence after surgery plus radiotherapy, early injection of low-dose 5-FU into the wound subcutaneous tissue should be applied as early as 4 weeks post-surgery, which is maintained for another five injections every 4 weeks until the sixth month post-surgery. Afterwards, 5-FU injection should be given whenever there is sign of pain, itching, and erythema to make sure that early management of recurrence is applied (see case 5).

For non-risk patients, or patient without previous surgery, an indication for low-dose 5-FU injection will be the minor level of erythema and the feeling of pain and itching. The injection should be given one more time after disappearance of these early signs.

Anti-indications of Low-Dose 5-FU Injection Therapy Combined with Steroids

Children are generally not the candidates for 5-FU-based chemotherapy in both keloid and HTS. In addition, female patients are recommended not to prepare for pregnancy during the treatment time period until 6 months after the cessation of the treatment. In addition, a blood cell count test is recommended every 2 months to monitor potential adverse effects on hematopoietic system. Close monitoring of steroid side effects is needed, and the cessation of the therapy is needed at once in case any side effect is confirmed.

Representative Case Reports

Case 1. Remodeling of Keloid into Normal-Looking Skin [7] (◘ Fig. 30.2)

A 53-year-old woman with 28 years of spontaneous formation and development of her chest keloid with previous history of cryotherapy and steroid injection. The keloid grew rapidly in the last several years with unbearable pain (++++)[1] and itching (++++). Physical examination revealed a big keloid in her chest skin with dimensions 10 cm wide, 7 cm high, and 0.3 cm thick along with severe erythema (++++), and hard tissue texture (++) (◘ Fig. 30.2a). The patient was first given nine intralesional injections of 5-FU (mostly 3.45 mg/ml) in 2% lidocaine every 2 weeks in order to control growth and abolish vascularity. The drug injections led to decreased erythema (+), thickness (0.15 cm), hardness (+), reduced itching (+), and also pain disappearance.

Afterwards, the patient received three injections of triamcinolone acetonide in lidocaine (8.3 mg/ml) every other week, resulting in flattened and softened scar with no pain and itching despite the fact that some minor elevated scar areas remained (◘ Fig. 30.2b). Due to re-increased erythema (++) caused by injected steroid, the patient received four injections of a mixture of steroid (7.58–7.35 mg/ml) and 5-FU (2.94–2.27 mg/ml) in lidocaine to achieve both drug effects simultaneously, and this further decreased erythema (+), while maintaining flattened and softened scar without symptom (◘ Fig. 30.2c). Because of improved symptom and physical sign, the patient was given a much lower dose of combined drugs (steroid: from 2.83 to 2.40 mg/ml, 5-FU from 2.27 to 1.42 to 0.96 mg/ml) for six times with 3–8-week intervals in order to prevent relapse and to remodel the scar. During this time, relatively high dose of drugs remained necessary in some small re-growing areas. When followed up 4 months later, it was surprising to find that some keloid areas became grossly invisible and normal-looking skin had appeared (◘ Fig. 30.2d).

Encouraged by this result, another five injections of low-dose combined drugs (steroids: 3.77 mg/ml, 5-FU: 1.42 mg/ml) were administered only to the remaining elevated scar areas with an interval of 4–8 weeks. After another 9-month treatment, scar portion further decreased, and normal-looking skin further expanded with skin color, surface, and texture close to those of normal skin (◘ Fig. 30.2e). After 3 years of tissue remodeling therapy, the treatment was completed and

1 Represents the level of pain, itiching or thickness of the scar, sort of semi-quantitative analysis.

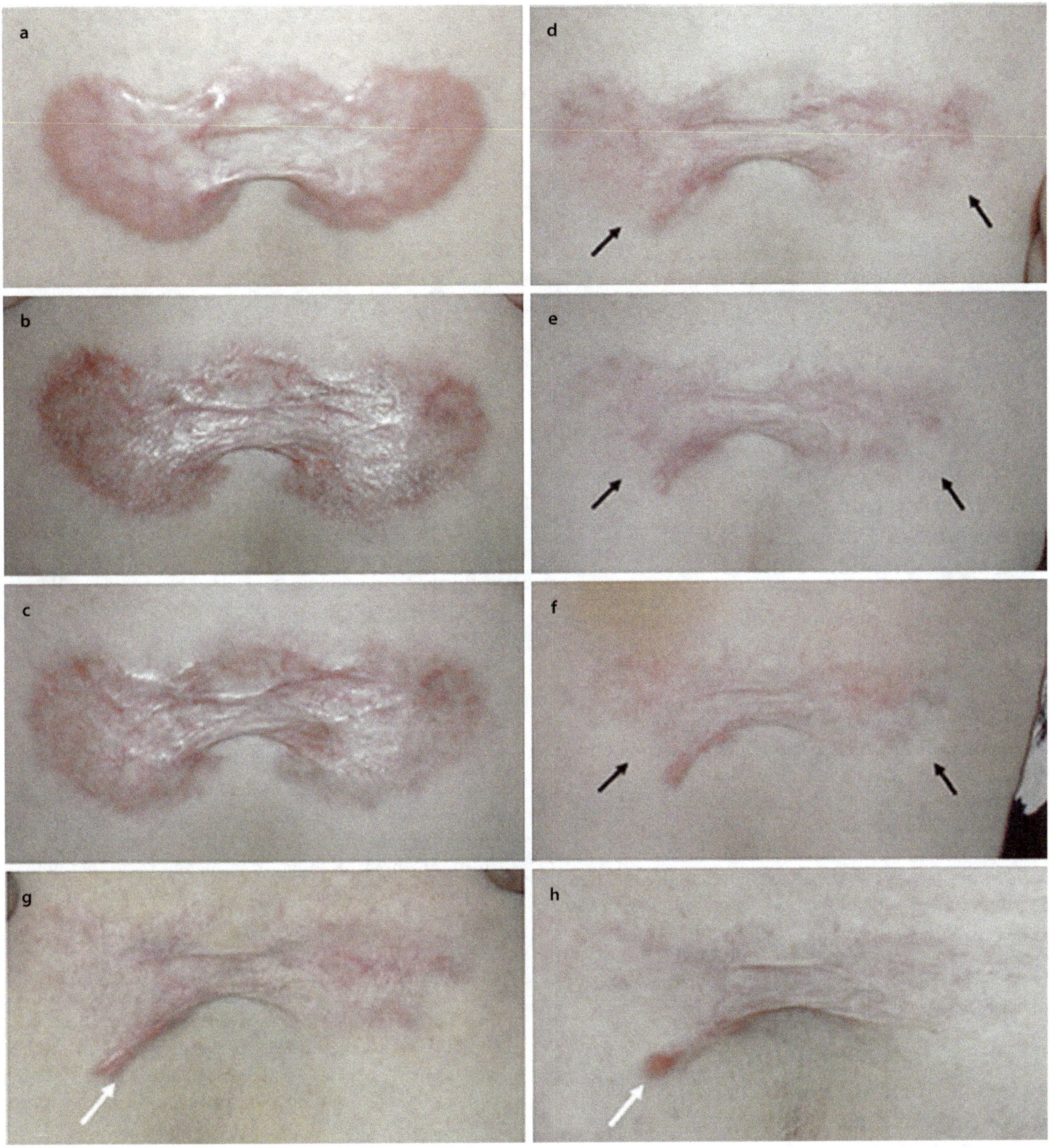

Fig. Case 1: Remodeling of keloid into normal-looking skin at various stages. Black arrows indicate the areas that are under continued tissue remodeling. White arrow indicates reoccurred keloid nodule. (See details in the text)

no further relapse was observed at 14 months post-therapy (Fig. 30.2f). Blood cell counts maintained normal during and after therapy.

Two years after the cease of the treatment, a small nodule with redness and pain and itching recurred at the left lower corner (Fig. 30.2g, white arrowed), and further injections with 5-FU (about 3 mg/ml) mixed with triamcinolone acetonide (about 9 mg/ml) were given at intervals of every 3–6 months for 2 more years and once a year for another 3 years. The complete cure of the scar was observed at 9 years after the initiation of the treatment except for an even smaller active nodule (Fig. 30.2h, white arrowed), which may deserve another therapy modality such as radiotherapy.

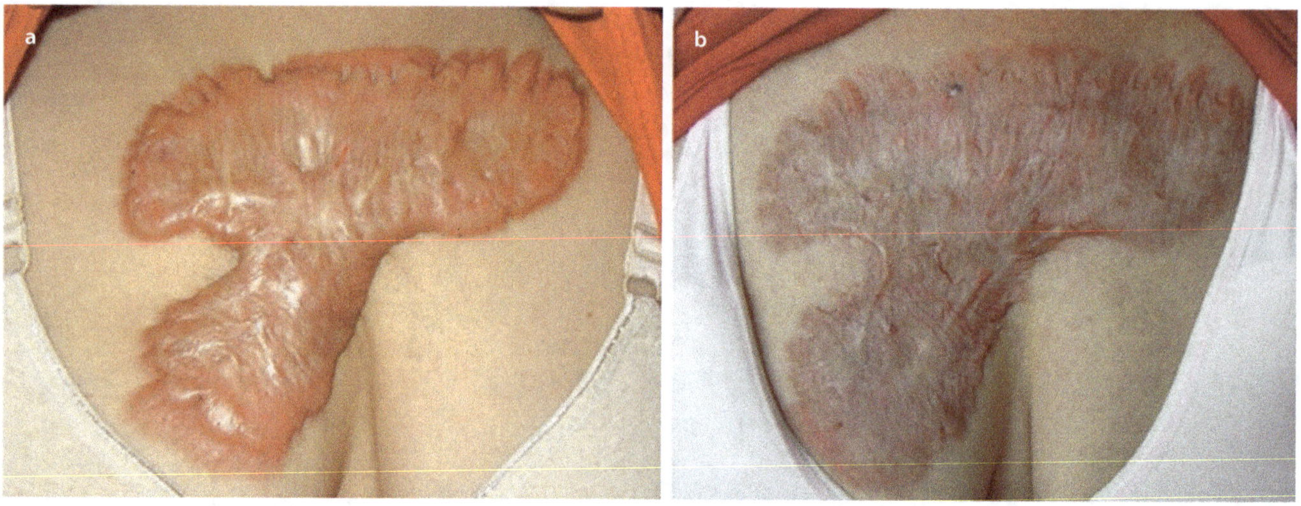

Fig. Case 2: Intralesional injection of low-dose 5-FU and steroids for the treatment of large-sized keloids before **a** and after **b** treat-ment. (See details in the text)

Case 2. Intralesional Injection of Low-Dose 5-FU and Steroid for a Large-Sized Keloid

A 50-year-old female patient visited the clinic with a chest keloid spontaneously forming for 5 years, which developed quickly along with the symptoms of pain and itching. The keloid revealed a size of 15 cm in width, 12 cm in length, and 0.5–1 cm in thickness with server erythema (◘ Fig. 30.3a). The patient was treated with intralesional injection of combined 5-FU and triamcinolone acetonide at low doses as described earlier. This big-sized keloid was divided into four regions, and the injectional therapy was given in a manner of region by region that lasted for 4 years and eventually resulted in a completely remodeled scar that was flattened and softened without erythema and symptoms (◘ Fig. 30.3b). Afterwards, the keloid was generally stable and inactive except for some minor nodules that needed occasional injection.

Case 3. Sufficient Therapy Is Essential for Curing Keloids

A 22-year-old female patient with a large-sized keloid (18 cm in length, 6 cm in width, and 0.5–1.5 cm in thickness) in the abdominal area visited the clinic for her keloid treatment (◘ Fig. 30.4a). The total keloid was roughly divided into three regions for one-by-one treatment. Due to high vascularity of the keloid, the patient was first given 5-FU injection alone at the dose about 3 mg/ml every 3–4 weeks for three times to reduce the vascularity via inducing endothelial cell apoptosis. Once the scar became darker with less erythema, combined 5-FU (2.6 mg/ml) and triamcinolone acetonide (7.5 mg/ml) was used for intralesional injection every 4 weeks. At the seventh-month posttreatment checkup, the top two-thirds of the keloid had already became softened and flattened with the disappearance of pain and itching and reduced erythema (◘ Fig. 30.4b). The patient was further treated for the rest of the keloid in a similar way and the total keloid area became completely softened and flattened without symptoms and with further reduced vascularity at the 24th-month posttreatment (◘ Fig. 30.4c). Then, reduced drug dose (2.6 mg/ml for 5-FU and 4.5 mg/ml for steroids) and prolonged injection interval (6–8 weeks) were applied to focus on remodeling keloid and improving tissue texture. At the 32th-month posttreatment, completely remolded keloid with tissue texture similar to normal skin and minimal level of redness was observed, except for a few isolated active keloid nodules which remained over-vascularized at the bottom region (◘ Fig. 30.4d). Afterwards, the treatment focused only on activated keloid nodules with an injection every 6–8 weeks and whole keloid was completely remodeled when observed at the 68th-month posttreatment except for a few nodules located at the stich markers that remained activated at the 63th-month posttreatment (◘ Fig. 30.4e). Following that time point, the nodule treatment remained and most nodules were completely remodeled after another 15 months of treatment with 3-month interval. The whole keloid has been completely remodeled, which became stably inactivated with whitened color and soften tissue texture when observed at the 78th-month posttreatment (◘ Fig. 30.4f). Afterwards, the whole keloid never reoccurred, and the treated nodules also completely inactivated after several more injections. After more than 6 years of treatment with low-dose 5-FU, the patient delivered a completely healthy child at 2 years post-

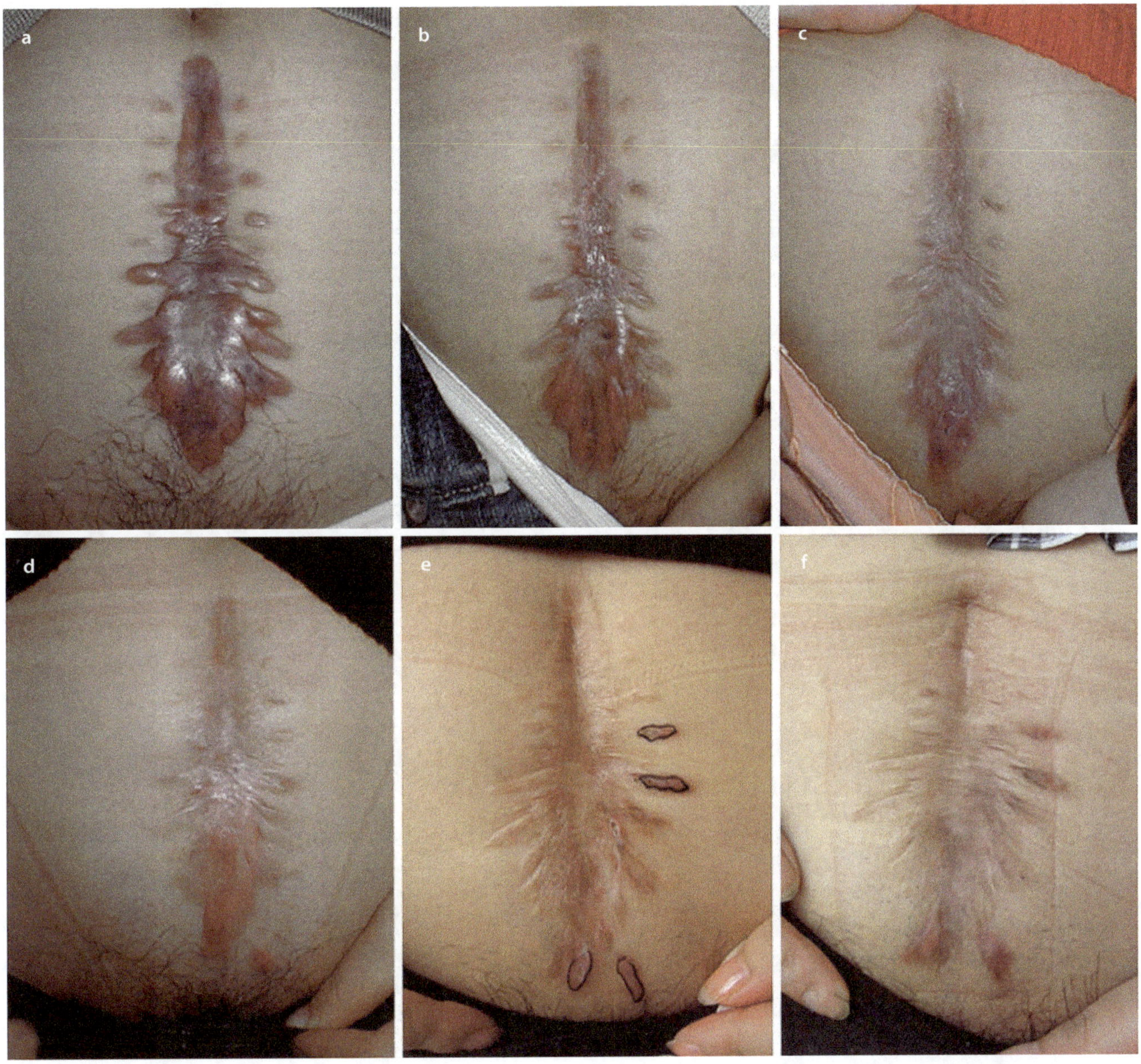

◘ Fig. Case 3: Sufficient therapy is essential for curing keloids with image presentation of an evolved keloid treated with low-dose 5-FU and steroid injection. (See details in the text)

cessation of the treatment. This exploratory treatment indicates the importance of sufficient treatment for preventing keloid reoccurrence.

Case 4. Low-Dose 5-FU for Preventing Keloid from Reoccurrence After Surgical Excision

A female patient who had a chest keloid (3 cm in width, 2 cm in height, and 0.5 cm in thickness) with severe pain and itching visited the clinic to request keloid treatment (◘ Fig. 30.5a). The patient received surgical excision of her keloid, and then the wound was irrigated with combined 5-FU (2.6 mg/ml) and triamcinolone acetonide (7.5 mg/ml) followed by primary wound closure with multiple tissue-layer suturing. A tension-reduction device was immediately applied on the closed wound and the patient was asked to keep wearing the device for at least 6 months after the surgery. The patient received radiotherapy within 24 hours post-surgery with a dose of 4 grays per time and per day for total 4 days. The patient was followed up every 4 weeks post-surgery with no sign of reoccurrence, and a linear white scar was observed at 13 months post-surgery without any sign of reoccurrence (◘ Fig. 30.5b).

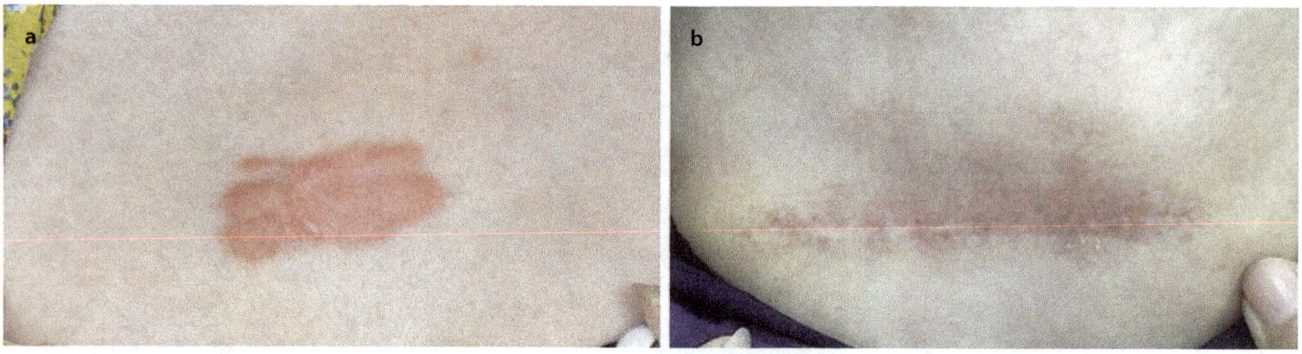

◘ **Fig.** Case 4: Low-dose 5-FU for preventing keloid from reoccurrence after surgical excision. **a** Before the surgery; **b** 13 months post-surgery. (See details in the text)

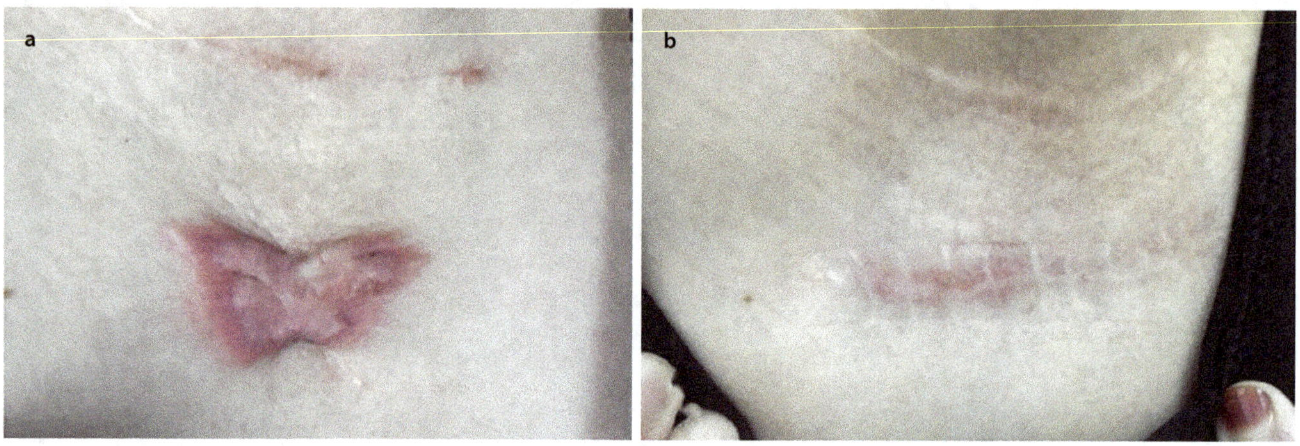

◘ **Fig.** Case 5: Low-dose 5-FU for combined chemoradiotherapy to prevent keloid from postsurgical reoccurrence. **a** Before the sur-gery; **b** 2 years post-surgery with multiple 5-FU injections. (See details in the text)

Case 5. Low-Dose 5-FU for Combined Chemoradiotherapy to Prevent Keloid from Postsurgical Reoccurrence

A female patient with multiple keloids on her neck, chest (◘ Fig. 30.6a), and left arm visited the clinic and requested keloid treatment. Her chest keloid (4 cm in width, 2 cm in height, and 1 cm in thickness) was heavily vascularized with severe pain, itching, and rapid growth (◘ Fig. 30.6a). The patient received surgical excision, wound irrigation, and closure and radiotherapy similarly as in case 4. However, relapse signs of itching and pain occurred early at 1 month post-surgery. Thus, the patient was given injection of low-dose 5-FU alone (about 3 mg/ml) at 1 month, 8 months, 10 months, 13 months, 16 months, and 19 months post-surgery and no further treatment after 19-month time point. At the 24th month post-surgery follow-up, a whitened linear mature scar was observed at the operational site with no sign of relapse (◘ Fig. 30.6b).

Conclusion

Intralesional injection of low dose 5-FU combined with steroids for keloid and HTS treatment has been practiced by the authors since 2002 with more than 10,000 cases and proven safe and effective. The use of low dose drugs is to keep this procedure safe and sustainable for long term therapy that is essential for reducing the post-therapy recurrence. Gradual adjustment of drug dose and injection interval time and the management of reoccurred keloids at the earliest possible time are the keys for the success of this procedure.

Take-Home Messages

- Intralesional injection of low dose 5-FU (1.5–5 mg/ml) combined with steroids has been used for keloid treatment with proved safety and efficacy.
- The working mechanism is to inactivate keloid fibroblasts and to gradually remodel keloid tissue, rather to cause keloid necrosis which is a trigger for keloid recurrence.
- The procedure can be used for treating primary keloids or for preventing recurrence of surgically removed keloids.
- Sustainable long-term treatment with adjusted drug dose and injection interval and early management of reoccurred lesions are the keys for keloid successful treatment and recurrence prevention.

References

1. Fitzpatrick RE. Treatment of inflamed hypertrophic scars using intralesional 5-FU. Dermatol Surg. 1999;25(3):224–32.
2. Mustoe TA, Cooter RD, Gold MH, Hobbs FD, Ramelet AA, Shakespeare PG, Stella M, Téot L, Wood FM, Ziegler UE, International Advisory Panel on Scar Management. International clinical recommendations on scar management. Plast Reconstr Surg. 2002;110(2):560–71.
3. Gold MH, McGuire M, Mustoe TA, Pusic A, Sachdev M, Waibel J, Murcia C, International Advisory Panel on Scar Management. Updated international clinical recommendations on scar management: part 2--algorithms for scar prevention and treatment. Dermatol Surg. 2014;40(8):825–31.
4. Gupta S, Kalra A. Efficacy and safety of intralesional 5-fluorouracil in the treatment of keloids. Dermatology. 2002;204(2):130–2.
5. Nanda S, Reddy BS. Intralesional 5-fluorouracil as a treatment modality of keloids. Dermatol Surg. 2004;30(1):54–6; discussion 56–7.
6. Davison SP, Dayan JH, Clemens MW, Sonni S, Wang A, Crane A. Efficacy of intralesional 5-fluorouracil and triamcinolone in the treatment of keloids. Aesthet Surg J. 2009;29(1):40–6.
7. Wu XL, Liu W, Cao YL. Clinical study on keloid treatment with intralesional injection of low concentration 5-fluorouracil. Zhonghua Zheng Xing Wai Ke Za Zhi. 2006;22(1):44–6.
8. Liu W, Wu X, Gao Z, Song N. Remodelling of keloid tissue into normal-looking skin. J Plast Reconstr Aesthet Surg. 2008;61(12):1553–4.
9. Song N, Wu X, Gao Z, Zhou G, Zhang WJ, Liu W. Enhanced expression of membrane transporter and drug resistance in keloid fibroblasts. Hum Pathol. 2012;43(11):2024–32.
10. Zhang Q, Yamaza T, Kelly AP, Shi S, Wang S, Brown J, Wang L, French SW, Shi S, Le AD. Tumor-like stem cells derived from human keloid are governed by the inflammatory niche driven by IL-17/IL-6 axis. PLoS One. 2009;4(11):e7798.
11. Uppal RS, Khan U, Kakar S, Talas G, Chapman P, McGrouther AD. The effects of a single dose of 5-fluorouracil on keloid scars: a clinical trial of timed wound irrigation after extralesional excision. Plast Reconstr Surg. 2001;108(5):1218–24.

28

Onion Extract

Julian Poetschke and Gerd G. Gauglitz

Contents

Background

Multiple studies on hypertrophic scar and keloid formation have led to a multitude of therapeutic strategies in order to prevent or attenuate keloid and hypertrophic scar formation. Until today preventing pathologic scarring remains undoubtedly more effective than treating it later on. Thus, avoiding all unnecessary wounds in any patient, whether keloid/hypertrophic scar-prone or not, remains an obvious but imperfect solution. Since delayed epithelialization beyond 10 to 14 days increases the incidence of hypertrophic scarring dramatically [1], achieving rapid epithelialization is mandatory for avoiding excessive scar formation. Particularly, wounds subjected to tension due to motion, body location, or loss of tissue are at increased risk of scar hypertrophy and spreading [2]. Thus, in case of any cutaneous injury, the goal for rapid primary closure of wounds under little to no tension cannot be overstated. In addition to gentle surgical techniques and suitable suture material, careful hemostasis, and intraoperative tissue treatment, the prevention of wound infections and delayed wound healing are extremely important for good scar healing. The incision should be made along the "Langer" lines of the skin and take esthetic subunits (especially in the face) into account. The patient himself or herself should expose fresh scars to little traction, pressure, and stretching, consistently protect them from the sun, and return early to the treating physician as growth increases. If there is a known tendency to formation of keloids and hypertrophic scars, early intralesional injection of triamcinolone acetonide into the fresh surgical wound after surgery may be considered. According to various studies, next to pressure garments, early and regular application of silicone-based products seems to lead to an improvement in scar quality and an accelerated reduction in redness. Current guidelines emphasize the importance of silicone gels and patches for preventive treatment (at the earliest from the 14th postoperative day for at least 2 months) to avoid excessive scars in high-risk patients.

Topical gels containing onion (*Extractum cepae*) extract have been available for more than 60 years treating, preventing, and reducing dermatologic scars and keloids [3]. *Extractum cepae* is reported to have anti-inflammatory, antimicrobial, antiproliferative, and regenerative activities [4]. Several clinical trials have indicated that *Extractum cepae* may prevent pathologic scarring and improves preexisting scars. It has been introduced as a preventional approach for unpleasant hypertrophic scars in current German scar guidelines in 2012 and in current international scar guidelines in 2014.

Onion Extract

Extractum cepae acts in an anti-inflammatory manner and is bactericidal. It is currently believed that the flavonoids (quercetin and kaempferol) in onion extract play the main role in reducing scar formation through inhibition of fibroblast proliferation and collagen production. A study by Phan and others suggested that these inhibitory effects may be mediated through inhibition of transforming growth factor-β (TGF-β1, −2) and SMAD proteins by quercetin [5, 6]. Specifically, the authors demonstrated that basal expression and activation of several key proteins in the IGF (insulin-like growth factor)-1 signal pathways were significantly reduced when keloid fibroblast cells were exposed to quercetin. The authors also analyzed keloid fibroblast cells treated with quercetin by means of immunoblotting and electron microscopic approaches. Fibronectin expression was suppressed by quercetin suggesting a strong inhibitory effect of this compound on production of fibronectin. Transmission electron microscopy was performed on keloid fibroblasts with and without quercetin. Keloid fibroblasts without quercetin showed markedly higher density of ECM fibers in a homogenous ECM, but no ECM deposition was seen in the fibroblasts treated with quercetin, indicating a strong effect of quercetin in the suppression of ECM production and deposition by keloid fibroblasts. In a follow-up study, Phan et al. treated keloid fibroblast cells with quercetin at different concentrations, and cells were then harvested and subjected to immunoblotting analysis. In the pathogenesis of keloids, both IGF-1 and transforming growth factor-β (TGF-β) signaling systems are usually overactive, stimulating fibroblast overproliferation and production of collagen and ECM. The data of Phan and colleagues suggested that quercetin could potentially have an anti-scarring effect by inhibiting the signaling pathway of IGF-1 and TGF-β systems.

It has been further demonstrated that several flavonoids inhibit the antigen-induced histamine release from human basophils, which may be of certain importance since there is evidence to the effect that histamine may accelerate collagen formation.

Today, an increasing body of literature and clinical experience are available testing the ultimate clinical benefit of onion extract-containing scar creams as monotherapy (◘ Fig. 24.1) or in combination with other measures (◘ Fig. 24.2). Study data on the efficacy of *Extractum cepae* for prevention and treatment of hypertrophic scars or keloids, however, remains inconsistent, and the quality of the studies is relatively poor.

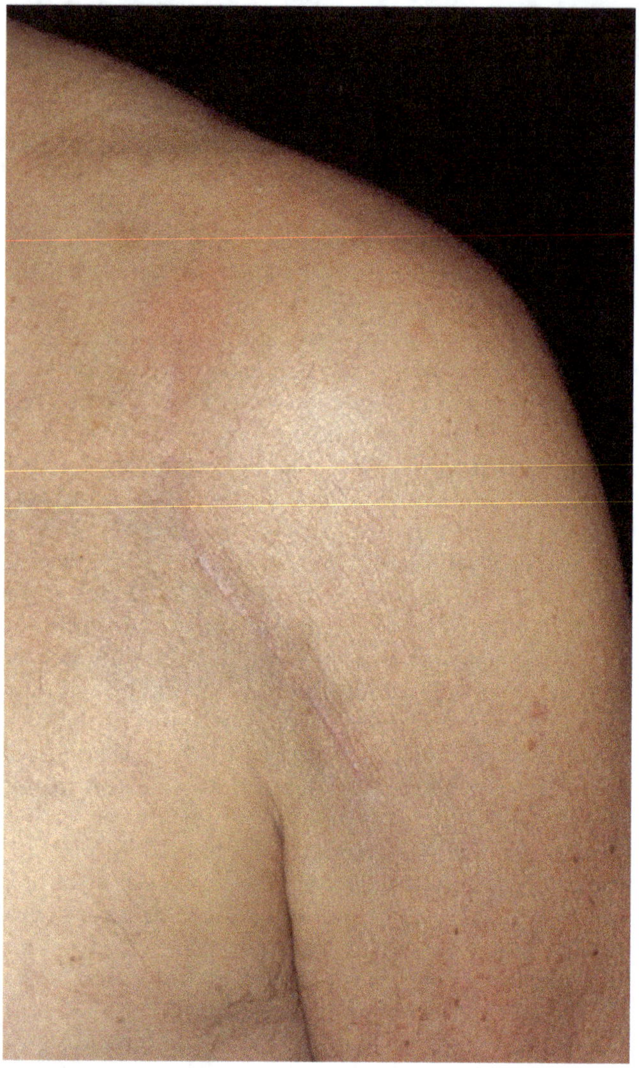

Fig. Upper half of the scar has been treated twice daily for 3 months with onion extract gel

Currently several onion extract-containing scar gel preparations do exists that are mainly based on combinations with either allantoin alone or allantoin and heparin.

Willital et al. evaluated the efficacy of *Extractum cepae* in combination with allantoin and heparin on early scars in an uncontrolled, multicenter, prospective observational study in 1268 subjects. In this study, the scar gel was used at least twice daily. The observational period was 4 to 5 months [7]. Data was recorded at start of treatment, after 2–3 months, and after 4–5 months. Even though the authors were able to show some benefit of regular application of an onion extract-containing gel and a considerably high patient satisfaction, the study was completely uncontrolled; did not use any consistent, recognized scar scale; and was thus highly susceptible to bias. For prevention of hypertrophic scars and keloids, a prospective, randomized, controlled non-blinded study on children with surgery on the thorax after 6-month use of a scar gel containing onion extract, allantoin, and heparin observed a less frequent development of excessive scars than in the untreated comparison group [8]. The therapy in the comparative group, however, remained largely unclear with the statement "normal wound therapy." This is of particular significance, as in a further comparative study on improving scar quality (erythema, pruritus, burning, pain, hypertrophy) between scar gels containing onion extract and a topical agent based on petrolatum, a specific effect of the ingredients could not be proven [9]. It must be considered, however, that the patient number in this study was low, the operations were not performed on specific predilection sites such as the thorax, and thus statistically significant results could have been expected only with very high patient numbers. For treatment of hypertrophic

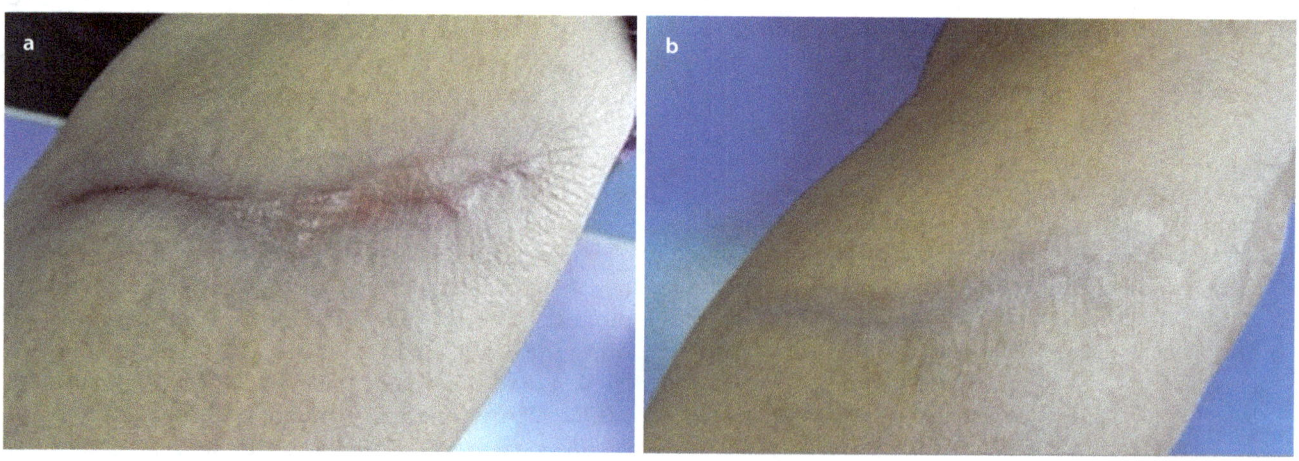

Fig. Before (**a**) and after (**b**) three sessions of fractional CO_2 every 4 weeks, in between onion extract-containing scar gel twice daily

scars and keloids, the benefit of a combination of intralesional triamcinolone and an onion extract combinational gel was reported as positive, with both monotherapy with triamcinolone alone and the combination with an additional topical agent containing onion skin extract resulting in statistically significant improvement. A calculation of statistical significance with respect to the differences of the therapy concepts was, nonetheless, not performed in the study [10].

In a prospective randomized controlled trial conducted in China, the use of onion extract was investigated in the prevention of scarring after laser removal of tattoos [11]. Local experience according to the authors found that nearly 25% of Chinese subjects with dark skin (Fitzpatrick types III–IV) developed scarring after laser removal of tattoos. A total of 120 subjects with 144 professional blue-black tattoos were randomized into the onion extract group or the control group. Subjects in the onion extract group applied onion extract to the treatment areas after reepithelialization twice daily in between laser treatment sessions, and subjects in the control group did not apply anything. A total of 52 subjects with 61 tattoos completed the study in the onion extract group. Seven tattoos (11.5%) in seven subjects developed scarring, four subjects (7.7%) had permanent hypopigmentation, and three (5.8%) had permanent hyperpigmentation. The control group comprised 55 subjects with 68 tattoos. Sixteen tattoos (23.5%) in 14 subjects developed scarring, 4 subjects (7.2%) had permanent hypopigmentation, and 5 (9%) had transient hyperpigmentation. According to this publication, the rate of scarring was statistically significantly lower in the onion extract group than in the control group.

It is currently recommended to apply the gel several times daily (usually two to three times a day) with mild massage of the scar tissue. In firm, mature scars use under occlusion or in combination with ultrasound may also be considered. In prophylactic postoperative use, treatment may be started shortly after removal of sutures. In the treatment of open wounds, scar prophylaxis using an onion extract gel should be delayed until complete epithelialization of the wound. Treatment usually continues over several weeks to months. While side effects are generally very low, treatment containing onion extract might be slightly irritating in facial areas, particularly in younger children.

Recently, an onion extract- and allantoin-containing patch has been introduced to the market. This product features an occlusive active release liner with an adhesive layer separated by a micro-air cushion seal. The so-called overnight intensive patch may be cut to size for small scars or placed side-by-side for larger scars. Its efficacy has been elucidated in an intraindividual randomized, observer-blind, controlled study in adults with post-dermatologic surgery scars [12]. Two scars per subject were randomized to no treatment or overnight treatment with the OIP for 12 to 24 weeks. Scar quality was assessed in a total of 125 subjects using the Patient and Observer Scar Assessment Scale (POSAS) and Global Aesthetic Improvement Scale. The authors found a decrease in observer-assessed POSAS from baseline, which was significantly greater for treated than untreated scars at week 6 and 24. The decrease in patient-assessed POSAS was further significantly greater for the treated scar than the untreated scar at week 12 and 24. Subject- and investigator-evaluated Global Aesthetic Improvement Scale scores were higher for the treated than the untreated scar at all visits. According to the manuscript, all subjects considered the global comfort of the OIP to be good or very good, and no safety concerns were identified. Also, no further studies have been published, testing this rather novel product, and current communications do confirm a high patient satisfaction due to the patient orientation application and a certain benefit for early scarring.

Conclusion

Scarring following surgery or trauma is difficult to predict, and both physicians and their patients are highly concerned with minimizing scar appearance and value even small improvements in scarring as clinically meaningful. Till to date, preventing pathologic scarring remains undoubtedly more effective than treating it. Next to specific surgical techniques and appropriate general aftercare of fresh wounds, a multitude of scar gels, creams, patches, and ointments are available and are being promoted for scarless wound healing. Next to silicone-based products, onion extract or cepalin has been highlighted as one potential anti-scarring agent over recent years. Although its underlying study data remains in part contradicting regarding its efficacy, onion extract-containing scar creams appear to positively influence scar texture, height, and associated symptoms compared to placebo or untreated control. Based on the recently published German guidelines on scarring, onion extract-containing scar creams may be considered as additional therapy for active hypertrophic scars and for postsurgical prophylaxis of excessive scarring.

Take-Home Messages

- Preventing pathologic scarring remains undoubtedly more effective than treating it.
- Next to silicone-based products, onion extract-containing creams have been shown to positively influence scar maturation if used shortly after wound healing.
- Data remains contradicting, but guidelines have incorporated onion extract in their recommendations on preventing unpleasant scarring.
- Onion extract-containing products are available as creams, ointments, gels, or patches.
- Therapy can be started after complete epithelialization of the wound and should continue for 12 to 24 weeks.
- Onion extract-containing products are safe, and side effects beyond irritation of the treated skin are extremely rare.

References

1. Mustoe TA, Cooter RD, Gold MH, Hobbs FD, Ramelet AA, Shakespeare PG, et al. International clinical recommendations on scar management. Plast Reconstr Surg. 2002;110(2):560–71.
2. Mutalik S. Treatment of keloids and hypertrophic scars. Indian J Dermatol Venereol Leprol. 2005;71(1):3–8.
3. Willital GH, Heine H. Efficacy of Contractubex gel in the treatment of fresh scars after thoracic surgery in children and adolescents. Int J Clin Pharmacol Res. 1994;14(5–6):193–202.
4. Sidgwick GP, McGeorge D, Bayat A. A comprehensive evidence-based review on the role of topicals and dressings in the management of skin scarring. Arch Dermatol Res. 2015;307(6):461–77.
5. Phan TT, Lim IJ, Chan SY, Tan EK, Lee ST, Longaker MT. Suppression of transforming growth factor beta/smad signaling in keloid-derived fibroblasts by quercetin: implications for the treatment of excessive scars. J Trauma. 2004;57(5):1032–7.
6. Phan TT, Lim IJ, Sun L, Chan SY, Bay BH, Tan EK, et al. Quercetin inhibits fibronectin production by keloid-derived fibroblasts. Implication for the treatment of excessive scars. J Dermatol Sci. 2003;33(3):192–4.
7. Willital GH, Simon J. Efficacy of early initiation of a gel containing extractum cepae, heparin, and allantoin for scar treatment: an observational, noninterventional study of daily practice. J Drugs Dermatol. 2013;12(1):38–42.
8. Maragakis M, Willital GH, Michel G, Gortelmeyer R. Possibilities of scar treatment after thoracic surgery. Drugs Exp Clin Res. 1995;21(5):199–206.
9. Chung VQ, Kelley L, Marra D, Jiang SB. Onion extract gel versus petrolatum emollient on new surgical scars: prospective double-blinded study. Dermatol Surg. 2006;32(2):193–7.
10. Koc E, Arca E, Surucu B, Kurumlu Z. An open, randomized, controlled, comparative study of the combined effect of intralesional triamcinolone acetonide and onion extract gel and intralesional triamcinolone acetonide alone in the treatment of hypertrophic scars and keloids. Dermatol Surg. 2008;34(11):1507–14.
11. Ho WS, Ying SY, Chan PC, Chan HH. Use of onion extract, heparin, allantoin gel in prevention of scarring in chinese patients having laser removal of tattoos: a prospective randomized controlled trial. Dermatol Surg. 2006;32(7):891–6.
12. Prager W, Gauglitz GG. Effectiveness and safety of an overnight patch containing Allium cepa extract and Allantoin for post-dermatologic surgery scars. Aesthet Plast Surg. 2018;42(4):1144–50.

29

Scar Formation: Cellular Mechanisms

Ian A. Darby and Alexis Desmoulière

Contents

Background

Tissue repair after injury is a complex phenomenon involving intricate and coordinated mechanisms. Even though during the last decade, many studies have increased our knowledge on the different cellular players involved in this process [16], many gray areas remain, particularly concerning the dialogue between different cell populations acting during wound healing and scar formation. Interestingly, an abnormal course of the inflammatory phase at the beginning of the healing process appears to have effects long after scar formation. In addition, the relationships between cells and the extracellular matrix remain a key aspect in understanding the normal development and remodeling of scars.

Introduction

The skin provides the primary protection against external injuries for the body and is also essential in the maintenance of general homeostasis. Located beneath the epidermis, the dermis represents the thickest compartment of the skin and is composed mainly of a dense extracellular matrix network of collagen fibers supporting the specific dermal appendages, including hair follicles, sebaceous glands, and sweat glands. Dermal (myo)fibroblasts play a major role in the synthesis and maintenance of the extracellular matrix as well as in the wound-healing process [4]. During healing, fibroblasts proliferate and migrate into the wound space, though the origin of these cells remains to be clearly elucidated. Moreover, research on progenitor cells present in the skin, which can differentiate into many different cell types, represents an interesting source of cells that may be able to promote (when correctly stimulated) wound healing, improve the repair process in impaired or difficult-to-heal wounds or be able to modify the process of excessive scarring. In this chapter, these different aspects will be expanded on, including the biochemical, cellular, and physical factors that are involved in regulating healing and scarring in skin wounds (e.g., cytokines, mechanical tension, and innervation).

General Mechanisms of Scar Formation

Immediately after wounding, the healing process commences leading to (partial) restoration of the injured tissue. Wound healing passes through three dynamic and interrelated phases which temporally overlap [3]. Based on morphological changes seen in the wound tissue during the course of the healing process, these phases are defined as the inflammatory phase, the proliferative phase (with the development of the granulation tissue) and reepithelialization phase, and the remodeling phase which includes maturation and scar formation. The inflammatory phase begins with capillary damage, where blood loss results in a clot forming, which consists of fibrin and fibronectin and stops further blood loss. The wound space is thus filled with a provisional matrix that provides a scaffold into which various cells can migrate. The initial source of chemokines in the wound is platelets that are present in the clot, and these degranulate and provide multiple factors that stimulate the recruitment of inflammatory cells, neutrophils, and macrophages. At the same time, fibroblasts and endothelial cells are attracted by growth factors that are chemotactic for these cells. The proliferative phase of healing which follows includes angiogenesis, the growth of new vessels into the wound. Angiogenesis is vital for tissue repair since it provides vascular perfusion of the wound, delivering oxygen and nutrients and thus contributing to cell proliferation, including the proliferation of fibroblasts. The wound is initially hypoxic, as it lacks normal perfusion, and hypoxia itself is an important stimulus for the release of growth factors, including those that regulate angiogenesis. During the proliferative phase, angiogenesis proceeds and eventually reestablishes a more normal level of perfusion. The regulation of angiogenesis may represent a target for improving wound repair, particularly in those cases where delayed or abnormal angiogenesis has been suggested to play a role in healing impairment. Fibroblasts present in the granulation tissue become activated and are then termed myofibroblasts. These myofibroblasts are responsible for the synthesis and deposition of extracellular matrix components which progressively replace the provisional matrix [6]. Myofibroblasts also show contractile properties, playing a major role in the contraction and maturation of the granulation tissue. Scar formation, which is the third phase of healing, involves progressive remodeling of the granulation tissue (◻ Fig. 3.1). A major role in this process is played by proteolytic enzymes, particularly the family of matrix metalloproteinases (MMPs) and their inhibitors (tissue inhibitor of metalloproteinases [TIMPs]). Synthesis of extracellular matrix is then reduced, though not completely stopped, and the components that make up the matrix are modified as the matrix is remodeled. Collagen type III, the major collagen present in granulation tissue, is progressively replaced by collagen type I, the main structural protein in normal unwounded dermis. Finally, elastin which is largely responsible for the elasticity of the skin and which is absent in granulation tissue also reappears. In deep human wounds, elastin fibers do not show complete regeneration after wound healing being both deficient and not showing normal structural

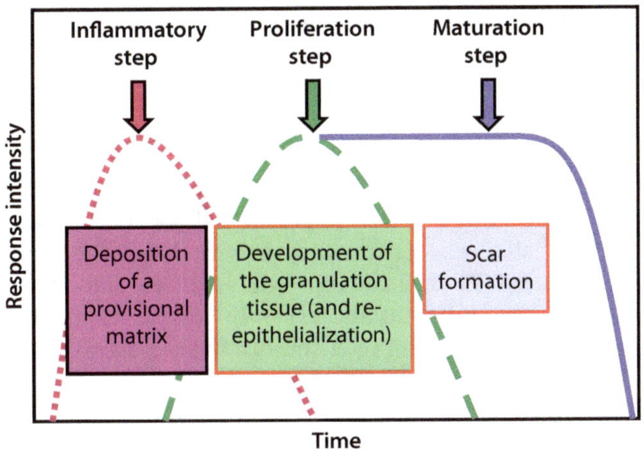

Fig. The various phases of the healing process. After dam-age, inflammation leads to the formation of granulation tissue dur-ing which myofibroblasts appear. A significant neoangiogenesis is also observed. A new epidermis can then develop over this granulation tissue. Subsequently, remodeling of this granulation tissue occurs via apoptosis of the cells present in the granulation tissue (myofibroblasts and vascular cells), and the extracellular matrix is gradually reorganized

organization. During the resolution phase of wound healing, apoptosis of both vascular cells and myofibroblasts results in a significant reduction in cell number in the granulation tissue. Whether myofibroblasts can reacquire a quiescent phenotype thus returning to a "normal" dermal fibroblast phenotype is still open to question.

Morphological and Biochemical Characteristics of Myofibroblast Phenotype

The earliest descriptions of myofibroblasts, based on their electron microscopic morphology, identified ultrastructural specializations showing some similarity to those of smooth muscle cells, in particular prominent bundles of cytoplasmic microfilaments. Further ultrastructural and molecular markers that define myofibroblasts have since been identified, including cell-cell and cell-matrix adhesions, stress fibers, and expression of α-smooth muscle actin [9]. Both in vivo and in vitro, the presence of fibroblasts exhibiting prominent microfilament bundles in their cytoplasm (known as stress fibers) can be observed; however, these cells do not necessarily contain α-smooth muscle actin-positive microfilaments. In vitro, these fibroblasts can also be shown to secrete a splice-variant form of fibronectin, ED-A fibronectin. These cells have been termed proto-myofibroblasts, and their stress fibers contain only β- and γ-cytoplasmic actin. Proto-myofibroblasts can exert tractional forces in connective tissue, and they may be induced by mechanical stress; however, to undergo full differentiation into myofibroblasts, they require stimulation with transforming growth factor (TGF)-β1 (see below). Fully differentiated myofibroblasts are then capable of exerting increased force due to contraction. The expression pattern of myofibroblasts and smooth muscle cells shows several differences. Smooth muscle cells express smooth muscle myosin heavy chain, smoothelin, and h-caldesmon, while myofibroblasts are generally negative for these markers. Desmin, an intermediate filament protein which is normally expressed in muscle cells, has also been used as a negative marker of myofibroblasts, since during normal wound healing myofibroblasts have been found to be desmin-negative. In some conditions of pathological scarring, myofibroblasts have been observed to be desmin-positive. Overall though α-smooth muscle actin is also expressed in smooth muscle cells and pericytes, it still represents the most reliable phenotypic marker of myofibroblast phenotype.

Given the important roles of myofibroblasts in tissue repair and scarring, in particular their role in contraction, the exact mechanisms regulating contraction in such tissues need to be clearly identified. Examination of spontaneous intracellular Ca^{2+} oscillations has shown that intracellular Ca^{2+} oscillations are coordinated between contracting myofibroblasts via adherens junctions but occur randomly between fibroblasts and non-contacting cells. Therefore the following model of mechanical coupling for myofibroblasts can be proposed: individual cell contraction is transmitted via adherens junctions leading to the opening of mechanosensitive ion channels in adjacent cells. The resulting Ca^{2+} influx induces a contraction that can feed back on the first cell and/or stimulate other contacting cells allowing the cells to work like a syncytium. This mechanism of coordination of myofibroblast activity may improve the remodeling of cell-dense tissue [8].

Cellular Origins of Myofibroblasts

Recruitment of fibroblasts from the local connective tissue is generally accepted to be the major source of myofibroblasts in the wound. Dermal fibroblasts that are located at the wound margins can acquire a myofibroblastic phenotype and then play a role in tissue repair. However, there is considerable heterogeneity in fibroblastic cell subpopulations. These fibroblast subpopulations are present in different locations within the skin and have specific activation and deactivation properties. At least three subpopulations have been identified in the dermis: superficial (or papillary) fibroblasts (the papillary dermis is approximately 300–400 μm in depth and is arranged as a ridgelike structure), reticular fibroblasts which are present in the deep dermis (which consists of thick collagen and elastin fibers that are arranged parallel to the surface of the skin), and fibroblasts which are associated with hair follicles. These cell subpopulations can be isolated for cell culture and then, depending on the age and nature of the skin sample, show distinct differences in phenotype in vitro.

It has been recently suggested that local mesenchymal stem cells may also be involved in the tissue repair process. These progenitor cells have been identified in the dermal sheath that surrounds the exterior of hair follicles, facing the epithelial stem cells. These cells are involved in regeneration of the dermal papilla and can also differentiate into wound-healing myofibroblasts after damage or injury.

Recent data has also suggested a role for circulating cells, termed fibrocytes, in the tissue repair process. Fibrocytes may enter damaged skin together at the same time as inflammatory cells and may then acquire a myofibroblastic phenotype. In burn wound, fibrocytes may infiltrate the wound where they both stimulate a local inflammatory response and additionally secrete extracellular matrix proteins, thus contributing to the pathological (hypertrophic) scarring that can be seen postburn injury.

Another bone marrow-derived circulating cell has also been suggested to play a role in tissue repair. Mesenchymal stem cells are bone marrow-derived nonhematopoietic precursor cells that may be present in both normal and damaged connective tissue, where they infiltrate the tissue and then contribute to the maintenance and repair of the tissue. Indeed, these cells have the capacity to seed into several organs and then differentiate into myofibroblasts, similar to those seen during wound healing. The degree to which damaged tissues or organs are infiltrated by these cells is dependent on the severity of tissue injury.

Lastly, epithelial- or endothelial-to-mesenchymal transition of either differentiated or malignant epithelium (or endothelium) can result in a phenotypic change to fibroblasts or myofibroblasts that are then responsible for extracellular matrix production. Although this mechanism is now accepted as playing an important role in fibrogenesis after tissue injury, it appears to play a less prominent role in normal tissue repair. Overall, myofibroblasts derived from circulating fibrocytes, mesenchymal stem cells, epithelial- or endothelial-to-mesenchymal transition, or bone marrow-derived cells may supplement local fibroblast recruitment and differentiation where their numbers are insufficient for the repair and remodeling process [14].

Regulation of Myofibroblast Phenotype

Wound healing and skin homeostasis are regulated by a number of cytokines and growth factors. Some growth factors act directly on granulation tissue formation and fibroblasts activity, while others have effects on vascular and epithelial cells. Of the factors with direct effects on fibroblasts, TGF-β1 is notable as it is a potent inducer of myofibroblast differentiation [18]. In addition to its role in inducing expression of α-smooth muscle actin, TGF-β1 also powerfully stimulates the synthesis of extracellular matrix proteins. TGF-β1 also favors the deposition of matrix by an effect on the balance between MMPs and their inhibitors, TIMPs, by reducing MMP activity while stimulating TIMP expression. The action of TGF-β1 on fibroblast to myofibroblast differentiation requires the presence of ED-A fibronectin, underlining the close relationship between growth factor activation, the extracellular matrix, and regulation of cellular function (◘ Fig. 3.2). It is interesting to note that granulocyte macrophage colony stimulating factor can also increase the number of myofibroblasts in vivo; however, this is most likely due to its activation and recruitment of macrophages which in turn increases the levels and availability of TGF-β1 [15]. Finally, microRNAs (miRNAs) have also been implicated in the induction of myofibroblasts in both fibrotic conditions and in cancer. Specifically, expression of miR-21 appears to be correlated with high levels of TGF-β1 stimulation of the myofibroblast phenotype. A recent study has suggested that the mechanism underlying this may be through effects on TGF-β1 inhibitory pathways. Improvements in our understanding of the effects of miRNAs in regulating fibrosis, potentially through actions on myofibroblast differentiation and activity, may allow miRNAs to be targeted in therapies aimed at inhibition of fibrosis and scarring.

Role of Myofibroblasts in Pathological Scarring and Fibrosis

In some cases, wound healing proceeds in a pathological course resulting in pathological scarring [17]. Such abnormal repair processes may be the result of impaired remodeling of the granulation tissue resulting in, for example, abnormal repair of the skin in the form of hypertrophic or keloid scars and to fibrosis in internal organs. In the case of excessive scarring in the skin such as hypertrophic scars, normal healing fails and the granulation tissue continues to expand, likely due to abnormal and excessive secretion of growth factors and/or to a lack of molecules that in normal healing are responsible for induction of apoptosis or remodeling of the

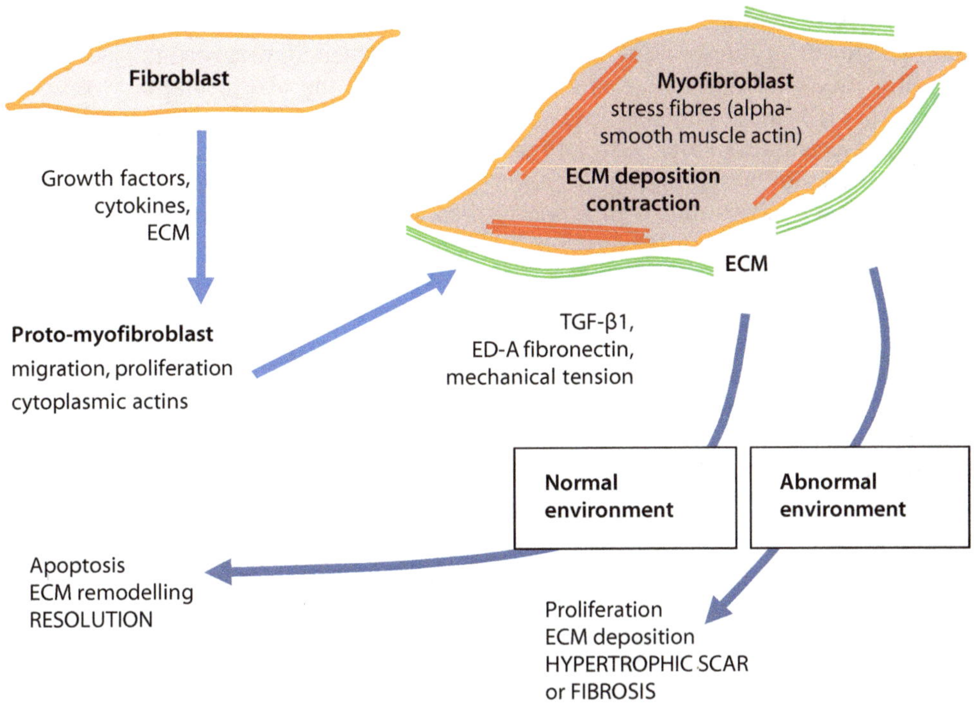

Fig. Illustration showing the evolution of the fibroblast phenotype during normal and pathological conditions. Changes observed in fibroblast phenotype as cells differentiate towards a myofibroblast phenotype begin with the appearance of proto-myofibroblasts. These cells possess stress fibers composed of β- and γ-cytoplasmic actins. These then evolve, at least in some cases, into fully differentiated myofibroblasts. These cells possess stress fibers containing α-smooth muscle actin. Soluble factors such as transforming growth factor-β1 (TGF-β1), extracellular matrix (ECM) components such as ED-A fibronectin, and/or the mechanical microenvironment are all involved in myofibroblastic differentiation. The myofibroblast may then disappear by apoptosis, while deactivation, leading to a quiescent phenotype, has not been clearly demonstrated at least in vivo. If the remodeling phase of the granulation tissue does not occur (with no apoptosis of the myofibroblasts and vascular cells present in the granulation tissue nor reorganization of the extracellular matrix), myofibroblasts may then persist, leading to pathological conditions characterized by excessive scarring

extracellular matrix. When the stimulus driving the response to injury persists in internal organs, excessive deposition of extracellular matrix then leads to organ fibrosis. As is observed in pathological healing in the skin, the occurrence of fibrosis and its chronic nature may be a consequence of an imbalance between matrix deposition and matrix degradation. The mechanism underlying this is most likely an imbalance in the levels of MMPs and their inhibitors, TIMPs.

Hypertrophic scars and keloids are both characterized by an abnormal accumulation of extracellular matrix; however, they represent two very different cutaneous pathologies. In the case of hypertrophic scars, these do not extend beyond the periphery of the lesion, while keloids do extend beyond the margins of the original lesion. α-Smooth muscle-positive myofibroblasts are abundant in hypertrophic scars, and these cells contract, inducing retraction of the scar, particularly when the scar tissue is located in a region that is subjected to mechanical tension. This is particularly the case when the scar is adjacent to joints including the shoulders, elbows, wrists, knees, and ankles. Conversely, retraction does not occur in keloids. The development of hypertrophic scars is frequently observed after severe burns, and it appears that prolonged inflammation contributes to the increased risk of hypertrophic scarring. Conversely chronic wounds, such as venous leg ulcers, can also show prolonged inflammation with the mixture of pro-inflammatory cytokines and MMPs leading to a failure of matrix deposition and repair. It is therefore suggested that after cleansing of the wound, treatment should be aimed at producing the most rapid recovery possible with the aim of limiting the time spent in the inflammatory stage of healing.

The Role of Mechanical Tension

Due to both their contractile nature and their intimate relationship with the extracellular matrix, myofibroblasts are sensitive to their mechanical environment, and mechanical signaling has been shown to play important roles in regulating the activity of myofibroblasts [10]. Differentiation markers of myofibroblasts, including stress fibers, ED-A fibronectin, and α-smooth muscle actin expression, appear earlier in granulation tissue that is subjected to increased mechanical tension. This has been shown in experiments using splinting of a full-thickness wound with a plastic frame and comparing this to unsplinted, normally healing granulation tissue. Additionally, mechanical forces can be altered by culturing fibroblasts on substrates of varying stiffness, and these experiments have shown alterations in fibroblast phenotype dependent on substrate compliance. In culture, fibroblasts grown on soft, compliant substrates do not show stress fiber expression, while increasing the stiffness of the substrate induces a rapid change in morphology and the appearance of stress fibers. In cultured fibroblasts, shear forces, from movement of fluid, are also able to increase TGF-β1 synthesis and thus stimulate fibroblast differentiation to a myofibroblast phenotype. Shear forces are able to affect fibroblast differentiation in the absence of other stimuli that are normally involved in their differentiation, for example, exposure to cytokines or pre-straining of the extracellular matrix which regulates TGF-β1 bioavailability. As mentioned above, the role of mechanical stress in stimulating myofibroblast activity has also been shown in experiments using mechanically stressed skin wounds in mice. These wounds are stretched or splinted, resulting in an increased mechanical load that in turn increases myofibroblast activity and results in increased scar formation. These models to some extent mimic hypertrophic scarring that is sometimes observed in humans. The mechanical environment of the wound and the tension present are thus essential factors that need to be taken into account and managed in order to reduce scarring. To this end controlled immobilization of the wound should be employed. Interestingly, devices that manage the mechanical environment and tension of the wound are now appearing on the market (e.g., Embrace® from Neodyne Biosciences, Inc. or Zip® from ZipLine Medical, Inc.).

Role of Innervation in Skin Healing

Recently it has been shown that innervation of the skin plays an important role in both normal and pathological wound healing. However, the precise roles of sensory and autonomic innervation during wound healing remain to be clearly established [12]. Keratinocytes, melanocytes, fibroblasts, and myofibroblasts have all been shown to express a variety of neurotrophins including nerve growth factor, neurotophin-3, brain-derived neurotrophic factor, as well as their receptors, and these promote cellular proliferation and differentiation. Neuropeptides including calcitonin gene-related peptide, substance P, and vasoactive intestinal peptide are able to modulate the activity of MMP-2 and MMP-9, both of which play important roles in granulation tissue remodeling and scar formation. Additionally, these neuropeptides also act on collagen type I and type III synthesis during skin wound healing, promoting dermal fibroblast adhesion and their differentiation into myofibroblasts. The effects of these neuropeptides on the composition of the extracellular matrix and its organization are certainly essential since it is well-established that the mechanical microenvironment, which is dependent on the organization of the extracellular matrix, can affect fibroblast to myofibroblast differentiation. Lastly, regulation of MMPs can also affect the subsequent activation of latent TGF-β1 which involves MMPs.

Injury to the skin induces the release of a number of inflammatory mediators, from both immune cells and sensory nerve endings. These include interleukin-1β, tumor necrosis factor-α, bradykinin, substance P, calcitonin gene-related peptide, nerve growth factor, and prostaglandins, and their release by these cells contributes to the "inflammatory soup" present in the wound. It has been suggested that changes in substance P levels may be involved in the aberrant wound-healing response seen in hypertrophic scarring. Furthermore, it has been observed that in cocultures of fibroblasts and neurites, the direct contact of these cells is able to induce myofibroblast differentiation leading to increased retraction of collagen lattices, mimicking the contraction seen in wound repair.

In keloids, nerve fiber density is significantly higher than in normal skin samples, and symptoms including itch, pain, abnormal thermal sensory thresholds to heat as well as cold, and pain associated with heat sensation are all reported suggesting the involvement of small nerve fibers in the pathogenesis of this disease. In hypertrophic scars, published data are inconsistent with either a decrease or an increase of the number nerve fibers having been reported. Nevertheless, in burn patients with chronic pain, abnormal cutaneous innervation has been reported. A recent pilot study has been published which compared healthy skin versus postburn scars from the same patient [2]. These authors examined the expression of genes involved in regulation of innervation and additionally looked at the intraepidermal density of nerve endings. Significant differences in the patterns of expression were observed when comparing healthy skin and postburn scars. Based on studies of a mouse model of hypertrophic scarring induced by mechanical loading, it has been suggested that innervation of the skin and the level of inflammation present may both play roles in the development of hypertrophic scars.

The role of the sensory nervous system in wound healing in the skin has been examined using several animal models of denervation. Surgical denervation has been employed, as has chemical denervation, and mice with genetic modifications resulting in denervation have also been used. Studies using surgical denervation have shown that wound healing is retarded in these animals, with a reduction observed in the number of inflammatory cells infiltrating the wound, delayed contraction of the wound, and a delay in reepithelialization. Another skin denervation model, which used chemical sympathectomy induced by intraperitoneal administration of 6-hydroxydopamine, also showed that denervation interfered with wound healing. 6-Hydroxydopamine-induced sympathectomy has also been shown to modify wound healing with an increase in wound contraction, a reduction in mast cell migration and delayed reepithelialization. These alterations in healing are associated with a decrease in neurogenic inflammation. Lastly, these studies have definitively shown that neuropeptides released by sensory fibers play an important role during wound healing, affecting the granulation tissue in particular.

Therapeutic Options

It has been recently shown, in human pulmonary fibrosis, that mechanical stretching of tissue can contribute to the development of fibrosis via mechanical activation of TGF-β1 [5]. Stretching of the extracellular matrix in the lungs, due either to breathing or to mechanical ventilation that is employed to support breathing in cases of lung injury or lung disease, may contribute to TGF-β1-driven disease progression. Since it is not possible to stop breathing to avoid mechanical TGF-β1 activation from established fibrotic tissue, therapeutic intervention might however be possible aimed at the cellular side of mechanical TGF-β1 activation. Thus, in organs that are subjected to mechanical stress, such as the lungs and skin, the role of TGF-β1 in excessive scarring and fibrosis is clearly crucial, and the mechanisms involved in activation of TGF-β1 represent an important therapeutic target.

The presence and activity of fibroblasts is vital for normal skin homeostasis, while the presence of myofibroblasts is crucial for tissue repair and has evolved to speed the process of normal tissue repair [1]. The importance of fibroblast activity in normal repair has been very well documented using in vitro models of dermal substitutes. For example, a living dermal equivalent (containing fibroblasts) that has been applied to skin graft beds was found to reduce pain, improve hemostasis, and also improve the mechanical and cosmetic properties of the graft, in particular, producing a normal undulating dermal-epidermal junction by 3–4 months after grafting and also leading to the presence of elastic fibers, which were detectable 6–9 months after grafting. Therefore, it seems apparent that tissue engineering approaches to normal repair require fibroblasts and myofibroblasts to be effective [7]. It is, however, very important to keep in mind that many different populations of fibroblasts exist and that these have different properties. These recent observations thus offer new perspectives for skin repair and for tissue engineering. In addition, promotion of normal reinnervation and adequate levels of neuropeptides during the healing process certainly appear to be crucial for improving skin healing and to avoid the occurrence of pathological repair processes and scarring [13]. Despite the existence of many areas that still require elucidation in myofibroblast biology, it seems clear that myofibroblasts are pivotal cells for the control of extracellular matrix deposition and remodeling during normal repair and are also important in pathological conditions such as excessive scarring. Myofibroblasts thus definitively represent an essential target to be considered when developing new therapeutic strategies.

Conclusion

Myofibroblasts are key cells during wound healing. It has become increasingly evident that a lack of myofibroblast apoptosis is a major mechanism leading to excessive scarring [11]. Blocking pro-survival mechanisms, particularly those linked to the mechanical environment, and modifying the myofibroblast phenotype to obtain cells able to remodel the excessive deposition of extracellular matrix certainly represent new ways to develop therapeutic options that could positively modulate scar formation.

Take-Home Messages

- Myofibroblasts play a major role during granulation tissue formation with transforming growth factor-β1 being the main soluble factor involved in myofibroblastic differentiation.
- Myofibroblasts, through mechanotransduction pathways, are very sensitive to their mechanical environment.
- Myofibroblast apoptosis and extracellular matrix remodeling are necessary for normal scar formation.
- Abnormal mechanical tension facilitates the development of hypertrophic scars.
- Normal innervation and neuropeptide secretion are necessary to maintain skin homeostasis and normal wound healing.

References

1. Bochaton-Piallat ML, Gabbiani G, Hinz B. The myofibroblast in wound healing and fibrosis: answered and unanswered questions. F1000Res. 2016;5:pii: F1000 Faculty Rev-752. https://doi.org/10.12688/f1000research.8190.1. eCollection 2016.
2. Buhé V, Trimaille A, Schollhammer M, Morvan F, Hu W, Egles C, Desmoulière A, Misery L. Heterogeneity of skin re-innervation after burns and factors involved in its regulation: a pilot study. Acta Derm Venereol. 2018;98(2):280–1. https://doi.org/10.2340/00015555-2826.
3. Darby IA, Laverdet B, Bonté F, Desmoulière A. Fibroblasts and myofibroblasts in wound healing. Clin Cosmet Investig Dermatol. 2014;7:301–11. https://doi.org/10.2147/CCID.S50046.
4. Darby IA, Zakuan N, Billet F, Desmoulière A. The myofibroblast, a key cell in normal and pathological tissue repair. Cell Mol Life Sci. 2016;73(6):1145–57. https://doi.org/10.1007/s00018-015-2110-0.
5. Froese AR, Shimbori C, Bellaye PS, Inman M, Obex S, Fatima S, Jenkins G, Gauldie J, Ask K, Kolb M. Stretch-induced activation of transforming growth factor-β1 in pulmonary fibrosis. Am J Respir Crit Care Med. 2016;194(1):84–96. https://doi.org/10.1164/rccm.201508-1638OC.
6. Girard D, Laverdet D, Desmoulière A. (Myo)fibroblasts and extracellular matrix in skin wound and aging. In: Quan T, editor. Skin aging and skin disorders. Boca Raton: Science Publishers; 2016. p. 41–60.
7. Girard D, Laverdet B, Buhé V, Trouillas M, Ghazi K, Alexaline MM, Egles C, Misery L, Coulomb B, Lataillade JJ, Berthod F, Desmoulière A. Biotechnological management of skin burn injuries: challenges and perspectives in wound healing and sensory recovery. Tissue Eng Part B Rev. 2017;23(1):59–82. https://doi.org/10.1089/ten.TEB.2016.0195.
8. Godbout C, Follonier Castella L, Smith EA, Talele N, Chow ML, Garonna A, Hinz B. The mechanical environment modulates intracellular calcium oscillation activities of myofibroblasts. PLoS One. 2013;8(5):e64560. https://doi.org/10.1371/journal.pone.0064560.
9. Hinz B, Phan SH, Thannickal VJ, Prunotto M, Desmoulière A, Varga J, De Wever O, Mareel M, Gabbiani G. Recent developments in myofibroblast biology: paradigms for connective tissue remodeling. Am J Pathol. 2012;180(4):1340–55. https://doi.org/10.1016/j.ajpath.2012.02.004.
10. Hinz B. The extracellular matrix and transforming growth factor-β1: tale of a strained relationship. Matrix Biol. 2015;47:54–65. https://doi.org/10.1016/j.matbio.2015.05.006.
11. Hinz B, Lagares D. Evasion of apoptosis by myofibroblasts: a hallmark of fibrotic diseases. Nat Rev Rheumatol. 2020;16(1):11–31. https://doi.org/10.1038/s41584-019-0324-5.
12. Laverdet B, Danigo A, Girard D, Magy L, Demiot C, Desmoulière A. Skin innervation: important roles during normal and pathological cutaneous repair. Histol Histopathol. 2015;30(8):875–92. https://doi.org/10.14670/HH-11-610.
13. Lebonvallet N, Laverdet B, Misery L, Desmoulière A, Girard D. New insights into the roles of myofibroblasts and innervation during skin healing and innovative therapies to improve scar innervation. Exp Dermatol. 2018;27(9):950–8. https://doi.org/10.1111/exd.13681.
14. Micallef L, Vedrenne N, Billet F, Coulomb B, Darby IA, Desmoulière A. The myofibroblast, multiple origins for major roles in normal and pathological tissue repair. Fibrogenesis Tissue Repair. 2012;5(Suppl 1):S5. https://doi.org/10.1186/1755-1536-5-S1-S5.
15. Pakshir P, Hinz B. The big five in fibrosis: macrophages, myofibroblasts, matrix, mechanics, and miscommunication. Matrix Biol. 2018;68–69:81–93. https://doi.org/10.1016/j.matbio.2018.01.019.
16. Rodrigues M, Kosaric N, Bonham CA, Gurtner GC. Wound healing: a cellular perspective. Physiol Rev. 2019;99(1):665–706. https://doi.org/10.1152/physrev.00067.2017.
17. Sarrazy V, Billet F, Micallef L, Coulomb B, Desmoulière A. Mechanisms of pathological scarring: role of myofibroblasts and current developments. Wound Repair Regen. 2011;19(Suppl 1):s10–5. https://doi.org/10.1111/j.1524-475X.2011.00708.x.
18. Zent J, Guo LW. Signaling mechanisms of myofibroblastic activation: outside-in and inside-out. Cell Physiol Biochem. 2018;49(3):848–68. https://doi.org/10.1159/000493217.

30

Treatment of Immature Scars with Botulinum Toxin

Alexandra Chambers

Contents

Background

Botulinum toxin type A (BoNTA) and occasionally of serotype B has been used for treatment of conditions associated with muscle spasm, hyperhidrosis and improving appearance of static rhytides.

The same neuronal effects and a muscle tension reduction at the site of injury were initially attributed to the benefits of BoNTA in a scar formation. However, a more detailed research into effects of BoNTA on wound healing suggested a variety of biologic effects of the toxin. New possibilities emerged for using BoNTA to modify early tissue repair mechanisms to promote more favourable outcomes and less noticeable scars.

Chapter Introduction

The Botulinum toxin A (BoNTA), and to a lesser degree type B (BoNTB), is used in clinical practice for the treatment of conditions associated with muscle spasms. The therapeutic indications include cervical dystonia, blepharospasm, strabismus, chronic migraine, and severe axillary hyperhidrosis. BoNTA is also approved for esthetic use in the treatment of facial wrinkles such as "crow's feet" and frown lines. In addition, there are many unlicensed off-label uses of BoNTA for the treatment of various other conditions.

The demand for BoNTA products is rapidly expanding due to ever-increasing esthetic applications, and there is a plethora of BoNTA formulations available across global markets. This can make it difficult to identify an adequate product for any specific application.

The most popular and well-tested products are Botox (onabotulinumtoxinA) and Vistabel (specifically for esthetic applications) that are manufactured by Allergan (USA). Dysport (abobotulinumtoxinA), marketed as Azzalure for cosmetic applications, is made by Ipsen Ltd. (UK) and Galderma Laboratories (USA). Xeomin (incobotulinumtoxinA) and its esthetic brand, Bocouture, are made by Merz Pharmaceutical (Germany).

Less known preparations include Evosyal made by Puretox (USA) and Linurase made by Phiderma (Canada). BoNTB preparations such as Myobloc (rimabotulinumtoxinB) are marketed by Solstice Neurosciences (USA). Other BoNTA products are available in Asian and Russian markets.

Although normally injected into the skin layer, several products for the topical delivery of BoNTA have become available recently. Examples include ANT-1207 (Anterios/Allergan), CosmeTox (USA), and RT001 (Revance, USA).

Each BoNTA product has a Botulinum toxin combined with a variety of other complex proteins, and each manufacturer uses a different assay to determine the potency of their batches. These differences make it difficult to compare clinical responses across products.

Recent studies have shown that BoNTA improves the appearance of established scars and can also positively affect the early stages of tissue healing for a more favorable mature scar. This chapter examines evidence of the BoNTA effects on early stages of scar formation and describes how this can be employed for controlling scar development as it occurs. Practical guidance on optimal doses of injections and on treatment protocols is described and evaluated. Choices of the BoNTA preparations used for immature scar treatment are also discussed.

Botulinum Exotoxin, Structure, and Mechanism of Action

Botulinum neurotoxin (BoNT) is an exotoxin of *Clostridium Botulinum* bacteria, which has several serotypes. In clinical practice, the serotypes A (BoNTA) and B (BoNTB) are most used for therapeutic, experimental, and esthetic purposes; however, due to their superior longevity of action, preparations of BoNTA have become the most popular.

Structure of BoNTA

The BoNTA molecule is made of a heavy (100 kDa) and a light (50kDA) polypeptide chain, linked together by a disulfide bond. The neurotoxin complex also includes associated nontoxic proteins: three hemagglutinin (HA) proteins and one non-HA protein. These play a role in transporting and protecting the toxin core.

Neuronal Mechanism of Action of BoNTA and Effects on Immature Scars

BoNTA impairs release of acetylcholine by disabling a soluble N-ethylmaleimide-sensitive factor attachment receptor (SNARE) protein. The latter facilitates acetylcholine release by mediating docking and fusion of synaptic vesicles with the inner surface of the axonal membrane at the sites of release.

BoNTA adheres by its heavy chain to cholinergic cell membrane surface structures such as ganglioside moieties, a vesicular protein (SV2) and synaptotagmin. Its light chain enters the neuronal terminal and reaches the cytosol (vesicles). It cleaves SNARE proteins: synaptosomal-associated protein (SNAP)-25, syntaxin, and vesicle-associated membrane protein (VAMP) also known as synaptobrevin II. The acetylcholine release into the synaptic cleft is impaired and the cholinergic mediation of neurons is blocked. Furthermore, BoNTA has also been shown to impair release of other neurotransmitters, such as glutamate, substance P (SP), and calcitonin gene-related peptide (CGRP).

The absence of the necessary mediator leads to a "chemical denervation" and temporary atrophy of the neuromuscular junction with a subsequent block of muscle contraction or reduction of exocrine glandular secretion.

Several studies involving animal and human subjects have tried to determine how reducing muscle contractility in the immediate vicinity to a fresh wound improves the esthetic result in scars. To date, findings have been inconclusive.

Immobilization of underlying musculature, reducing tension of the wound and skin (similar to the use of a surgical Z-plasty), has resulted in more favorable scarring according to Ziade M et al. (2013). Patients in this research were injected within 3 days following facial surgery, and results were assessed using a visual analogue scale. However, no statistically significant differences were found between the two groups in this study when using other assessment methods [1].

In another example of effects of BoNTA on the early stages of wound healing, researchers Lee B-J et al. (2009) [2] used a rat wound model. In this study, each of 15 animals was its own control. The results showed significant differences in wound size between BoNT-treated and untreated control wounds. Also observed were less infiltration of inflammatory cells, fewer fibroblasts, and a lower expression of transforming growth factor (TGF)-β1 (as compared to the control wounds).

TGF-β1 is a cytokine that has multiple mediatory actions in tissue healing, and it is involved in the formation of fibrotic tissue and hypertrophic scars. The finding that BoNT-treated wounds show a lower amount of TGF-β1 may be the result of the chemoimmobilization of the muscle as well as of a direct effect of BoNTA on the expression of TGF-β1 in fibroblasts and fibroblast proliferation.

It is known that a muscle paralysis due to the inhibition of acetylcholine exocytosis is reversible by natural SNARE protein recovery. After application of BoNTA, it takes 2 weeks to 4 months for neurotransmission to recover. Therefore, its period of action is definitely within the timeframe of early scar formation. Nevertheless, the effects of BoNTA on tissues are more complex than just reducing tension and decreasing TGF-β1.

Nonneuronal Mechanisms of Action of BoNTA and Effects on Immature Scars

More research into Botulinum toxin demonstrates that its biological effects on various cells and tissues are much more complex than previously understood [3]. The BoNT receptors and intracellular targets are not unique for neurotransmission, as several of these receptors and targets have been found in neuronal and nonneuronal cells.

BoNTA, for example, can attach to some other cell-surface proteins and, through them, modulate the function of a variety of human cell types [3]. These proteins include E-cadherin, fibroblast growth factor receptor 3 (FGFR3), and vanilloid receptors. Indeed, epidermal keratinocytes, dermal fibroblasts, sebocytes and vascular endothelial cells, adipocyte-derived mesenchymal stem cells, and many other cells including macrophages and neutrophils have receptors capable of binding and cleaving the BoNTA molecule. Therefore, the effects of BoNTA at the nonneuronal level have an impact on inflammatory and immunological cascades, neurosensory signaling, cellular inhibition and proliferation, vascular and tissue differentiation, and growth (or atrophy). Familiarity with these effects is useful in understanding how BoNTA is helpful for tissue healing and scar development.

Effects of BoNTA on the Inflammatory Cascade

Both pro- and anti-inflammatory effects by BoNTA have been demonstrated in animal models and cell cultures. Those effects are expressed on additional binding sites for BoNTA and its carrier proteins. These have been identified at the RMS 13 receptor sites of skeletal muscle cells, TIB-152 of lymphoblasts, Detroit 551 of fibroblasts, and SH-SY5Y of neuronal cells. BoNTA alone does not induce inflammatory responses; it only does so in a complex with the Neurotoxin Associated Protein (NAP). The latter is responsible for the release of pro-inflammatory cytokines such as IL-6, IL-8, MCP-1, and TNF- α at these sites [4]. This last reference suggests that it is NAP that determines the pro-inflammatory effects of BoNTA at the time of the toxin application.

The inflammatory phase of a wound healing lasts approximately 2–4 days. It is marked by an abundant release of cytokines, growth factors (such as platelet-derived growth factor (PDGF)), interleukin-1 and interleukin-8 (IL-1 and IL-8), chemokines, and hormones. These all work to sustain activation of the target cells and promote migration of the inflammatory cells.

PDGF and transforming growth factor-β (TGF-β) released by Alpha granules of platelets attract neutrophils and macrophages. The latter scavenges the wound site, and the former produces transforming growth factor (TGF), tissue growth factor-α (TGF-α), and epidermal growth factor (EGF). These give rise to fibroblast and keratinocyte migration, signaling the start of the proliferative phase of healing.

Once the heavy and light chains of BoNTA have reached their targets, inflammation starts downscaling. They reduce lymphocyte proliferation and migration and decrease cytokine expression. This is seen a few days after wounds have been treated with BoNTA [2, 3].

BoNTA has also demonstrated the ability to decrease inflammatory enzyme cyclooxigenase-2 (COX-2) and prostaglandin E2 receptors [5] in animal models and cell cultures. It also decreases the infiltration of monocytes and macrophages while blocking expression of interleukins-1B (IL-1β). Moreover, it is able to suppress nitric oxide and tumor necrosis factor-α (TNF-α) via inhibition of specialist receptors on macrophages [6].

Inflammation in tissues is often associated with pain and itching. BoNTA reduces pain by local muscle spasm relief and by blocking cholinergic and other neuropeptide sensory transmission. However, it is now known that BoNTA has effects at sites distant to the injection location, as well as at a central level. In addition to the local uptake of BoNTA in the synaptic terminal, a distinct retrograde transport pathway results in accumulation of BoNT toward the neuronal soma. This retrograde channeling facilitates remote action of BoNTA at the dorsal root ganglion and the spinal cord, and it is believed to explain the efficacy of BoNTA used for the control of pain [7]. In addition to neurons, the glial cells such as Swann's and astrocytes are also receptive to BoNTA, which suggests yet another pain modulation mechanism.

BoNTA also has been shown to reduce infiltration by cutaneous lymphocytes and decrease acanthosis, processes associated with intense itching (most commonly mediated by histamine). BoNTA affects chemotaxis of mast cells, affecting their migration and histamine release and IL-4 expression. The histamine acts as the main mediator of H1-H4 receptors, responsible for activation of the target molecules within the sensory neurons that code pruritic signals. BoNTA also downregulates transient receptor potential channel type V1 (TRPV1) and type A (TRPA1), responsible for histamine-mediated and non-histamine-dependent itch, respectively [8].

It is believed that the ability of BoNTA to moderate a florid inflammatory response and control itch and pain may explain its off-label use in treating scar hypertrophy and keloid formation. A recent double-blind randomized study concluded that BoNTA was as effective as steroids when injected into keloid scars, but patients additionally reported the alleviation of pain and itching after use of the former [9].

In experiments, BoNTA has demonstrated properties inhibiting the overgrowth of a variety of cells, including malignant proliferation in breast, prostate, and colon cancers. It has been theorized that this is the same mechanism as the one that provides its inhibitory effects on fibroblast proliferation. This has motivated the use of BoNTA on the unchecked growth of the cells leading to keloid deposition.

Effects of BoNTA on Fibroblasts and Keratinocytes

BoNTA has a direct effect on dermal cells such as fibroblasts and keratinocytes and through them can positively mediate dermal tissue remodeling. This is an important characteristic for reversing the effects of skin aging, assisting in wound epithelization, and reducing scar formations.

Fibroblasts and their differentiated subset, myofibroblasts, are the main components of the proliferation phase in wound healing. The transforming growth factor-beta 1(TGF-β1) prompts some of the fibroblasts to differentiate into myofibroblasts, possessing a retractile protein alpha-SM (α-SM), similar to those in smooth muscle cells. Myofibroblasts create bridging connections and promote the approximation and retraction of wounds. They do this by creating a matrix that further promotes the migration of additional fibroblasts and keratinocytes [10]. BoNTA seems to interrupt the differentiation of fibroblasts to myofibroblasts by blocking TGF-β1 signaling and in so doing reduces excessive wound retraction and scar thickening [11].

Fibroblasts are also responsible for angiogenesis in a healing wound. This is mediated by fibroblast growth factor (FGF) and vascular endothelial growth factor (VEGF), both of which also promote epithelization and collagen synthesis. Epithelial growth will happen either from the basement membrane or from the edges of the wound by migrating keratinocytes. BoNTA acts to increase migration, proliferation, and differentiation of keratinocytes and the expression of epidermal growth factor (EGF). Collagen type III is mainly produced in this stage, actively promoted by IL4 mediators. Subsequently collagen type III degrades, and it is replaced by collagen type I with reorganized orientation of the fibers. This adds strength to the resulting scar.

BoNTA influences the ratio of collagen I to collagen III by increasing or inhibiting its degradation by matrix metalloproteinases (MMPs) [12]. Excess of collagen synthesis by fibroblasts can determine scar hypertrophy and keloid formation, whereas lack of collagen matrix can predispose to a weak scar with atrophy [13].

Effects of BoNTA on Vascular Endothelium

BoNTA has been shown to have protective effects on dermal flap survival in animal models even with adverse conditions such as nicotine exposure, oxidative stress, or preexisting diabetes. BoNTA reduced accumulation of reactive oxygen species and prevented oxidative damage to endothelial cells. It increased the blood flow in dermal vasculature by dilating lumen of the blood vessels. The model skin flaps also had increased production of vascular endothelial growth factor (VEG) and expression of platelet endothelial cell adhesion molecules 1, CD31 and CD34 lymphocyte subsets, interleukin (IL)-1, and tumor necrosis factor (TNF) [14].

Clinical Application of BoNTA for Treatment of Scars

The time frames of the various stages of wound healing are not precise and can be overlapping. The vascular stage lasts for roughly 24 to 48 hours after trauma, and the inflammatory phase runs 2 to 4 days. The proliferative phase starts from roughly day 3, peaks around day 7, and finishes after 2 to 4 weeks. Finally, scar maturation (often referred to as remodeling) can take up to 12 months.

The usefulness of BoNTA in the management of immature scars (by definition, less than a year old) can be summarized as follows:

- Reduces local muscle contractility, allowing better approximation of the edges of healing wounds
- Moderates the inflammatory response at the site of the injury via suppression of inflammatory cytokines and neuropeptides
- Reduces pain and itching in healing wounds (these effects can be both peripheral at the site of the scar and central through a retrograde uptake of the toxin)
- Inhibits excessive proliferation of fibroblasts and their increased differentiation under TGF-β1 into myofibroblasts and so downgrades the over-proliferative scarring and retraction of the wound bed
- Mediates MMP enzymatic activity in controlling expression of collagen fibers, optimizing collagen I to III ratios, and preventing fibrosis and scar thickening

Timing of BoNTA Injections

The most efficacious timing of BoNTA application remains to be determined. For example, some researchers advocate injecting the toxin before surgery [15, 16] for better titration of BoNTA dose and improving local circulation via inhibition of norepinephrine. In other studies, BoNTA have been applied intraoperatively [17] at the time of wound closure or within the first 24 hours [2, 18–20]. Several clinicians have reported using the toxin after 72 hours [1], while others injected BoNTA at the time of suture removal (7 to10 days) [21]. In another study, BoNTA was only used at the time of a scar revision [22].

As can be seen, there are a wide variety of protocols proposed in the literature for the timing of BoNTA injections. That said, in the context of the discussion in Sect. 2, there are good reasons to prefer a single, early application of BoNTA from the onset of an injury. This timing is the one that has the best potential of benefitting from all the additional effects of BoNTA.

Choosing BoNTA Preparation

The majority of published studies have used BoNTA preparations, including ona-, abo-, and incobotulinumtoxinA. However, BoNTB had been reported to also have beneficial results in wounds healing in a study involving facial reconstruction surgery [17]. Most other published studies use BoNTA, namely, the brand preparations such as Botox, Dysport, and Xeomin. Quantitative reporting on conversions of BoNTA unit rate and levels of toxin spreading is mainly based on these three products. Given the availability of the data, it would seem prudent to continue using the well-tested products when planning a scar treatment.

Reconstituting BoNTA

Currently BoNTA preparations are manufactured in lyophilized powder form. There have been some attempts at creating liquid preparations; however, these are not widely available.

Normal saline is most commonly used for the reconstitution of the toxin. Gassner et al. (2000) [18] have recommended mixing BoNTA with lidocaine and epinephrine, the former for immediate efferent block and the latter for the reduction of toxin diffusion.

Preparing BoNTA with bacteriostatic normal saline (BNS) reduces the discomfort of injections. Various dilution proportions have been tried, but the most common volume of saline used per 100 U of BoNTA was 1.5 to 2.5 ml. For keloid and large surface scars, the volume of BNS can be doubled.

Dose of BoNTA for Scar Treatment

A dose titration for a novel application of any medicine is always a challenge, and the amount of BoNTA required for the treatment of scars seems to be much lower than traditional doses used for immobilizing muscles and treating wrinkles. The most popular BoNTA doses tried in various studies have been 5 U [21], 7 U [18, 19], and 10 U [2]. In the main, however, these studies do not provide a rationale for their choices.

One reference, however, performs a preliminary systematic study of BoNTA dosages to determine optimum outcomes. Quantities of 5 U, 15 U, and 25 U of BoNTA were used on the postoperative wounds of rhytidectomy patients [20]. For the specific approach of this study, the best results were obtained with the use of about 15 units of BoNTA. That said results might vary significantly if other parameters are adopted. Facets that could be investigated going forward could include modifying the injection protocol. For example, these results suggest that increasing the number of injection points might achieve a more uniform reduction in scar width.

This last study seems to correlate to in vitro experiments demonstrating the dose dependencies of keratinocytes and endothelial cell function when subjected to the effects of BoNTA [25]. Doses lower than 20 units were found to support proliferation of endothelial cells but higher than 20 units impaired keratinocyte and endothelial migration and growth, these being responsible for epithelization and angiogenesis, respectively.

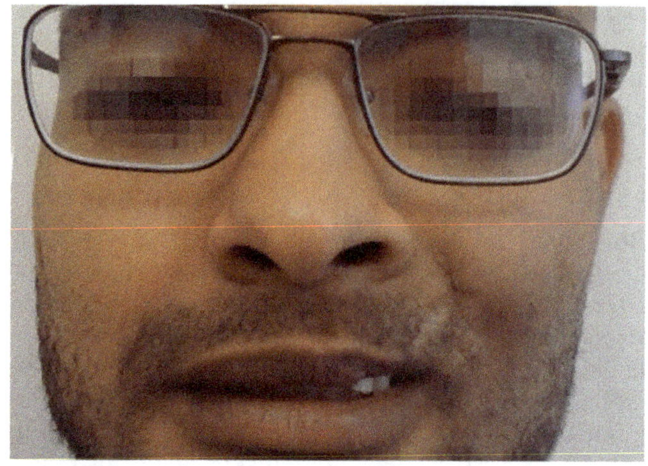

◘ **Fig.** A post-traumatic hypertrophic scar, restricting articu-lation of the patient

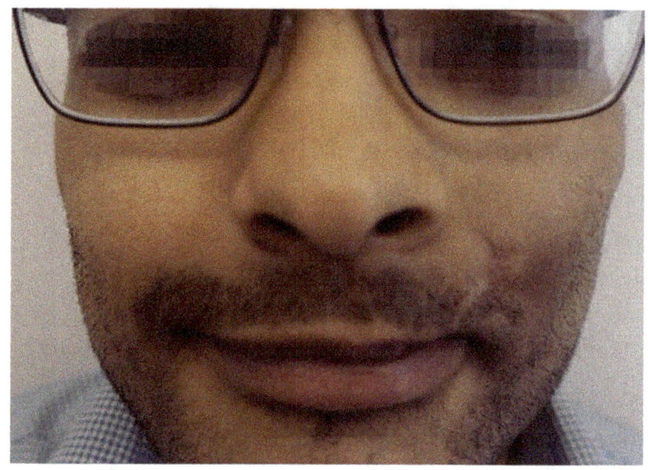

◘ **Fig.** The scar is reduced in size and more pliable following a single session of BoNTA injections

BoNTA for Treatment of Keloid and Hypertrophic Scars

The treatment of pathologically healed wounds such as keloid and hypertrophic scars is a difficult and often fruitless task. BoNTA has demonstrated some promising results for reducing stiffness, hardness, and pain characteristic for these types of scars; see ◘ Figs. 26.1 and 26.2.

Studies based on repeated monthly application of BoNTA, involving multiple injections of the toxin covering the entire surface of a scar, have shown some effectiveness [23, 24]. In these cases, the maximum concentration of 35 U was diluted to enable full coverage of the scar area. The injection volume was reduced into a microdroplet to ensure distribution was mainly in the skin and the superficial muscle layer [24].

Summary of Practical Guidelines for the Application of BoNTA in the Treatment of Scars

In summary, a practical clinical approach for the treatment of scars is to administer BoNTA reconstituted in 1.5 to 2.5 ml of bacteriostatic normal saline (BNS). Injections should be made using a superficial intradermal technique. The expectation is that the toxin will travel in the vertical and horizontal plane, reaching superficial muscles and even distant central locations by retrograde uptake. Leaving a 1 cm margin from the freshly sutured wound (see ◘ Fig. 26.3) and 1 cm between injection points (see ◘ Fig. 26.4) would seem to be adequate based on reported BoNTA diffusion distances. The total dose of BoNTA should remain below 20 U. A one-off treatment is likely sufficient to promote better healing of the wound and to achieve more favorable scarring.

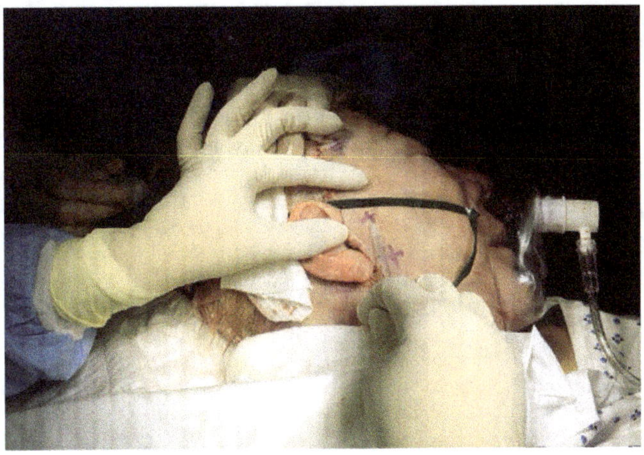

Fig. BoNTA is injected immediately after closure of the facelift wound, about 1 cm anterior to the margin

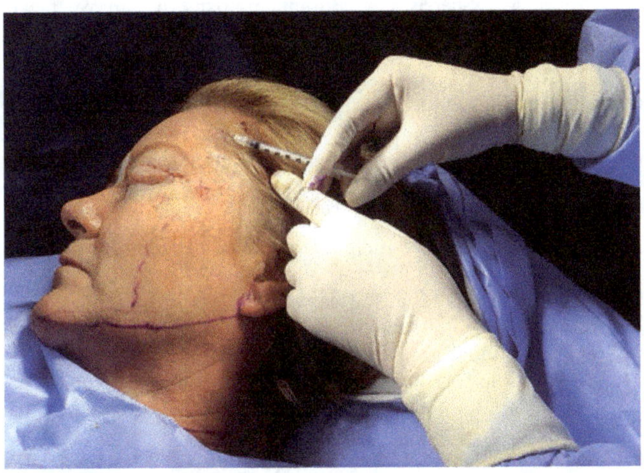

Fig. BoNTA injections spaced evenly 1 cm apart after upper blepharoplasty and eyebrow lift surgery

For scars already displaying features of keloid or hypertrophic change, reconstituting 20 U of BoNTA in 3 to 5 ml of BNS is recommended. An example of this is shown in Fig. 26.5. Injections, delivered in microdroplets, should be applied to cover the whole surface of a pathological scar (similar to a mesotherapy technique). Monthly repeated treatments, consisting of three to eight sessions, are advised.

Conclusions

The scope of using of Botulinum toxin for various conditions is ever expanding, and the benefits it provides for tissue healing and immature scar management are gaining recognition and acceptance. Clearly, the complex effects of BoNTA on various cells and tissues are still

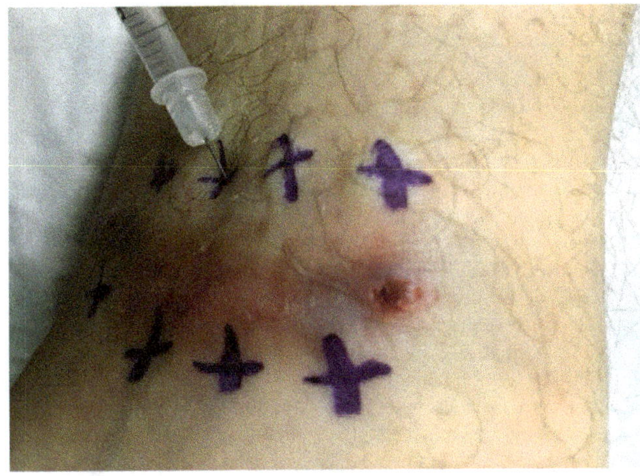

Fig. BoNTA injections should cover the entire surface of the early keloid scar and the adjacent normal skin

not fully understood, and we continue to discover more about its full range of biological effects and useful applications. This chapter concludes with a description of practical approaches for the use of BoNTA in managing scarring in a clinical environment.

Take Home Message

- Effects of BoNTA on wound healing are multifaceted and not restricted just to the underlying muscles relaxation and a wound tension reduction. The toxin exerts influence on various cells and tissues involved in tissue repair following an injury. BoNTA can alter inflammatory reactions, cellular proliferation, mediation and inhibition
- Early application of BoNTA, within 24–72 hours of initial injury seems to ensure a less conspicuous scar
- All well known commercially available BoNTA preparations seem to be effective for that purpose
- A dose of 15 -20 units of BoNTA demonstrated to be sufficient to benefit for a wound of a traditional rhytidectomy length (15–20 cm). The preparation injected in equal amounts of 1–5 U spaced evenly along the length of the wound 1cm from the border. Injection points can be spaced either along the both sides of the wound or a just unilaterally.
- Dilution of the BoNTA for wound treatment was 1.5 -2 ml of Bacteriostatic Normal Saline for 100 u of the Botox (or equivalent in case of other products). For larger surface wounds BoNTA could be diluted in a double amount of saline to provide a sufficient volume for coverage, as the dose of up to 20 u is still applicable in these cases

References

1. Ziade M, Domergue S, Batifol D, Jreige R, Sebbane M, Goudot P, Yachouh J. Use of botulinum toxin type a to improve treatment of facial wounds: a prospective randomised study. J Plast Reconstr Aesthet Surg. 2013;66(2):209–14.
2. Lee BJ, Jeong JH, Wang SG, Lee JC, Goh EK, Kim HW. Effect of botulinum toxin type a on a rat surgical wound model. Clin Experiment Otorhinolaryngol. 2009;2(1):20.
3. Grando SA, Zachary CB. The non-neuronal and nonmuscular effects of botulinum toxin: an opportunity for a deadly molecule to treat disease in the skin and beyond. Br J Dermatol. 2018;178(5):1011–9.
4. Wang L, Sun Y, Yang W, Lindo P, Singh BR. Type a botulinum neurotoxin complex proteins differentially modulate host response of neuronal cells. Toxicon. 2014;82:52–60.
5. Chuang YC, Yoshimura N, Huang CC, Wu M, Chiang PH, Chancellor MB. Intravesical botulinum toxin a administration inhibits COX-2 and EP4 expression and suppresses bladder hyperactivity in cyclophosphamide-induced cystitis in rats. Eur Urol. 2009;56(1):159–67.
6. Yoo KY, Lee HS, Cho YK, Lim YS, Kim YS, Koo JH, Yoon SJ, Lee JH, Jang KH, Song SH. Anti-inflammatory effects of botulinum toxin type a in a complete Freund's adjuvant-induced arthritic knee joint of hind leg on rat model. Neurotox Res. 2014;26(1):32–9.
7. Fonfria E, Maignel J, Lezmi S, Martin V, Splevins A, Shubber S, Kalinichev M, Foster K, Picaut P, Krupp J. The expanding therapeutic utility of botulinum neurotoxins. Toxins. 2018;10(5):208.
8. Gazerani P. Antipruritic effects of botulinum neurotoxins. Toxins. 2018;10(4):143.
9. Shaarawy E, Hegazy RA, Abdel Hay RM. Intralesional botulinum toxin type a equally effective and better tolerated than intralesional steroid in the treatment of keloids: a randomized controlled trial. J Cosmet Dermatol. 2015;14(2):161–6.
10. Li B, Wang JH. Fibroblasts and myofibroblasts in wound healing: force generation and measurement. J Tissue Viability. 2011;20(4):108–20.
11. Lee SD, Yi MH, Kim DW, Lee Y, Choi Y, Oh SH. The effect of botulinum neurotoxin type a on capsule formation around silicone implants: the in vivo and in vitro study. Int Wound J. 2016;13(1):65–71.
12. Oh SH, Lee Y, Seo YJ, Lee JH, Yang JD, Chung HY, Cho BC. The potential effect of botulinum toxin type a on human dermal fibroblasts: an in vitro study. Dermatol Surg. 2012;38(10):1689–94.
13. Chambers A. Unified approach to the treatment of hypertrophic and atrophic scars: a pilot study. Am J Cosmet Surg. 2016;33(4):176–83.
14. Kim TK, Oh EJ, Chung JY, Park JW, Cho BC, Chung HY. The effects of botulinum toxin a on the survival of a random cutaneous flap. J Plast Reconstr Aesthet Surg. 2009;62(7):906–13.
15. Mahboub T, Ahmed Sobhi MD, Habashi H. Optomization of presurgical treatment with botulinum toxin in facial scar management. Egypt J Plast Reconstr Surg. 2006;30:81–6.
16. Lebeda FJ, Dembek ZF, Adler M. Kinetic and reaction pathway analysis in the application of botulinum toxin a for wound healing. Journal of toxicology. 2012;2012.
17. Flynn TC. Use of intraoperative botulinum toxin in facial reconstruction. Dermatol Surg. 2009;35(2):182–8.
18. Gassner HG, Sherris DA, Otley CC. Treatment of facial wounds with botulinum toxin a improves cosmetic outcome in primates. Plast Reconstr Surg. 2000;105(6):1948–53.
19. Gassner HG, Brissett AE, Otley CC, Boahene DK, Boggust AJ, Weaver AL, Sherris DA. Botulinum toxin to improve facial wound healing: a prospective, blinded, placebo-controlled study. In: Mayo clinic proceedings, vol. 81(8): Elsevier; 2006. p. 1023–8.
20. Chambers A. Effects of botulinum toxin a observed during early scar formation following Rhytidectomy: controlled, Double-Blinded Pilot Study. Am J Cosmet Surg. 2018;18:0748806818794528.
21. Goodman GJ. The use of botulinum toxin as primary or adjunctive treatment for post acne and traumatic scarring. J Cutan Aesthet Surg. 2010;3(2):90.
22. Wilson AM. Use of botulinum toxin type a to prevent widening of facial scars. Plast Reconstr Surg. 2006;117(6):1758–66.
23. Xiao Z, Zhang F, Cui Z. Treatment of hypertrophic scars with intralesional botulinum toxin type a injections: a preliminary report. Aesthet Plast Surg. 2009;33(3):409–12.
24. Wu WT. Skin resurfacing with Microbotox and the treatment of keloids. In: Botulinum toxins in clinical aesthetic practice: CRC Press; 2011. p. 204–19.
25. Gugerell A, Kober J, Schmid M, Buchberger E, Kamolz LP, Keck M. Botulinum toxin a: dose-dependent effect on reepithelialization and angiogenesis. Plast Reconstr Surg Glob Open. 2016;4(8).

31

Minimally Invasive Technologies for Treatment of HTS and Keloids: Pulsed-Dye Laser

Sebastian P. Nischwitz, David B. Lumenta, Stephan Spendel, and Lars-Peter Kamolz

Contents

Background

Hypertrophic scars and keloids can be a major medical concern with varying impact.

Depending on the literature one chooses, prevalence between 30% and 70% for postsurgical hypertrophic scarring is reported; looking at burn injuries, the numbers even range from 60% to 90%. Keloids on the other hand, show a prevalence of about 4–14% in Afro-Americans. Given the fact, that the number of people developing significant scars after surgery or trauma ranges in the lower hundred millions every year, one can easily imagine, that scars can be more than an unavoidable side effect after trauma and pathologic scars are not rare.

Besides the cosmetic appearance and the psychological impact (especially after burns), those pathologic scars tend to be responsible for physical and functional impairing symptoms like pruritus, erythema, (neuropathic) pain, and in extreme cases even restriction of movement. The therapy has a wide variety from topical applications to complete surgery – all being covered in this book.

Since the management of cutaneous scars has and often still does rely on personal preference and experience, rather than large-scale and high-quality studies, to date no standard-of-care for the optimal therapy could be established, at least not based on solid scientific evidence.

Many treatment modalities are accompanied by high recurrence rates and with variable effect, which emphasizes the value of and need for minimally invasive technologies. This and the following chapters introduce and focus on several laser technologies as minimally invasive technologies in the treatment of hypertrophic scars and keloids.

On the following pages, the pulsed-dye laser (PDL) is delineated and its significance in the treatment of hypertrophic scars and keloids discussed.

Historical Development

Among the wide variety of available treatment options, laser applications are considered more recent technologies. Medical use of the physical properties of light dates back to ancient times, when Egyptians, Greeks, and Romans used some form of heliotherapy thousands of years BC. However, none other than Albert Einstein first described the stimulated emission of radiation, the base of laser technology, in 1917 [1]. In 1955, 38 years later, the manuscript of the first functioning precursor of a laser, the *MASER* was published by Gordon, Zeiger, and Townes [2]. Schawlow and Townes, who filed the first US patent for a laser in 1960, altered the ***M****icrowave* ***A****mplification by* ***S****timulated* ***E****mission of* ***R****adiation*-device (MASER) to visible *L*ight wavelengths (LASER).

In the same year, Maiman built the first functioning laser, which used a synthetic pink ruby crystal as active medium [3]. In the early 1960s, the laser was first used for medical purposes in humans [4], and Townes along with two others (Prokhorov and Basov) were awarded the Nobel Prize in Physics for their work based on the MASER (1964). In 1981, Schawlow (along with Bloembergen) shared this honor for his contribution in the development of the laser spectroscopy.

After the development of the first laser, different kinds of light amplification devices have been developed using all kinds of active media.

The first dye laser was introduced in 1966 by two teams more or less simultaneously: the Americans Sorokin and Lankard at the Thomas J. Watson Research Center, as well as the German Schaefer at the University of Marburg developed the apparatus. While Sorokin and Lankard published the invention [5], Schaefer's manuscript was rejected. After resubmission, the journal *Applied Physics Letter* asked Sorokin to review the manuscript, who finally made a publication possible [6], and also acknowledged Schaefer as the first to describe the dye laser's advantage of adjustable wavelengths.

In 1983, Anderson and Parrish described the principle of selective photothermolysis, which enabled further research to adapt and better understand the medical possibilities of the laser and its tissue interactions [7]. First results of the use of the pulsed-dye laser (PDL) in Naevi flammei were published in the same year [8]. Also in that year, hypotheses for the application of lasers for the treatment of hypertrophic scars were made public [9].

Alster and colleagues were the first to issue their positive results in the treatment of hypertrophic scars ($n = 14$; [10]) and keloidal post-sternotomy scars ($n = 16$; [11]) with the 585 nm PDL.

Of note is that these positive results of the PD laser have so far failed to be reproduced in subsequent studies, and only minimal improvements in scar texture have been reported.

Technique of a Laser

The following section outlines the principle of a laser with a focus on the basics and the most relevant properties for a clinical understanding.

The mode of action of a laser is based on the emission of light by active medium molecules in an excited state, as described by Einstein [1]. This requires an energy source that is able to excite these molecules. To enhance this effect of excitation and reach higher energy levels, an additional resonator is used. These three components are the key elements of a laser (◘ Fig. 31.1).

Atoms in the active medium, which can be of solid (e.g., ruby crystal), liquid (dye), or gaseous (CO_2) state, are excited by supplying them with energy from the energy source. Depending on the used active medium, the time of decay varies until the atoms return to their ground state. The longer the time of decay, the more time remains for an incoming photon to interact with the excited atom, which in turn makes it return to its ground state and emits an additional photon of the same wavelength and frequency (◘ Fig. 31.1, Detail). This doubling ignites a chain reaction leading to the required high intensity of a laser. The resonator, which can be embodied by (various numbers of) plane or curved mirrors, in between the photons are reflected, enhances this effect additionally. One of these mirrors is subtotal-reflective, creating an exit for a part of the photons. In lasers that use dye as active medium, the resonator holds another function. Being equipped with a dispersive element (grid, filter, prism), the wavelength of the emitted light becomes tunable, as described by Schaefer as adjustable wavelengths (see ► Sect. 31.2).

The main difference between laser and regular light lies in its coherence, which allows a monochromatic (just one specific wavelength), high energetic, low divergent emission of light. It can also be applied as continuous wave or in short pulses of up to a femtosecond (one quadrillionth of a second), which allows for a temporal selective application.

Tissue Interaction of Laser

The effect and clinical impact of a laser is determined by its interaction with the irradiated tissue. The interaction can basically be distinguished in reflected, scattered, and absorbed photons. While reflective light is predominantly relevant for diagnostic use of lasers, scattering limits the depth of focusing of the laser beam by attenuation. The therapeutic effort is caused by the absorption of light, which can be used for various therapeutic effects. Due to the relevance for the present topic, we only deal with the photothermal effect; other effects can be comprehensively looked up in laser textbooks (see Further Reading).

Since every tissue component shows a different absorption coefficient, which equals the reciprocal of the distance that a photon can travel in that component until it is absorbed, therefore, every tissue component reacts differently to a specific type of light. While, for example, bilirubin and melanin show good absorption of visible light, water (H_2O), the main component of human soft tissue, has its absorptive maximum in infrared wavelengths (◘ Fig. 31.2).

The penetration depth of a laser also depends on the wavelength; the higher the wavelength, the higher the penetration depth in the visible spectrum (blue to red).

The photothermal effect describes the transformation of electromagnetic energy (light) to heat by absorption and thereby photoexcitation of matter. Photothermal therapy is the most common application of laser therapy.

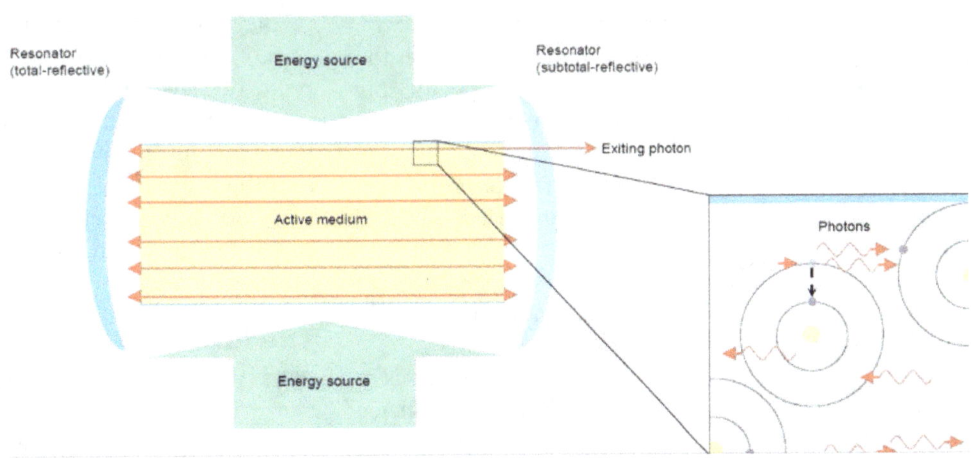

◘ **Fig.** The working principle of a laser is dis-played (simplified). An *energy source* causes excitation in atoms of the *active medium* that, amplified by the *resona-tor*, leads to a chain reaction with the photons ultimately exiting through the subtotal-reflective resonator. The detailed view shows photons interacting with excited electrons of the active medium and emission of additional photons of the same energy

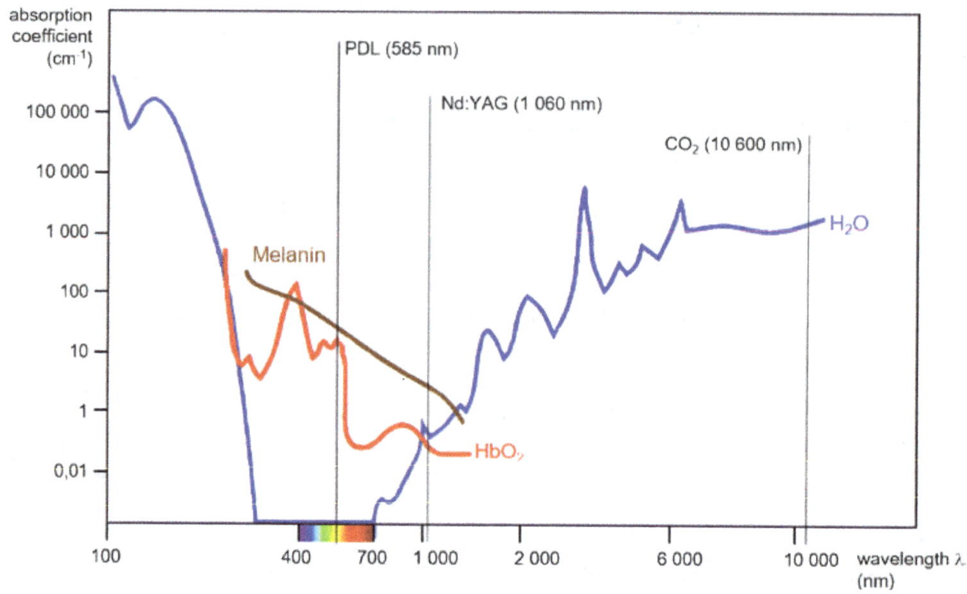

Fig. The wave-length-dependent absorption coefficients of H_2O, oxygenated hemoglobin (HbO_2) and melanin are displayed; the wavelengths of pulsed dye (PDL), Nd:YAG, and CO2 laser are presented exemplary. The wavelength of visible light ranges from about 400 to 700 nm. (Design: Dr. med. univ. Hanna Luze, Graz, Aus-tria. © All rights reserved)

The absorptive properties of the irradiated tissue together with the properties of the used laser determine the exact location and effect of the irradiation. The more energy the irradiated matter absorbs, the more heat is produced, therefore explaining the correlation between the absorption coefficient and the different laser wavelengths.

Depending on the temperature reached, edema and apoptosis induction (≥ 45 °C), coagulation, and denaturation of proteins (≥ 60 °C), and even ablation and cutting by vaporization (≥ 100 °C) can be induced.

Another important aspect determining the amount of damage is the fluence. It is given in J/cm^2 and describes the energy deposited on a certain area over a certain amount of time. This makes it an excellent parameter suitable for description of a treatment protocol.

Selective Photothermolysis

Selective photothermolysis describes a principle that enables selective damage to wavelength-specific pigments within the skin without harming the surrounding or above lying tissues.

The photothermolysis-induced damage is not only transmitted by direct local interaction, but also by heat diffusion additionally irradiating surrounding tissue layers; this principle is of particular importance for calculating selectivity and precise interaction of the laser with adjacent tissue layers.

A basic condition for selective photothermolysis is for the desired target to have a higher absorption coefficient than the surrounding tissues. By pulse-wise-specific irradiation of the target tissue a higher thermal energy is deposited in the target pigment with the higher absorptive coefficient than the surrounding tissue, and directs damaging temperatures only to the target pigment. Due to the pause in between the pulses, there is enough time for the target tissue to cool down by heat diffusion before applying another pulse. On the one hand, depending on the exposure time of the pulses, the amount of damage is relatively well-adjustable to the target area. On the other hand, the wavelength of the chosen and applied light determines the target area. For instance, light of around 580 nm (red light) is predominantly absorbed by hemoglobin, while water has its absorption maximum in the infrared wavelengths and melanin absorbs light throughout the visible region of the electromagnetic spectrum with a decrease toward higher wavelengths. The selectivity of the physical properties allows for a certain approximation of the beam to the target area including a pulse-dependent diameter of several millimeters around it. The downside of this specificity results in a relatively narrow therapeutic spectrum for each type of laser. Due to the monochromatic property of a given laser (emission of light of just one wavelength) and from a technical point-of-view, this leads to different therapeutic targets requiring individual lasers of a different spectrum. This latter fact has made the PDL with its active medium dye and the tuneability (see ► Sects. 31.2 and 31.3) predestined for exploiting this physical principle generating various targets with the same active medium.

The PDL and Its Application on Hypertrophic Scars and Keloids

The PDL is based on the principle of selective photothermolysis and was developed to damage and destroy small cutaneous vessels without harming epidermal structures. Being initially developed with a wavelength of 577 nm, the current models mostly work on a spectrum of 585 or 595 nm. Small cutaneous vessels absorb energy at these specified wavelengths. Consequently, the vessels are destroyed, ultimately leading to hypoxemia by diminution of the vascular supply. Then, by allegedly reported secondary effects, disulfide bonds are dissociated, collagen production is reduced, and expression of enzymes such as matrix metalloproteinases is induced [11, 12], leading to a loosening and restructuring of the fibrous structure in hypertrophic scars and keloids. However, there is no ultimate and scientifically proven consensus about the exact mechanisms promoted by PDL.

Hypertrophic scars and keloids often show significant characteristics like erythema and pruritus, which can be caused by hyperemia. Destruction of small cutaneous vessels can therefore significantly reduce these symptoms.

The mentioned restructuring procedures may be responsible for the observed improvement of pliability and height [13].

The properties of PDL and its modes of action also suggest the application in the prevention of hypertrophic scars, since some authors suggest an early laser application after surgery [14, 15].

In support of this theoretical recommendation (early use after surgery) is that the PDL proved to be less effective in thicker scars (>1 cm) due to its restricted penetration depth.

Side effects are relatively rare and include edema, scab formation, and pigmentary disorders (temporary often, permanent rarely), but also range from hypotrophic to hypertrophic scarring [16], but may be related to the therapeutic context of PDL application.

While most PDL work with 585 nm, more recently the 595 nm long-pulsed dye laser has been introduced. Longer pulses have been promoted on the basis of a more effective destruction of larger vessels by higher deposition of energy, and less posttreatment hyperpigmentation. In contrast to that, 585 nm lasers have reportedly ameliorated the scar texture; it remains to be seen if this also applies to the next generation of 595 lasers.

All in all, no scientifically solid high quality studies exist, and the above-mentioned studies do not support the development of definite recommendations for a PDL protocol on hypertrophic scars or keloids. The only common denominator seems to be the minimum requirement of greater than two PDL applications every 4–12 weeks across the scanned literature.

Selected Studies and Evidence

The first publications of hypertrophic scars treated with the PDL date back to 1994. Alster presented 14 cases of patients suffering from hypertrophic and/or erythematous scars after trauma or surgery [10]. After treatment with one or two sessions of 585 nm PDL within a 6-week interval, they showed an improvement in erythema and scar flattening of 57–83% as evaluated by two different and independent observers. The fluence used in this study was 6.5–6.75 J/cm^2.

One year later, in 1995, Alster and Williams described another series of patients (n = 16) that had developed keloidal or hypertrophic scars after a median sternotomy [11]. Those patients had half of the scars treated with a similar protocol (mean fluence: 7.00 J/cm^2, two sessions, 6–8 weeks apart) and afterwards evaluated by two independent, blinded observers. Significant amelioration of pruritus, tenderness, burning, scar height, pliability, and erythema was observed 6 months after laser treatment, as compared to untreated scars.

Subsequently, no study was able to reproduce these initially promising results. While several studies described changes in scar erythema, pliability, height, and volume, very few demonstrated a statistical significance (also due to the low number of scars treated). Significant improvement in Vancouver Scar Scale scores and pigmentation could be shown by Bowes et al. [17] and Chan et al. [18] for patients treated with PDL compared to no treatment intra-individually, respectively. Alster further showed a significant reduction in pruritus by adding intralesional injection of triamcinolone [19] in contrast to Wittenberg et al. who could not observe a significant reduction of pruritus in hypertrophic scars treated with PDL over patients treated with silicone gel sheeting [20].

Another study by Asilian et al. could reach a significant participant-subjective, inter-individual overall improvement from baseline and a reduction of erythema in patients treated with PDL, intralesional injection of triamcinolone, and 5-fluoruracil compared to the controls treated with the intralesional injection alone [21].

Ouyang et al. (2018) reached significant improvement in height, vascularity, pliability, and Vancouver Scar Scale in 56 patients with fresh (immature), red hypertrophic scars [22], suggesting an early application and possible prevention strategy in conjunction with a recommendation of an international panel of experts [23].

To summarize, data on PDL treatment in hypertrophic scars and keloids is scarce. Studies were conducted with no or insufficient control groups, no standardized treatment protocols, small numbers of participants, or lack of differentiation between the scar types treated.

The exact mechanisms of PDL application in hypertrophic scars or keloids remain elusive and precise recommendations cannot be made on the given evidence.

Nonetheless, PDL may serve as effective additional (second-line) therapeutic strategy given the relatively low side-effect spectrum; application in fresh pathologic, erythematous, itching scars and use for preventive strategies can be considered. PDL use is limited by its low penetration depth (thick scars) and higher amount of melanin as concurrent absorber (darker skin types).

Clinical Relevance

Since most of the published research demonstrated inconclusive results of the use of PDL for hypertrophic scars and keloids, no solid recommendation can be derived from the given literature. Hypertrophic scars tend to involute over time, and without the evidence served by adequate control groups in published research, it remains difficult to support them. Since medical device regulations will require more published research in the future (notably for device registration in the European Union), future therapeutic registration or re-registration might add in encouraging industry to support more science-driven studies.

Active hypertrophic scars as seen with the clinical sign of erythema or symptom of pruritus can be treated by PDL with a low level of side effects but only if used in conjunction with other more proven methods.

Limiting factors are thick scars (>1 cm) and dark skin types. As a result the PDL can play a role in the prevention of pathologic scars. Future studies should aim toward more standardized research with an adequate selection of control groups (e.g., intra-individual comparison), and are still necessary to reach the actual potential of the PDL.

Conclusion

This chapter dealt with the minimally invasive treatment of hypertrophic scars and keloids with the pulsed-dye laser. Being the first chapter about laser technology, an introduction on lasers, their functioning, and an outline of the temporal development were given. We then explained the principle behind the PDL, called selective photothermolysis, and clarified its relevance in the treatment of pathologic scars. Lastly, selected studies in terms of clinically applied PDL were presented, the evidence was analyzed, and the clinical relevance delineated.

The reader should now be able to sort the relevance of PDL for treatment of hypertrophic scars and keloids in the whole arsenal of treatment methods for pathologic scars.

Summarizing, we want to emphasize one more time that laser technology itself is a rather new technology, which certainly holds many advantages – not least its minimal invasiveness and low side-effect profile. With only few studies available, we refrain from giving absolute recommendations. We rather want to encourage the reader, if interested in this topic, to help creating more evidence and perform further research on this specific topic. PDL holds potential, that still is to be grasped comprehensively.

Take-Home Messages

- Pulsed-dye laser is based on a principle called selective photothermolysis.
- Its wavelength ranges from 585 to 595 nm.
- PDL's main targets are cutaneous vessels that are coagulated by the irradiation.
- PDL should be applied a minimum of two times every 4–12 weeks.
- PDL application can reduce symptoms like pruritus or erythema.
- PDL should NOT be used for thick scars (>1 cm) and/or in dark skin types.
- PDL should only be used in combination with other treatment modalities to achieve the most effective treatment.
- The low risk and side-effect profile makes the PDL a valuable alternative for the prevention of pathologic scars.
- Long-term outcome and high-quality intervention studies are necessary to provide proper evidence for PDL application in hypertrophic scars and keloids.

References

1. Einstein A. Zur Quantentheorie der Strahlung. Phys Zeitschrift. 1917;18:121–8.
2. Gordon JP, Zeiger HJ, Townes CH. The maser – new type of microwave amplifier, frequency standard, and spectrometer. Phys Rev. 1955;99(4):1264–74.
3. Maiman TH. Stimulated optical radiation in ruby. Nature. 1960;187:493–4.
4. Goldman L, Igelman JM, Richfield DF. Impact of the LASER on nevi and melanomas. Arch Dermatol. 1964;90:71–5.
5. Sorokin PP, Lankard JR. Stimulated emission observed from an organic dye, chloro-aluminum phthalocyanine. IBM J Res Dev. 1966;10:162–3.
6. Schäfer FP, Schmidt W, Volze J. Organic dye solution laser. Appl Phys Lett. 1966;9:306–9.

7. Anderson R, Parrish J. Selective photothermolysis: precise microsurgery by selective absorption of pulsed radiation. Science. 1983;220(4596):524–7.
8. Strempel H, Klein G. New approach in the laser therapy of nevus flammeus. Z Hautkr. 1983;58(13):967–74.
9. Castro DJ, Abergel RP, Meeker C, Dwyer RM, Lesavoy MA, Uitto J. Effects of the Nd:YAG laser on DNA synthesis and collagen production in human skin fibroblast cultures. Ann Plast Surg. 1983;11(3):214–22.
10. Alster TS. Improvement of erythematous and hypertrophic scars by the 585-nm flashlamp-pumped pulsed dye laser. Ann Plast Surg. 1994;32(2):186–90.
11. Alster TS, Williams CM. Treatment of keloid sternotomy scars with 585 nm flashlamp-pumped pulsed-dye laser. Lancet. 1995;345(8959):1198–200.
12. Dierickx C, Goldman MP, Fitzpatrick RE. Laser treatment of erythematous/hypertrophic and pigmented scars in 26 patients. Plast Reconstr Surg [Internet]. 1995;95(1):84–90; discussion 91–2. Available from: http://europepmc.org/abstract/MED/7809272.
13. Gauglitz GG, Potschke J, Clementoni MT. Therapy of scars with lasers. Hautarzt. 2018;69(1):17–26.
14. Karmisholt KE, Haerskjold A, Karlsmark T, Waibel J, Paasch U, Haedersdal M. Early laser intervention to reduce scar formation - a systematic review. J Eur Acad Dermatol Venereol. 2018;32(7):1099–110.
15. Brewin MP, Lister TS. Prevention or treatment of hypertrophic burn scarring: a review of when and how to treat with the pulsed dye laser. Burns. 2014;40(5):797–804.
16. Raulin C, Kimmig W, Werner S. Laser therapy in dermatology and esthetic medicine. Side effects, complications and treatment errors. Hautarzt. 2000;51(7):463–73.
17. Bowes LE, Nouri K, Berman B, Jimenez G, Pardo R, Rodriguez L, et al. Treatment of pigmented hypertrophic scars with the 585 nm pulsed dye laser and the 532 nm frequency-doubled Nd:YAG laser in the Q-switched and variable pulse modes: a comparative study. Dermatol Surg. 2002;28(8):714–9.
18. Chan HHL, Wong DSY, Ho WS, Lam LK, Wei W. The use of pulsed dye laser for the prevention and treatment of hypertrophic scars in Chinese persons. Dermatol Surg. 2004;30(7):987–94.
19. Alster T. Laser scar revision: comparison study of 585-nm pulsed dye laser with and without intralesional corticosteroids. Dermatol Surg. 2003;29(1):25–9.
20. Wittenberg GP, Fabian BG, Bogomilsky JL, Schultz LR, Rudner EJ, Chaffins ML, et al. Prospective, single-blind, randomized, controlled study to assess the efficacy of the 585-nm flashlamp-pumped pulsed-dye laser and silicone gel sheeting in hypertrophic scar treatment. Arch Dermatol. 1999;135(9):1049–55.
21. Asilian A, Darougheh A, Shariat F. New combination of triamcinolone, 5-fluorouracil, and pulsed-dye laser for the treatment of keloid and hypertrophic scars. J Isfahan Med Sch. 2012;32(7):907–15.
22. Ouyang HW, Li GF, Lei Y, Gold MH, Tan J. Comparison of the effectiveness of pulsed dye laser vs pulsed dye laser combined with ultrapulse fractional CO2 laser in the treatment of immature red hypertrophic scars. J Cosmet Dermatol. 2018;17(1):54–60.
23. Mustoe TA, Cooter RD, Gold MH, Hobbs FDR, Ramelet A-A, Shakespeare PG, et al. International clinical recommendations on scar management. Plast Reconstr Surg. 2002;110(2):560–71.

Permissions

All chapters in this book were first published in TSM, by Springer; hereby published with permission under the Creative Commons Attribution License or equivalent. Every chapter published in this book has been scrutinized by our experts. Their significance has been extensively debated. The topics covered herein carry significant findings which will fuel the growth of the discipline. They may even be implemented as practical applications or may be referred to as a beginning point for another development.

The contributors of this book come from diverse backgrounds, making this book a truly international effort. This book will bring forth new frontiers with its revolutionizing research information and detailed analysis of the nascent developments around the world.

We would like to thank all the contributing authors for lending their expertise to make the book truly unique. They have played a crucial role in the development of this book. Without their invaluable contributions this book wouldn't have been possible. They have made vital efforts to compile up to date information on the varied aspects of this subject to make this book a valuable addition to the collection of many professionals and students.

This book was conceptualized with the vision of imparting up-to-date information and advanced data in this field. To ensure the same, a matchless editorial board was set up. Every individual on the board went through rigorous rounds of assessment to prove their worth. After which they invested a large part of their time researching and compiling the most relevant data for our readers.

The editorial board has been involved in producing this book since its inception. They have spent rigorous hours researching and exploring the diverse topics which have resulted in the successful publishing of this book. They have passed on their knowledge of decades through this book. To expedite this challenging task, the publisher supported the team at every step. A small team of assistant editors was also appointed to further simplify the editing procedure and attain best results for the readers.

Apart from the editorial board, the designing team has also invested a significant amount of their time in understanding the subject and creating the most relevant covers. They scrutinized every image to scout for the most suitable representation of the subject and create an appropriate cover for the book.

The publishing team has been an ardent support to the editorial, designing and production team. Their endless efforts to recruit the best for this project, has resulted in the accomplishment of this book. They are a veteran in the field of academics and their pool of knowledge is as vast as their experience in printing. Their expertise and guidance has proved useful at every step. Their uncompromising quality standards have made this book an exceptional effort. Their encouragement from time to time has been an inspiration for everyone.

The publisher and the editorial board hope that this book will prove to be a valuable piece of knowledge for researchers, students, practitioners and scholars across the globe.

List of Contributors

Wouter B. van der Sluis
Nirvana S. S. Kornmann
Robin A. Tan
Johan P. W. Don Griot
Magda M. W. Ulrich
Clarisse Ganier
Rei Ogawa
M. El Kinani
Thomas A. Mustoe
Osama Farrukh
Chenyu Huang
Eric Van den Kerckhove
Yating Yang
A. Pijpe
L. van Haasterecht
M. E. H. Jaspers
Marguerite Guillot Masanovic
Michelle E. Carrière
Juhee Lee
Alia Sadiq
Docteur N. Frasson
Margriet E. van Baar
Julian Poetschke
Yaron Har-Shai
Peter Moortgat
Wei Liu
Ian A. Darby
Alexandra Chambers
Sonia Gaucher
F. Duteille
Ioannis Goutos
Zhaozhao Wu
Mieke Anthonissen
Xiaoli Wu
K. L. M. Gardien
Paul P. M. van Zuijlen
P. Moortgat
Luc Téot
Annekatrien L. van de Kar
Jihee Kim
Nonhlanhla P. Khumalo
Gerd G. Gauglitz
Lior Har-Shai
Alexis Desmoulière
Yanan Du
R. E. van Meijeren-Hoogendoorn
ML. Groot
Ardeshir Bayat
Ulrike Van Daele
Zheng Gao
E. Middelkoop
Jill Meirte
Lingling Xia
Tine Vanhullebusch
Koen Maertens
Sebastian P. Nischwitz
David B. Lumenta
Stephan Spendel
Lars-Peter Kamolz

Index

www.ingramcontent.com/pod-product-compliance
Lightning Source LLC
LaVergne TN
LVHW081031210926
848485LV00004B/994
* 9 7 8 1 6 3 9 8 9 4 7 8 9 *